Child and adolescent mental health services

An operational handbook

Second edition

Child and adolescent mental health services

An operational handbook

Second edition

Edited by Greg Richardson, Ian Partridge and Jonathan Barrett

RCPsych Publications

For Dr Tom Pitt-Aitkens
– who understood the importance
of 'the good authority'

RCPsych Publications is an imprint of the Royal College of Psychiatrists,
17 Belgrave Square, London SW1X 8PG
http://www.rcpsych.ac.uk

British Library Cataloguing-in-Publication Data.
A catalogue record for this book is available from the British Library.
ISBN 978 1 904671 80 0

Distributed in North America by Publishers Storage and Shipping Company.

The views presented in this book do not necessarily reflect those of the Royal College of
Psychiatrists, and the publishers are not responsible for any error of omission or fact.

The Royal College of Psychiatrists is a charity registered in England and Wales (228636) and in
Scotland (SC038369).

Printed by Bell & Bain Limited, Glasgow, UK.

Contents

Tables, boxes and figures

Figures

Contributors

Sue Bailey, MBChB, MRCPsych, FRCPsych, OBE, Consultant Adolescent Forensic Psychiatrist, Adolescent Forensic Services, Bolton, Salford & Trafford Mental Health Partnership, and Professor of Adolescent Psychiatry at the University of Central Lancashire

Margaret Bamforth, MBChB, FRCPsych, MA (Clinical Education), Consultant Child and Adolescent Psychiatrist, 5 Boroughs Partnership NHS Trust

Mandy Barker, CQSW, DMS, Social Worker, formerly Service Manager of York Deaf Child and Family Service.

Jonathan Barrett, MBBS, MMedSc, MRCGP, MRCPsych, FHEA, Consultant and Honorary Senior Lecturer in Child and Adolescent Psychiatry, Cringlebar, West Leeds CAMHS, NHS Leeds

Rosie Beer, Retired Consultant in Child and Adolescent Psychiatry, Leeds

Tom Berney, MBChB, DPM, FRCPsych, FRCPH, Honorary Consultant Developmental Psychiatrist, Northumberland, Tyne & Wear NHS Trust

Sarah Bryan, BHSc (Hons) OT, Senior Occupational Therapist, York

Chris Butler, Chief Executive, Leeds Partnerships NHS Foundation Trust

Geraldine Casswell, BSc, MSc Clin Psy, M Psychotherapy, Consultant Child Clinical Psychologist, Lime Trees CAMHS, North Yorkshire & York Primary Care Trust

Enys Delmage, MBChB, MRCPsych, Specialist Registrar in Adolescent Forensic Psychiatry, Adolescent Forensic Services, Bolton, Salford & Trafford Mental Health Partnership

Fiona Gospel, BSc, DClinPsych, Consultant Clinical Psychologist, Lime Trees CAMHS, North Yorkshire & York Primary Care Trust

Lesley Hewson, MBChB, MRCPsych, FRCPsych, Consultant Child and Adolescent Psychiatrist, Bradford District Care Trust

Matthew Hodes, MBBS, BSc, MSc, PhD, FRCPsych, Senior Lecturer in Child and Adolescent Psychiatry, Division of Neurosciences and Mental Health, School of Medicine Imperial College London

Jackie Johnson, RMN, BSc, CAMHS Community Nurse, Lime Trees CAMHS, North Yorkshire & York Primary Care Trust

Nick Jones, Consultant Nurse, Lime Trees CAMHS, North Yorkshire & York Primary Care Trust

Tony Kaplan, MBChB, FRCPsych, Consultant Child and Adolescent Psychiatrist, New Beginning Young People's Crisis Recovery Unit, Edgware Hospital, Barnet, Enfield & Haringey Mental Health NHS Trust

Juliette Kennedy, MBBS, MRCPsych, Specialist Registrar in Child and Adolescent Psychiatry, Yorkshire and the Humber Postgraduate Deanery

Steve Kingsbury, MBBS, MRCPsych, Consultant Child and Adolescent Psychiatrist, Hertfordshire Partnership Trust

Sebastian Kraemer, MBBS, FRCPsych, Consultant Child and Adolescent Psychiatrist, Whittington Hospital, London

Clare Lamb, MBBS, MRCPsych, FRCPsych, Consultant Child and Adolescent Psychiatrist, North Wales Adolescent Service

Phil Lucas, Consultant Child and Adolescent Psychiatrist

Tim McDougall, Lead Nurse, Cheshire & Wirral NHS Foundation Trust

Norman Malcolm, MBChB, MRCPsych, Consultant in Child and Adolescent Psychiatry, Bradford District Care Trust

Mary Mitchell, MA, BM, MRCPsych, Consultant Child and Adolescent Psychiatrist, Leigh House Hospital Winchester, Hampshire Partnership NHS Trust

Ruth Norton, MBBS, MRCPsych, MedSci Clinical Psychiatry, Consultant Child and Adolescent Psychiatrist, Oakwood Young People's Centre, Sheffield

Ian Partridge, MA, MSc, CQSW, Social Worker, formerly at Lime Trees CAMHS, York

Greg Richardson, MBChB, DCH, DPM, FRCPsych, Consultant Child and Adolescent Psychiatrist, Lime Trees CAMHS, North Yorkshire & York Primary Care Trust

Sophie Roberts, BMedSc, MBBS, MRCPsych, Consultant Child and Adolescent Psychiatrist, Lime Trees CAMHS, North Yorkshire & York Primary Care Trust

Angela Sergeant, RMN, RGN, MSc, ENB 603, Consultant Nurse in Child and Adolescent Psychiatry, Leigh House Hospital, Winchester, Hampshire Partnership Trust

Christine Williams, Consultant Child Clinical Psychologist, Lime Trees CAMHS, North Yorkshire & York Primary Care Trust

Anne Worrall-Davies, MBChB, MMedSc, MRCPsych, Senior Lecturer in Child and Adolescent Psychiatry, University of Leeds, and Honorary Consultant in Child and Adolescent Psychiatry, NHS Leeds

Barry Wright, Consultant Child and Adolescent Psychiatrist, Lime Trees CAMHS, North Yorkshire & York Primary Care Trust

Kate Wurr, MBChB, MRCPsych, Consultant and Honorary Senior Lecturer in Child and Adolescent Psychiatry, Cringlebar, West Leeds CAMHS, NHS Leeds

Ashley Wyatt, CAMHS Commissioning Manager, Leeds

Ann York, MBBS, MRCPsych, Consultant Child and Adolescent Psychiatrist and Clinical Team Leader, Child and Family Consultation Centre, Richmond Royal, Surrey, and Honorary Senior Lecturer, St George's Hospital Medical School, London, South West London & St George's Mental Health NHS Trust

Abbreviations

ADHD	attention-deficit hyperactivity disorder
BMA	British Medical Association
BMI	body mass index
BSL	British Sign Language
CAMHS	child and adolescent mental health service(s)
CAPA	Choice and Partnership Approach
CBT	cognitive–behavioural therapy
CGAS	Children's Global Assessment Scale
CHI–ESQ	Commission for Health Improvement Experience of Service Questionnaire
CORC	CAMHS Outcomes Research Consortium
CPD	continuing professional development
CRB	Criminal Records Bureau
CSIP	Care Services Improvement Partnership
DSM	*Diagnostic and Statistical Manual for Mental Disorders*
ECHR	European Convention on Human Rights
GMC	General Medical Council
GP	general practitioner
ICD–10	*International Classification of Mental and Behavioural Disorders*, tenth revision
ICT	information and communication technology
LSD	lysergic acid diethylamide
NCG	National Commissioning Group
NHS	National Health Service
NIASA	National Initiative for Autism: Screening and Assessment
NICE	National Institute for Health and Clinical Excellence
NIMHE	National Institute for Mental Health in England

NSF	National Service Framework
NTA	National Treatment Agency for Substance Misuse
OCD	obsessive–compulsive disorder
PACE	Promoting Action on Clinical Effectiveness
PTSD	post-traumatic stress disorder
QINMAC	Quality Network for Multi-Agency CAMHS
QNIC	Quality Network for In-patient CAMHS
RCT	randomised controlled trial
SCIE	Social Care Institute for Excellence
SDQ	Strengths and Difficulties Questionnaire
SEAL	Social and Emotional Aspects of Learning
WTE	whole time equivalent

Preface

'"Lucky we know the forest so well, or we might get lost," said Rabbit...and he gave the careless laugh which you give when you know the Forest so well that you can't get lost.'

A. A. Milne, *The House at Pooh Corner*

This second edition is a 'how to do' text and an update of the evidential and operational base for child and adolescent mental health services (CAMHS) delivery, and about organising intervention into the lives of children and their families, into their functioning and relationships. It is a parochial rather than a universal text – it addresses CAMHS in a particular country, the UK and primarily England, at a particular time, although we hope the principles of service delivery will have a more universal resonance. Service delivery is bound by the interacting contexts of healthcare delivery, attitudes to mental health, attitudes to children and broader social mores, locally and regionally, and the wider social, political and economic context as well as the tension between a demand for and supply of clinical provision. This book describes ways of delivering services to young people and their families within, and with full awareness of, those contexts.

This book is about the operation of services for children and young people who have been identified as having mental disorders or psychological problems. It is not about the emotional well-being of all children, although it recognises and acknowledges factors in our society that influence that emotional well-being. The difference between treating mental disorder and ensuring emotional well-being are clarified by the two questions those of us interested in the welfare of children need to address.

1   How do we as a society support, respect and develop self-esteem in those who in turn will do the same for their children? This question belongs in the arena of nurturing the mental health of the community, of society.

2   How do those of us working in CAMHS assess and manage those children and their families who are suffering because of their mental disorder or psychological difficulties?

Unfortunately, the answers to these two questions have become confused. In 2009, the Department of Health published *Healthy Lives, Brighter Futures*, a strategy for young people's health, claiming that 'Children and young people are healthier today than they have ever been' – a claim that may be true of physical health, but is at odds with the 2007 UNICEF report that made uncomfortable reading for the UK. What is particularly distressing is that in a wealthy society such as ours, young people view their families and peers as unsupportive, and although society does an average job of protecting their health and safety, they are the highest risk takers; they appear not to value themselves. The UNICEF report points out that 'levels of child well-being are not inevitable but policy susceptible', i.e. the structures and policies of state have a major impact upon how children and young people grow and develop. Sadly, our society seems to be going down the identify, pathologise and treat route, rather than learning from other countries how to make their children happier and more content. The result is an ever increasing expectation of CAMHS to address all this 'pathology'. There is a real danger that if we in CAMHS believe that we are the only route to emotional well-being, focusing too tightly on our own operation, success criteria, language and professional ideology as we 'know the forest so well', we will ultimately be blamed when the emotional well-being of children becomes 'lost'.

Mental health professionals may come to view emotional well-being merely as the absence or removal of pathology rather than the development of a nurturing mentally healthy society. After all, mental health professionals use measures of ill health as indicators for poor emotional well-being and they rarely see emotional well-being in their everyday work! The avoidance of lung cancer was never informed by thoracic surgeons who spent their careers removing cancerous lungs. We must therefore ensure that we also apply the systemic, relational and interactional underpinnings of our work in CAMHS to society as a whole.

Child and adolescent mental health services must be clear about the most socially healthy form of intervention and, as it concerns children's and families' lives, must operate within a framework formed as much from societal research as individual intervention research. Intervention should always be considered carefully in terms of both its individual and social benefit, and kept to the minimum. It is to social policy, which encourages and facilitates an environment conducive to mental health and emotional well-being, that societal intervention should be targeted, supporting a healthy environment rather than identifying pathology in individuals and treating it. A consequence of pathologising children to justify intervention is that parenting becomes an anxiety-driven activity, wherein the anxiety is temporarily managed by reference to the 'expert'; the parent needs a 'parenting programme', all developmental difficulties and hiccups require professional advice and intervention. Dependency is both legitimised and encouraged, and the circularity of learned helplessness is reinforced. The emotional well-being of the community is undermined. Child and adolescent mental health services should be challenging this 'mission creep'. To use a Titanic analogy, by questioning what we are doing, we may avoid the iceberg instead of spending our time dealing with the anxieties of the passengers about hitting the iceberg, their dietary allergies or the behaviour of their children. Our success in these areas may become a justification for providing more treatment as we are treating better, while we ignore the main threat to the child.

Resilience on the part of both parent and child is in danger of being undervalued and underplayed; the reality of developmental difficulties as normal and healthy, a part of the process of the mastery of developmental tasks, is often ignored. The wise words of an experienced and skilled primary school teacher to a class of 5-year-olds – 'it's OK to get it wrong, it shows we're learning' – are forgotten. It is not surprising to find that Sir Michael Rutter, at the end of a career that has developed immensely our understanding of child mental health and the emotional well-being of children and families in society, has been studying and researching resilience. As in most things professional, we should follow his lead.

A child is influenced and feels valued if they feel respected as an individual by their family, their school, their peers and their community. We need to develop ways of running our society that promote such mutual respect and resultant emotional well-being rather than concentrate on correcting pathology. We need to ask who influences and is involved in the promotion of children's mental health, as these are the people who may be most helpful at nurturing emotional well-being among the children with whom they work. We must always be aware that intensive input doesn't always mean productive output. In the USA, boys at high risk of delinquency felt counselling had been helpful, but 30 years later had worse outcomes than those who had had no intervention (McCord, 1992), and intensive support of vulnerable groups produced a worse outcome in the children (Bickman, 1996). Interventions for emotional well-being therefore must be societal, not targeted at those we have pathologised.

Thirty years ago Rutter *et al* (1979) identified factors contributing to the success of pupils in schools:

- admission of all abilities
- ethos of consultation with the pupils and strong leadership by the head
- class sizes of fewer than 20.

However, arguments about selective entry continue despite the fact that selective entry tends to make the majority feel not good enough by assessing all functioning on academic or, occasionally, sporting excellence. Our education system still doesn't seek out young people's skills and develop them. We do recognise the difference a head can make, but are there enough good ones around, and are they remunerated adequately? After all, in state education there has never been any attempt to get class sizes under 20.

Addressing the UNICEF report's indicators might go a long way to improving children's emotional well-being.

1   Improve material well-being. Reduction of child poverty has been a long-term aim, but it is in danger of becoming a meaningless aspiration when

social mobility is falling and inequality in wealth distribution is rising. We need to ensure that families with children, who are an enormous financial drain, are adequately remunerated for their child rearing.

2　Improve health and safety. As a society, we are quite good at trying to reduce infant deaths, but perhaps we need to be more assertive in our approach to antenatal care, a bit like the care programme approach where the least adherent with antenatal care are targeted to ensure the well-being of their unborn children. *Every Child Matters* (HM Government, 2004) is trying to keep children safe, but maybe we need a higher threshold for deciding who is safe to care for children.

3　Gear education to children's strengths and abilities.

4　Strongly support parents in staying together so that they feel able and confident to support and value their children.

5　Provide information about, and reward children for being involved in, a healthy lifestyle, including the provision of balanced emotional, social and sex education in school, as part of the Social and Emotional Aspects of Learning (SEAL) programme (Department for Children, Schools and Families, 2005).

6　Make children feel better about themselves by making their parents and teachers feel better about themselves by concentrating on their achievements rather than on what they are doing wrong. Getting the media to turn that round will be a major task.

These issues remain outside the remit of CAMHS; however, we must consider our negative impact as a maintaining factor. We will serve children better if we can avoid pathologising them or their families as this increases the unfairness with which they are treated. What is unfair to children is being witness to domestic violence, having parents suffering the effects of alcohol and drug misuse, having parents who put their needs before the children's, having their parents use them as tools in domestic and marital disputes, being abused and neglected. These are potentially more important factors than poverty, in that they generate a 'poverty of aspiration' resulting in the ultimate unfairness to children of having them treated by CAMHS so that they can continue to live in intolerable and damaging situations. Children's mental disorders are often the healthiest way of coping with the environment in which they find themselves. As John Pierce put it, 'you talk to any child who is depressed and you find they have damn good reason to be' (personal communication, 1985); fluoxetine and cognitive–behavioural therapy (CBT) are effective in treating children with depression, but should we do nothing about why the child is depressed? The fact that the UNICEF report found young people in England to be the most emotionally unhappy in Europe cannot be down to an increased level of illness but must reflect how they feel treated and valued by society. Child and adolescent mental health service interventions are not going to sort that out, and neither should they try. The solutions to the problems lie elsewhere and the indiscriminate use of CAMHS interventions collude with the problem.

Some 13 years ago the NHS Health Advisory Service (1995) defined mental health as the ability to:

- develop psychologically, emotionally, intellectually and spiritually;
- initiate, develop and sustain mutually satisfying personal relationships;
- become aware of others and to empathise with them;
- use psychological distress as a developmental process, so that it does not hinder or impair further development.

Every Child Matters (HM Government, 2004) converted these into the more realistic sound societal targets of being healthy, staying safe, enjoying and achieving, making a positive contribution and achieving economic well-being, with which we can perhaps begin to draw the boundaries between the specific work of CAMHS and the wider context of facilitating an emotionally nurturing society. Unfortunately, many of the links on the *Every Child Matters* website (Department for Children, Schools and Families, 2009*a*), and many community initiatives, are for those already in some sort of difficulty, so they are orientated towards pathology rather than nurturing. For example, part of the Healthy Schools initiative (Department for Children, Schools and Families, 2009*b*) is SEAL, but even that is advertised as being a method of addressing social, emotional and behavioural difficulties, rather than emphasising school as an emotionally nurturing, self-esteem building environment. Even the success of Healthy Schools programmes in schools tend to be measured by factors such as exclusions or bullying, probably because measuring global improvements in well-being is more difficult. The creeping in of counselling as part of the package is particularly worrying as there is nothing more stigmatising and marginalising than being counselled, the very antithesis of a systemic approach to the development of emotional well-being. So it is unfortunate that mini mental health teams in each school are now being developed, again a reversion to a medical model of identifying pathology, referring the children with it and their then receiving therapy. This is the real danger of mental health professionals being involved in trying to improve the emotional well-being of all young people in the country. Sure Start (www.dcsf.gov.uk/everychildmatters/earlyyears/surestart/aboutsurestart/aboutsurestart/) is also a community-based model for developing emotional well-being, but again tends to be targeted at areas designated as deprived or in need rather than an universal service, which is the only way it won't become stigmatised.

There are effective interventions for children's mental disorders and it is our responsibility to use them. The National Institute for Health and Clinical Excellence (NICE) regularly provides the most up-to-date available advice on managing conditions based on the evidence. Unfortunately, randomised controlled trials (RCTs) are notoriously difficult to interpret in children's psychological conditions. First, one has to have cooperative children and families, and often the major task is gaining that cooperation and working in partnership with them: core skills of any CAMHS professional. Second, comorbidity is common and often an exclusion factor. Third, it is highly likely that different interventions are more or less effective at different stages of a young person's development, for example family therapy is more effective for young people with anorexia nervosa under 19 years of age and with a history of less than 3 years, after which individual therapy is more effective. Similarly, antidepressants seem to have different effects at different ages. Fourth, being in a trial has its own beneficial effects: the methylphenidate trial in the USA demonstrated that it was more effective than any other treatment including routine treatment. However, routine treatment included treatment with methylphenidate (MTA Cooperative Group, 1999a,b). Fifth, many children with mental disorders have been treated by CAMHS using evidence-based treatments (as well as others), but it seems the effects are not as great as in clinical trials. It is as if a new evidence-based treatment will suddenly change this. Perhaps we need to be a little more circumspect about specific treatments and concentrate on the genuineness, warmth and empathy of the therapist.

We require a well-trained workforce, targeted interventions, a fully professional (mental health) assessment for those who really need it, and a dedicated research fund to look at effective interventions, resource use and outcomes; however, even with our current responsibilities there are insufficient staff, and far less than in other European countries (Kelvin, 2009) to undertake all that work. Throwing minimally trained therapists at young people and their families will not radically improve CAMHS or improve the emotional well-being of the population. An increase in workforce is required, but let's be clear about what we want those people to do and ensure they are properly trained to do it.

This book uses the tiered system as it's foundation for the delivery of CAMHS, and in this second edition we recognise that it has not been fully or correctly understood or implemented. It has been increasingly subject to confusion, the term 'Tier 3 CAMHS' being misleadingly used to describe a comprehensive multidisciplinary CAMHS, which should always include both Tier 2 and Tier 3. The tiered system was designed as a structure and strategy for comprehensive CAMHS that describes function, not people. It recognised the fundamental significance of Tier 1 and stresses that all CAMHS professionals have a role and responsibility in supporting Tier 1. It is in Tier 1 that the emotional well-being of the community is most likely to be addressed by supporting those people working every day with children who, often unknowingly, have such a major impact on their emotional development. This role has been taken on to a large extent by the primary mental health worker, who in many services provides a very useful access point to CAMHS. They are trained CAMHS professionals working in a locality who are in regular contact with local schools, general practitioner (GP) surgeries, and Social Service departments, so they are aware of the environments in which children they are consulted about live. They therefore provide CAMHS advice to professionals, but also pick up and undertake initial assessments on young people who may require more specialist CAMHS intervention. They are a local, knowledgeable, accessible, environmentally aware resource for young people and families, and those who are working with those children and families (Hickey *et al*, 2007). The role certainly cannot be left to junior and less experienced CAMHS members. To fulfil their work they need to be integrated with a comprehensive CAMHS that has all its professionals working at Tier 2 and Tier 3.

A comprehensive CAMHS can and should impact upon, rather than merely respond to or manage, demand; however, to do so it needs to be clear, confident and authoritative in what it does. Child and adolescent mental health services need to explicitly, in negotiation with partner agencies and commissioners, define their boundaries by stating both what they do and how they do it, and by clearly defining what they do not do. Child and adolescent mental health services should be clear about areas where it is unhelpful or damaging to respond to the demand. Running CAMHS, like being a parent, is simple, but that should never be confused with being easy. The importance of context, developmental, systemic and organisational, must pervade all our work. Tom Pitt-Aikens's notion of the 'good authority' recognised the difficulties of doing the right thing in the face of various contextual pressures (Pitt-Aikens & Thomas Ellis, 1989). It forces us to address the central question of any form of intervention, what we are doing and why, and how we are doing it. It is the same question we use in addressing families, and we must address it to ourselves.

The lack of clarity in purpose, the misuse of the tiered system, conflicting departmental targets, economic pressures and lack of understanding of service produce real problems for those commissioning and providing CAMHS. The usual case is that providers develop their own services in line with perceived need and the evidence base, perform their commissioners' jobs for them and do a very good job of it. Unfortunately, when commissioners come under pressure from national and financial pressures, they request existing CAMHS to tender to provide such services. Clinicians' time is then taken from service delivery to prepare complex tender documents correcting naive service specifications when in reality there is a rarely an alternative to provide a comprehensive CAMHS. Sadly, the shortsightedness of some commissioners and provider organisations has lead to CAMHS becoming staffed by low-paid and poorly trained personnel in the mistaken belief that anybody can look after mentally disordered children. Poor commissioning has also meant that expensive in-patient beds are being increasingly provided in the independent sector, without close relationships with community CAMHS. So uninformed commissioning is dismembering services which can only operate effectively if they are integrated.

Good practice by its very nature involves engagement, collaboration, information sharing and working together. Like the majority of parents, most professionals care and want to do their best for those with whom they work; this book is aimed at assisting them in their task through all the contextual difficulties discussed above. We have the responsibility for the baby in bathwater and although not throwing baby and bathwater into a whirlpool of unrealistic expectations, we need to understand when the bathwater will be healthy for the baby and when it has passed its usefulness and the baby will do better without it!

Ian Partridge and Greg Richardson

References

Bickman, L. (1996) A continuum of care: more is not always better. *American Psychologist*, **44**, 69–76.

Department for Children, Schools and Families (2005) *Social and Emotional Aspects of Learning: Improving Behaviour, Improving Learning*. TSO (The Stationery Office).

Department for Children, Schools and Families (2009*a*) *Every Child Matters* (http://www.dcsf.gov.uk/everychildmatters/about/). Department for Children, Schools and Families.

Department for Children, Schools and Families (2009*b*) Healthy Schools (http://home.healthyschools.gov.uk/Default.aspx). Department for Children, Schools and Families.

Department of Health (2009) *Healthy Lives, Brighter Futures. The Strategy for Children and Young People's Health*. TSO (The Stationery Office).

Hickey, N., Kramer, T. & Garralda, M. E. (2007) Is there an optimum model of practice for the newly developed child and adolescent primary mental worker posts? *Journal of Mental Health Training, Education and Practice*, **2**, 10–18.

HM Government (2004) *Every Child Matters: Change for Children*. TSO (The Stationery Office).

Kelvin, R. (2009) *Proposed Recommendations for growth in NTNs, Consultant Workforce and Non-Medical Multidisciplinary Teams for 2009–2012*. Faculty of Child and Adolescent Psychiatry, Royal College of Psychiatrists.

McCord, J. (1992) The Cambridge-Somerville study: a pioneering longitudinal-experimental study of delinquency prevention. In *Preventing Antisocial Behaviour: Interventions From Birth Through Adolescence* (eds J. McCord & R. E. Tremblay), pp. 196–206. Guilford Press.

MTA Cooperative Group (1999*a*) A 14 month randomised clinical trial of treatment strategies for attention-deficit/hyperactivity disorder. *Archives of General Psychiatry*, **56**, 1073–1086.

MTA Cooperative Group (1999*b*) Moderators and mediators of treatment response for children with attention-deficit/hyperactivity disorder. *Archives of General Psychiatry*, **56**, 1088–1096.

NHS Health Advisory Service (1995) *Together We Stand: Commissioning, Role and Management of Child and Adolescent Mental Health Services*. HMSO.

Pitt-Aikens, T. & Thomas Ellis, A. (1989) *Loss of the Good Authority: The Cause of Delinquency*. Viking.

Rutter, M., Maughan, B., Mortimore, P., *et al* (1979) *Fifteen Thousand Hours*. Open Books.

UNICEF (2007) *An Overview of Child Well-being in Rich Countries: A Comprehensive Assessment of the Lives and Well-being of Children and Adolescents in the Economically Advanced Nations*. Innocenti Report Card 7. UNICEF.

CHAPTER 1

Introduction

Ian Partridge and Greg Richardson

'The world is disgracefully managed, one hardly knows whom to complain to.'
Ronald Firbank, *Vainglory*

Purpose and scope of the book

Child and adolescent mental health services (CAMHS) comprise a small, unusual specialty often ill understood by those who work within, those trying to use and those trying to commission them. In an attempt to make order out of the possible chaos, *Together We Stand* (NHS Health Advisory Service, 1995a) offered a review of and a strategic framework for, the organisation and management of CAMHS. This strategic approach was sanctioned by the House of Commons Health Committee (1997) and provided the benchmarks against which CAMHS have been measured (Audit Commission, 1999). Unfortunately, since the publication of the first edition of this book, the application of the principles and strategic approaches that informed *Together We Stand* has been subject to individualistic variation.

The tiered system has been bastardised or 'moved on' over the past 10 years to an incomprehensible 'lingo' in which many writers assume all 'specialist' or 'core' CAMHS operate at Tier 3, and Tier 2 has been confined to limbo, beneath the dignity of so-called 'senior professionals' of whatever discipline. The differing interpretations have resulted in the very confusion about services that the tiers were intended to overcome, so the risk of the confusion that reigned prior to 1995 has reoccurred, indeed it has been amplified. There is a serious risk that CAMHS will again become marginalised as they cannot be understood and are subject to changes and targets from those in power who do not understand their functioning, as advisors to government ministers have no real understanding of what the tiers are about. The tiered system is an integrated approach in which CAMHS professionals work across tiers: it is not and cannot function as a hierarchical system in which 'senior clinicians' are seen to operate at Tiers 3 and 4 only. The creation of 'Tier 2 teams' is a contradiction in terms, and reinforces the hierarchical attitude that only senior staff work at Tier 3 and above, which undermines both an integrated approach and true multidisciplinary working. It is worth restating the following.

- Tier 1 is the services provided by people who in the normal course of their professional lives have an effect on children's mental health (e.g. teachers, social workers). There have been tremendous developments in Tier 1 in recent years with the establishment of Sure Start (Department for Children, Schools and Families, 2009), Healthy Schools (www.healthyschools.gov.uk) and organisations such as Connexions (www.connexions-direct.com), and CAMHS have an onerous responsibility in supporting their work through consultation and advice.
- Tier 2 is an integral part of 'specialist CAMHS' or 'CAMHS proper' and is where individual CAMHS professionals practice their individual skills as part of the multidisciplinary CAMHS. Professionals operating at Tier 2 must be able to undertake a full and competent assessment, and that assessment needs to be holistic in assessing the many difficult predicaments the child and family may find themselves in. Just looking for a diagnosis that leads to a treatment package is too simplistic. Any CAMHS professional who doesn't have the skills to work on their own is a waste of CAMHS resources. Primary mental health workers provide a very effective bridge and gateway between Tier 1 and community CAMHS; one of the most effective and reassuring interventions for Tier 1 professionals is consultation (Wyatt & Richardson, 2006; details available on request from the author) and this should be an integral part of any CAMHS professional's work.
- Tier 3 includes teams within a 'specialist' or 'core' CAMHS, with a team structure and approach targeted at particular problems (e.g. an eating disorders team or an attentional problems team). Therefore, Tiers 2 and 3 constitute CAMHS secondary care.
- Tier 4 is very specialist services such as in-patient care, a mental health liaison service to a paediatric service or a service for deaf children with mental health problems.

The tiers are clearly laid out in the document that spawned them (NHS Health Advisory Service, 1995a) and the tendency to use the term Tier 3 for specialist, core or community CAMHS seems to arise from some CAMHS professionals requiring a status reflection of their own self-importance. This handbook sticks to the clear system advocated in *Together We Stand*, in which CAMHS is composed of staff working in Tiers 2–4, and Tier 3 are specialist teams within a CAMHS such as a bereavement team or a learning disability team. In this book, CAMHS refer to generic services for child and adolescent mental health problems provided by the National Health Service (NHS) or independent health providers. Teams refer to specific groups of CAMHS professionals working on specific tasks within a generic CAMHS (e.g. an eating disorders team or an attentional problems team), but which may also involve inter-agency working with staff who are not employed by health services (e.g. social workers in a looked-after children's team).

It is important to have an effective and properly resourced national CAMHS for mental disorders as mental health problems affect 10–20% of children (Fombonne, 2002) and appear to be becoming more prevalent. With a finite supply, this ever-growing demand on CAMHS has rightly stimulated the development of community-based initiatives in which effective working with and into Tier 1 is an essential function of provision. All CAMHS professionals must work across all tiers, all must have a 'consultant' function, and all services must be able to identify not just what they do but what they do not do. Expansion of services into ever more specialist niches may do wonders for individual or disciplinary imperialism, but there is a danger of devaluing and undermining so-called 'bread and butter' provision with a consequent impact on the mental health of the wider community. A useful CAMHS will have negotiated with commissioners and partner agencies what it's priorities must be.

Child and adolescent mental health services must be responsive to change whether in terms of identified need, legal structures, governmental policy, clinical practice or priorities, while maintaining stability and continuity in service delivery. It is a mature service that recognises that reorganisation and refocusing for its own sake as a mere reactive impulse to any new stimulus results in chaos, uncertainty and dissatisfaction.

This second edition describes how the strategic framework described in *Together We Stand* (NHS Advisory Service, 1995a) can be put into practice by further developing and updating the principles of clinical management to the delivery of CAMHS. This is not a text describing clinical work at any one tier, although the provision of any service must be thoroughly informed by a relevant understanding of clinical need and practice. It is a description of how the nuts and bolts of the organisation of CAMHS delivery can be put together at each tier and between tiers to provide a robust, patient-centred, clinically effective service. The handbook addresses the interface between all tiers and the development of effective operational structures that allow for professional functioning in an integrated fashion. The settings in which such practices operate have been extended in this edition. The book concludes with the reflections of a Chief Executive who identifies not only what he expects of a service, but also what a service can legitimately expect of him.

The handbook remains geared to those from all disciplines working in CAMHS as well as those responsible for their organisation. The editors consider that the handbook will be helpful to commissioners, as it details how services should be organised to ensure value for money when commissioning CAMHS at whatever level (Morley & Wilson, 2001). The text is underpinned by research evidence as well as government policy, but also by reference to experience, achievement and opinion.

This is not a textbook for Tier 1 professionals looking to develop services for children with mental health problems. However, the importance of the support of Tier 1 and the interface between Tier 1 and other CAMHS provision is emphasised in Chapter 13. The development of formal links as well as informal understanding of relative functions is part of the relationship building that is at the core of the effective operation of CAMHS.

The developing role of the voluntary sector and client interest/support/ pressure groups has affected the nature of service provision. Fortunately, patient partnerships are inevitable in CAMHS as it is not possible for CAMHS to make any useful intervention without full patient and family participation in managing the difficulty presented. However, more formal links must be developed and effective networks established with such groups so that they can truly become partners in service delivery. The voluntary sector has developed differently in different parts of the country, with different agencies taking different priorities; it is therefore difficult to be prescriptive. However, commissioners should certainly involve voluntary agencies when planning and developing CAMHS for which they are responsible.

Principles considered

Multi-agency, multiprofessional liaison, cooperation and management

Children come into daily contact with any number of different professionals who influence their mental health. Any agency that purports to be interested in the mental health of children must work with all professionals, whatever agency, voluntary or statutory, or profession they come from. Child and adolescent mental health services must therefore work with all other agencies involved with children. Similarly, a competent CAMHS cannot hope to meet children's needs without the input of different disciplines, each offering differing perspectives and knowledge bases. The management of each agency and service must understand the need to work with other agencies and services to ensure integrated services. Professional and organisational boundaries, which encourage professional and organisational imperialism have no place in a service that puts children and their families at its centre.

Systemic approaches

Children thrive in some systems and do badly in others (Rutter *et al*, 1979). Viewing pathology as lying within the child so that they are assessed individually and out of context does not serve the child well, and can often lead to stigmatisation and foster low self-esteem, not to mention absolving adults involved with the child from any need to change their behaviour. This handbook takes a systemic approach and looks at organisational matters that promote mental health, as well as the organisation of individual interventions geared to the needs of the child in the predicament in which they find themselves. This does not mean that children with individual problems such as autism or anorexia nervosa do not require management packages tailored to their needs, but those packages must be provided in a manner and within an organisational structure that systemically supports their mental health. This handbook remains based on the premise that a systemically healthy CAMHS will be more effective than a collection of non-interacting mental health professionals.

Clear structure, terms of reference and operational policy

In order to meet the generally increasing demand upon services and to meet ever proliferating targets and guidance, the organisational structure of any CAMHS must be explicit in terms of both the service that can be offered and the service that cannot. This will involve a degree of prioritisation and, at times, rationing, as we identify that which we are not able or qualified to do. This position is often muddied by the creation of waiting lists in acceptance of the out-of-date mechanics of responding to referrals rather than managing and restructuring the referral process as described in Chapters 11 and 12. Child and adolescent mental health services need to move away from the linear notion of referrals, which is clearly inadequate as only 10–25% of children with mental disorders and mental health problems are referred to such a service (Fombonne, 2002). A system is required that involves work with children and families based upon need through multi-agency and multiprofessional liaison, cooperation and management. Those who commission or need to use a service or team within CAMHS have the right to know how that service or team operates. It also helps the service or team to understand its own function and for the induction of new members for it to have developed a clear operational policy.

Integration between tiers

The advantage of the tiered structure and multidisciplinary working is to move away from medical model-based systems, defined by finished consultant episodes (a period of admitted care under a consultant within an NHS trust) and face-to-face contacts, with the consequent medicalisation of child and family development, to a system where intensity of input is geared to complexity of need. The tiered system is one of organisational structure that supports such a method of service delivery, each CAMHS professional having the potential to work at, or with, more than one tier.

Different services will have both different resource levels and different skill mixes, and this will affect their provision. A CAMHS will need to have sufficient professionals within it to provide a comprehensive Tier 2 service and to form a comprehensive range of Tier 3 teams. However, each of the identified clinical needs can be managed at different positions within the tiered system, depending upon local circumstances. The effective management of CAMHS is dependent on recognition of the interface between the tiers and a close working integration of them all. In clinical terms, a linear approach to the tiered system will result in its failure, whereas a systemic understanding will allow it to function effectively.

Integration of organisational structure

Although CAMHS are generally small, they are sufficiently different from other health service provisions that they require their own discrete managerial and organisational structure and commissioning processes. Only then will there be allowance for the greater sophistication and specificity in understanding of service delivery and consequent financial management, including effective costing, of the different aspects of service provision, which will be essential when 'Payment by Results' (Department of Health, 2009) is introduced. An example of the need for an understanding of CAMHS complexity and the integration of all tiers is in the commissioning and provision of Tier 4 in-patient services. The need for such services may decline with effective community provision at Tiers 1, 2 and 3, but they will still be required, albeit possibly with fewer beds. In the short term, such services may appear both over-expensive and over-staffed, thereby offering the scope for financial savings in times of cutbacks. However, if locality CAMHS withdraw resources from Tier 4 provision, such provision will disappear and not be there on the few occasions when it is required. Such disinvestment by the NHS is indeed happening, and so between 2001 and 2006 the independent sector had moved from providing a quarter to a third of in-patient provision (O'Herlihy *et al*, 2007). The integration of the tiers rather than fragmentation of CAMHS by separating the tiers will allow for a full provision of services for young people from their communities through to the most specialist provision.

Caring for the carers

A service that does not care for itself is likely to have difficulty caring for others – a fact often overlooked within the caring professions. Working in CAMHS is a tiring and often emotionally draining experience. There must be formal lines of responsibility, accountability and supervision in place, as well as access to training, so that people feel professionally secure and supported by the organisation and their colleagues; this is described in Chapter 7. A sense of perspective must be maintained so that we do not take ourselves too seriously. There is a place for insensitivity, black humour, prejudice, irritation, frustration and irrationality – all those defence mechanisms essential to our sanity. There is a myth of the objective, detached professional who can shed personality, beliefs and values on entering a professional arena – it is a myth that can lead to burn-out and professional underfunctioning. Child and adolescent mental health services work with reality rather than ideals. A simple structural entity can aid this process, namely the staff room or common room. This should be a place wherein the shackles of professional responsibility can be loosened in the comfy cushion of shared coffee or lunch, a place where folk can meet and discuss the problems bothering them, and gain advice and support in their ongoing practice, or just let off steam and be unreasonable and uncaring.

Evidence-based practice

The Children Act 1989 requires that any intervention into a child's or family's life should result in a demonstrably better situation for the child than not intervening. This is a principle, along with the Hippocratic injunction of 'first, do no harm', that can and should inform our clinical practice. In CAMHS we are faced with a wide range of what can broadly be termed 'mental health problems' causing considerable psychological distress and morbidity, although we face a small range of specific diagnosable mental illnesses (Meltzer *et al*, 2000), and public perspectives of referral to a CAMHS will tend to focus upon the latter. Any service provision for distressed members of society cannot be an exact science, ratified by double-blind randomised controlled trials (RCTs) as many problems often occur together and are difficult to disentangle, but all need addressing to alleviate the distress: the care, support and treatments offered are as much an art as a science.

Referral to a CAMHS may result in the labelling and stigmatisation of the child and family, as well as in the deskilling of the parent. A systemic understanding must always inform our knowledge of the evidence base. Our work should, of course, be focused, problem-solving, collaborative and, where possible, short term. Beyond this, we should always consider the effect of any CAMHS intervention, which starts in the mind of the child and family long before their first consultation with the referrer. When considering a CAMHS response, those processes preceding referral must be weighed in the balance of mental health pros and cons, so that the response is geared to positive mental health rather than increasing mental health problems.

Services described

Throughout this book, the above principles are paramount and guide the service delivery described. To avoid repetition, the following principles can be considered to guide the authors of all the chapters in both the management of the service and the development of effective clinical provision.

- The CAMHS is based on multidisciplinary working.
- It represents a responsive service that offers advice and support, and that avoids stigmatisation and the disempowering of families; that is, a service that is child- and family-centred and that dovetails with services from other agencies.
- The CAMHS takes on board the social, educational, emotional and medical needs of the young person and family.
- The service provides clear information to other services and agencies about routes of referral and consultation.
- There is a clear operational policy for each professional, team and service that details skills, accessibility and comprehensiveness.

This handbook was conceived as a manual for those wishing to put their CAMHS in order. Inevitably, it takes a CAMHS perspective. However, the need for CAMHS to work with other agencies and for them to understand CAMHS is overwhelming and the principles underlying the handbook dictate a multi-agency perspective.

The services described in this book are based within the legislative framework of England, much of which also pertains to Scotland, Northern Ireland and Wales. There will be differences in details, as a result of initiatives in the devolved UK (e.g. National Assembly for Wales, 2001). However, the principles of CAMHS delivery will remain the same if services are based on need and effectiveness rather than professional or legal nicety.

Any service exists, as indeed do patients, in a context and, as such, both influence and are influenced by relational factors, be they internal (within a CAMHS) or external (e.g. government or trust policy). Organisational change within the NHS has no discernible end-point, so this handbook is heavily informed by reference to 'what works' for both provider and recipient of CAMHS provision, but will clearly have to develop as government policies, societal mores and research dictates.

References

Audit Commission (1999) *Children in Mind*. Audit Commission Publications.

Department for Children, Schools and Families (2009) Sure Start children's centres (http://www.dcsf.gov.uk/everychildmatters/earlyyears/surestart/whatsurestartdoes/). DCSF.

Department of Health (2009) What is Payment by Results? (http://www.dh.gov.uk/en/Managingyourorganisation/Financeandplanning/NHSFinancialReforms/DH_4065236). Department of Health.

Fombonne, E. (2002) Case identification in an epidemiological context. In *Child and Adolescent Psychiatry* (eds M. Rutter & E. Taylor), pp. 52–69. Blackwell.

House of Commons Health Committee (1997) *Child and Adolescent Mental Health Services*. TSO (The Stationery Office).

Meltzer, H., Gatward, R., Goodman, R., *et al* (2000) *Mental Health of Children and Adolescents in Great Britain*. TSO (The Stationery Office).

Morley, D. & Wilson, P. (2001) *Child and Adolescent Mental Health: Its Importance and How to Commission a Comprehensive Service. Guidance for Primary Care Trusts*. YoungMinds.

National Assembly for Wales (2001) *Child and Adolescent Mental Health Services: Everybody's Business*. Primary and Community Healthcare Division.

NHS Health Advisory Service (1995) *Together We Stand: Commissioning, Role and Management of Child and Adolescent Mental Health Services*. HMSO.

NHS Health Advisory Service (1995b) A strategic approach to commissioning and delivering child and adolescent mental health services. In *Together We Stand: Commissioning, Role and Management of Child and Adolescent Services*, pp. 59–69. HMSO.

O'Herlihy, A., Lelliott, P., Bannister, D., *et al* (2007) Provision of child and adolescent mental health in-patient services in England between 1999 and 2006. *Psychiatric Bulletin*, **31**, 454–456.

Rutter, M., Maughan, B., Mortimore, P., *et al* (1979) *Fifteen Thousand Hours*. Open Books.

CHAPTER 2

CAMHS in context

Greg Richardson and Ashley Wyatt

'The farther backward you can look, the farther forward you are likely to see.'
Winston Churchill (1874–1965)

Introduction

Over the years, CAMHS have had disparate masters and homes. Local Authority-based child guidance clinics and health service-based in-patient units came together in 1974. At that time, there was recognition that mental health services for children and adolescents should be based in the community rather than in institutions (Department of Health and Social Security, 1975). Now that they are based in health services, the idea and functioning of multidisciplinary services and teams can represent a mystery to doctor-led, referral-based health systems and those responsible for commissioning such services. Child and adolescent mental health services have often been prey to strategic and resource neglect, but idiosyncratic clinical practice has often been of an outstanding nature. With the acceptance of a tiered strategy for CAMHS, there has been increased coordination, an influx of resources and increased scrutiny (Department for Children, Schools and Families & Department of Health, 2008).

Publications in the field of social care (e.g. *Children in the Public Care*; Department of Health & Social Services Inspectorate, 1991), a precursor of *Quality Protects* (Department of Health, 1999), education (e.g. *Getting in on the Act*; Audit Commission, 1992) and health (e.g. *With Health in Mind*; Kurtz, 1992) were calling attention to children 'in need', children with 'educational and behavioural difficulties' and children with 'mental health problems'. They overlapped considerably. Traditionally, health services were interested only if a child had a mental health problem, Social Services were interested only in children in need, and education services were interested only in children with emotional and behavioural difficulties, but children's developmental needs cannot be subdivided into different educational, social and health boxes without a similar dismembering of the child.

It was only in the early 1990s that the need to work across agencies achieved some political recognition as 'care in the community' was failing for lack of it. In 1993, as part of the Health of the Nation initiative, *Working Together for Better Health* (Department of Health, 1993) showed government recognition of health being dependent on 'healthy alliances' across agencies.

To those using formulations that looked at the constitutional, family and environmental factors affecting children at their developmental stage this was nothing new, but it was quite a shift for medically based illness services.

Outcomes and economics

With a greater questioning of not just the organisation but also the legitimacy and funding of the welfare state, medical practice needed to be more systematic in its outlook in terms of interventions, outcomes, costs and effectiveness. The reorganisation of the NHS in the early 1990s had the expressed objective of making it more accountable to patient, taxpayer and government. An interest in the management of CAMHS became legitimate and sadly overdue as the problems were already well recognised (NHS Health Advisory Service, 1995), many still being evident (Box 2.1). In CAMHS, there is a great deal of overlap in the work that team members do, which has raised challenges in the economics of CAMHS organisation and costing. For example, with the development of community psychiatric nursing, a briefer, task-focused way of working has provided the basis for a service that responds more readily and rapidly to children and families' difficulties; however, to provide a comprehensive and responsive service, the skills and experience of other service members must be available. To demonstrate the need for such a multidisciplinary service, the measurement of outcomes is essential and this is now driven by the CAMHS Outcome Research Consortium (CORC). Interventions are now expected to have an evidence base and directories of the evidence base are now appearing (Fonagy *et al*, 2002; Mental Health Foundation, 2002; Wolpert *et al*, 2006) as well as young people being informed about what might be helpful to them (CAMHS Evidence-based Practice Unit, 2007).

A strategic framework

This coalescence of historical factors led to a survey of service provision for the mental health of children and young people, which recognised the poor organisation of and the poor coordination across services (Kurtz *et al*, 1994), hence the need for a strategy (Box 2.2). The publication the following year of *Together We Stand* (NHS Health Advisory Service, 1995) provided a strategic framework for the organisation and comprehension of CAMHS. This has provided a springboard for CAMHS throughout the country to differentiate their four-tier functioning and clarify their operation at each of the tiers. However, by 1999 limited progress had been made (Audit Commission, 1999).

The tiered model

The tiered model is now generally accepted as the way to describe and understand CAMHS. A filter 'guards' entry to each tier. The first filter

Box 2.1 Problems in the management of CAMHS

- The enthusiasms of therapists and teams traditionally drove interventions, which were often effective because of that enthusiasm. The concept of tailoring interventions to needs is increasingly dependent on the evidence available, rather than overriding therapeutic ethos.
- Multi-agency working within a service or team made the members of that team hostage to the fortunes of the managers of their agency. Social workers have been withdrawn from CAMHS all over the country, while other Social Services departments have demonstrated high levels of commitment to local CAMHS.
- Multidisciplinary services and teams were easily rendered dysfunctional by pressures from disciplinary hierarchies. This contributed to the many institutional, professional and personal factors that disrupt the trust, mutual respect, sense of responsibility, role clarity, communication, commitment and clarity of purpose that a properly functioning multidisciplinary service or team requires.
- Some services do not have a strategy, operational policies, business plans or measurement of what they are doing and whether it is effective, so their focus and functioning are unclear.
- Even within the health service, different professions are frequently managed separately. For example, community nurses may have separate management from clinical psychologists, who may be separate from psychiatrists.
- In the competitive world of health provision, overlaps in desirable areas are developing (e.g. the in-patient management of anorexia nervosa), and gaps in provision for the most difficult problems (e.g. children who are violent) are becoming more evident.
- Poorly managed services, which cannot take a strategic view, are soon overwhelmed by the demanding nature of the work and become demoralised. The only defences then are long waiting lists, complex referral pathways that alienate the community they purport to serve and dissatisfy commissioners, or to say the referred problem is not 'appropriate'.
- Young people and families do not feel involved in planning of interventions and services for them.

separates children, young people and their families from the first tier of professionals who work directly with them. Children with mental health problems and mental disorders primarily present their distress and behaviour to parents, teachers, health visitors and other workers within the community and a few to GPs. These professionals operate the second filter by deciding when it is necessary to involve a more specialist service from Tier 2. It is here that a referral system may get in the way of good mental health. Those referred to a CAMHS often feel blamed, stigmatised, incompetent, bewildered and frightened; the referral process may seriously assault their mental health. The direct input of Tier 1 professionals may be considerably more helpful to the mental health of a young person and family than referral to Tier 2, and supporting them in that task is a major role for CAMHS. Tier 2 consists of specialist mental health workers – community

Box 2.2 The requirements of a strategy

- Multi-agency collaboration and service provision
- Availability of information about services for young people and families
- Support for those professionals who are the first point of contact for children and families
- The way of working of the CAMHS should promote mental health and prevent further mental health problems
- Mental health service provision up to the age of 18 and transitional services for those requiring ongoing mental healthcare
- Improved provision for children with learning disabilities who also have emotional, behavioural and mental health problems
- Improved provision for children looked after by the local authority and leaving care
- Involvement of young people and their families in the planning and provision of services
- The provision of better quality, and management control over, services through improved single-agency and joint commissioning
- Outcome measurement

psychiatric nurses, clinical psychologists, psychotherapists, child and adolescent psychiatrists, social workers and occupational therapists – who are usually organised in a CAMHS working individually with young people and their families. A service will also have a number of Tier 3 teams, but these are not the sole components of a comprehensive CAMHS, where a number of those professionals work together for a specific task such as in a family therapy team or an eating disorders team. Tier 4 provides specialist services for a very small, but clearly defined group such as those with sensory deficits (e.g. deafness) or those requiring in-patient psychiatric care. The advantages of this tiered approach to service provision are restated in Box 2.3.

The inter-agency nature of CAMHS

The NHS Health Advisory Service (1995) report both clarified the functioning of CAMHS and called attention to the fact that mental health problems in children and young people 'may arise from a young person's difficulties in coping with life, developmental difficulty, the impact of sensory handicap or an educational difficulty or from social difficulties'. These problems are caused by, and present, in all areas of a child's functioning. Parents, teachers, health visitors and social workers have an important role in the maintenance of mental health. Education, Social Services, health services and the voluntary sector must work together, as children's mental health needs cannot be addressed separately. A multi-agency approach has to be at the core of services for children and young people with mental health

Box 2.3 The advantages of a tiered approach

- The functioning of CAMHS is easier to understand; managing and evaluating services becomes clearer and simpler. The Audit Commission (1999) and the CAMHS mapping process use the tiered system as a basis for their work on CAMHS.
- Resource input is related to complexity of need and appropriately filtered.
- The links required between tiers are clarified. Those between Tiers 2 and 3 and to Tier 4 services are often difficult because of geographical distances and the sometimes insular perspectives of Tier 4 facilities. Links between these, as espoused by the care programme approach (Department of Health, 1990), are essential for integrated care pathways for young people requiring such specialist resources.
- Clarification of professional functioning gives confidence in role fulfilment in each tier (Tier 3 teams often provide the glue that holds a service together).
- Specific areas of service deficit are highlighted.
- Planning is facilitated because it is easier to identify areas where the service needs to develop or change its focus.
- Integration with other agencies that have such tiered structures is enabled. Indeed, staff such as educational psychologists and behaviour support staff do Tier 2 work in the education services, as do social workers in the Social Services. Similarly, each agency has its own Tier 3 and Tier 4 teams.

needs. Health-based CAMHS have a major contribution to make to that multi-agency functioning.

Current context

The Department of Health, the Department for Children, Schools and Families, the Department for Education and Skills, and Her Majesty's Government have produced initiative after initiative over the past few years. It is often difficult to know which initiative is building on a previous policy and which is replacing a previous policy. Reading them all with all other guidance and outputs from non-governmental agencies as well as research would preclude any contact with children or families. Child and adolescent mental health services are increasingly subject to more and more government directives geared towards children's social, educational and health needs, which make it difficult for services to know whether they are meeting all the targets. The integration of the many current initiatives represents a considerable task, especially as there is increasing confusion between the interventions made by CAMHS and fellow professionals working to treat and manage mental or developmental disorders, and societal changes made to improve psychological well-being in the child population as a whole. This differentiation has become confused in the *National CAMHS Review* (Department for Children, Schools and Families & Department of Health, 2008), where what is nominally a review of

CAMHS is being asked to encompass 'improving the mental health and psychological well-being of children and young people'. Fortunately, the review is very thorough and provides required reading for anyone working with children's mental health needs in the second decade of the 21st century. The emotional well-being of children is the remit of society as a whole, whereas CAMHS are only responsible for those who have developed mental health problems. The review seems to assume that if CAMHS are properly resourced and organised then emotional well-being will improve throughout the population. The analogy is that drugs and surgery may improve the health of individuals, but it is measures such as clean water, proper diet and immunisation that have improved the health of populations. We need to seek the advice of sociologists in countries that have done far better in the UNICEF (2007) report, not mental health professionals on what will improve the mental health of young people in the UK.

Management of mental disorder

The government's Green Paper *Our Healthier Nation* (Department of Health, 1998) recognised the need for inter-agency working, so there is top-of-the-country ownership for such collaboration that has been espoused by government edicts if not practice for many years. The *National Service Framework for Mental Health* applied primarily to adults of working age, but some of the principles of healthcare delivery apply equally to children and young people (Department of Health, 2001), although the 5-year review paid scant regard to this age group (Department of Health, 2004). The *National Service Framework for Children* has provided considerable impetus for development in CAMHS (Department of Health & Department for Education and Skills, 2004), especially Standard 9, which states that:

> 'All children and young people from birth to their eighteenth birthday, who have mental health problems and disorders have access to timely, integrated, high quality multi-disciplinary mental health services to ensure effective assessment, treatment and support, for them, and their families.'

There are clear expectations that CAMHS will provide services for all those requiring them up to the age of 18, will provide cover 24 hours a day, 7 days a week, and will integrate the care of the learning disabled into their services, although the latter is taking a long time to come to fruition (Wright *et al*, 2008). The factors that increase children and young people's vulnerability to mental health problems are being increasingly recognised and addressed, for example the effects of secure settings on mental health (Department of Health, 2007), the effects of parental smoking (BMA Board Of Science, 2007), proper nutrition (Crawley, 2005, 2006) and unintentional injury (Audit Commission & Healthcare Commission, 2007), all of which must be considered when an individual child is being assessed. On an international scale, the World Health Organization (2005) has provided guidelines on the development of CAMHS.

Improving psychological well-being

Child mental health and psychological well-being are the responsibility of all in a civilised society. In response to the appalling death of Victoria Climbié (Department of Health & Home Office, 2003), the whole purpose of *Every Child Matters* (HM Government, 2004) was to establish criteria that would make children and young people emotionally healthy through:

- being healthy
- staying safe
- enjoying and achieving
- making a positive contribution
- economic well-being.

The measures that were put in place were rightly more wide ranging than just an increase in funding to CAMHS in the Priorities and Planning Framework between 2003 and 2006, to fund improved access to universally comprehensive CAMHS. Possibly because *Every Child Matters* is really about ensuring agencies work together for the purposes of safeguarding children, so it is a highly developed attempt at prevention rather than a nurturing measure, the result has been that despite the fact that 'it is a law that everyone must make these aims top priorities for all children and young people', we do not appear to be making progress on these aims (UNICEF, 2007). The UNICEF report made uncomfortable reading for us in the UK. It is prefaced by a definition of a civilised society that:

> 'the true measure of a nation's standing is how well it attends to its children – their health and safety, their material security, their education and socialization, and their sense of being loved, valued, and included in the families and societies into which they are born.' (UNICEF, 2007)

Unfortunately, the UK's standing is the lowest of all 21 countries (Table 2.1).

We clearly need to understand why children are feeling so badly about themselves and their lives compared with their counterparts in other countries. However, this is not primarily a CAMHS responsibility. The report points out 'levels of child well-being are not inevitable but policy susceptible'; it makes no comment about the susceptibility to mental health professional interventions.

Commissioning

Commissioning by primary care organisations has the potential to ensure a more useful CAMHS design, but at present has made little useful impact, possibly because their agendas are large and CAMHS very small and difficult to understand. Commissioning has been abandoned in Wales and one wonders how much money that has freed up for use in provider services. A broader strategy may have to be visualised to encompass comprehensive

Table 2.1 UK's score for the six dimensions of child well-being

Dimension	Score
Material well-being	18/21
Health and safety	12/21
Educational well-being	17/21
Family and peer relationships	21/21
Behaviours and risks	21/21
Subjective well-being	20/20
Average	18.2/21

Data from UNICEF, 2007.

CAMHS than will come into the purview of a primary care organisation. The development of children's trusts, led by the Local Authority, but with input from other agencies such as primary care trusts, represents a further recent development. These will increasingly provide a structure for all children's services (including CAMHS) to work towards a common set of aims set out in the local Children's and Young People's Plan.

Despite calls for greater integration of services, CAMHS are in danger of being pulled in two conflicting directions. If they are part of children's trusts as part of the spectrum of children's services operating within an overall Children and Young Peoples' Plan, they will increasingly receive and be expected to respond to referrals from all parts of children's services, often because of the common assessment framework. If they are part of a more traditional health service economy (and increasingly in the future as part of a foundation trust) in which CAMHS referrals continue to come mainly from other health services, they may be seen as increasingly out of touch with generic children's services and of limited use to them. Most CAMHS manage this potential split by responding to the degree of need and by consultation, but there is a danger that their managerial masters may wish them to favour their employing organisation's priorities.

The future

Structure and strategy

Nationally, regionally and locally there are considerable pressures for change in CAMHS to ensure comprehensive provision and ready access. Resources have been made available nationally to drive these changes, but there is a danger that those resources are now being leached away by the provider organisations that were given money specifically for CAMHS and are now taking money out of CAMHS budgets to use elsewhere. However, the National Child and Adolescent Mental Health Service

Mapping Exercise (www.childhealthmapping.org.uk/), which is undertaken annually, should record any depletion of CAMHS staff. Close cooperation between strategic health authorities, Local Authorities, health and social care trusts, and primary care organisations will be required to ensure the child and adolescent population and their families benefit from those increased resources. In the past, CAMHS have largely determined, from their own perspective, how they allocated their resources. In the future, it is increasingly likely to be other commissioning processes and partners who set out what they require of CAMHS to support their own services. Voluntary and independent providers may be keen to provide mental health services and local CAMHS may be commissioned to provide the consultation required by these services. Child and adolescent mental health services may have to go through a tendering process in order to be funded to provide a service that commissioners consider meets the needs of the population. This is likely to lead to the skill set required being more clearly articulated, with outcome measures being a required benchmark of the service being commissioned.

A common language across agencies should enable working together to find a way of sharing information; this has been possible in safeguarding children (HM Government, 2004, 2008) and should not be an impossible task. There should be involvement of users and carers in the development of services in line with good clinical practice. Children and young people and their families should be able to follow pathways of care without encountering the barriers of inter-agency, inter-professional and inter-tier boundaries. The aim should be to provide a service that is accessible, multidisciplinary, comprehensive, integrated with other agencies, accountable, and open to development and change (NHS Health Advisory Service, 1995).

Great effort should also be made in finding ways of working with Tier 1 professionals that lighten their load and do not make them feel burdened with an extra task; the British Medical Association (BMA) has described their role with regard to the mental well-being of children (BMA Board of Science, 2006). There should also be a move towards the standardising of Tier 4 provision.

The direction CAMHS will go in in the next 5–10 years is uncertain, as the medical 'seeing patients' model vies with the improvement of the well-being of children and young people model, the danger being that failure in the latter may bring CAMHS into disrepute, the alternative being the pathologising of more children so that CAMHS can intervene with them. However, there are perhaps a number of tests that can be applied to the service in the future to ascertain which model is more influential.

- Where are the majority of CAMHS referrals coming from – universal children's services such as schools or children's centres, or health services such as GPs or paediatricians?
- Is a significant proportion of specialist CAMHS time being devoted to the provision of consultation or training to other children's services

staff, or is the vast majority of effort expended on direct work with children and families?

- Do CAMHS see themselves as primarily part of mental health services or primarily part of children's services?
- Is the term 'CAMHS' used mainly as a shorthand for 'specialist CAMHS' (those whose focus is exclusive to mental health problems) or as a shorthand for 'comprehensive CAMHS', services having an impact on the emotional health of children – most of the professionals within which are not mental health specialists?
- Do specialist CAMHS use the same language as other children's agencies to describe the mental health/emotional health difficulties of children?
- Has the traditional perception of CAMHS by other children's services as difficult to access, and providing 'magical solutions' if they can be accessed, been modified to any significant extent?

The *National CAMHS Review* reported at the end of 2008 (Department for Children, Schools and Families & Department of Health, 2008). Much of the document concerned the 'emotional health' responsibilities of universal and targeted children's services. The review clearly expects specialist CAMHS to undertake case work within NHS waiting limits, to increase the resources allocated to vulnerable groups, as well as to increase the level of consultation and training to other children's services. The document is not clear as to how to prioritise between these competing demands, but the increasing focus provided to 'mental health and psychological well-being' is to be welcomed.

Transitions

Transitions between services because of age or nature of disability or illness are fraught with difficulty, but have to be addressed if young people are not going to have serious, anxiety-inducing interruptions in their care pathway. Those with neurodevelopmental difficulties such as attention-deficit hyperactivity disorder (ADHD) or autism-spectrum disorders are at particular risk as they do not traditionally fall into the purview of adult psychiatric services (Lamb *et al*, 2008). In future, the transition of a young person's care to adult mental health services when required must be clearly planned through discussion between CAMHS and adult mental health services, and occur at an age between 16 and 18 that best meets the young person's mental health needs The expectation that CAMHS deal with all young people under 18, which has not been funded in England or Scotland, although the Welsh assembly intends to fund this in Wales, but has not yet done so, has thrown into focus the difficulties young people have in moving between CAMHS and adult mental health services. A rigid cut-off of the 18th birthday for admission to a CAMHS bed is not in young people's interests, as some under-18s may be better cared for on an adult ward close to home and some over-18s may be better cared for in a CAMHS bed that better meets their developmental needs.

Transitions are further complicated by the fact that some services such as early intervention psychosis services deal with an overlapping age range, 16–35, and certain organisations target transitional age groups for their work (Garcia *et al*, 2007). The difficulties of such transitions, and how they might be managed, have been the subject of recent guidance (Department of Health, 2008). In the interests of the welfare of young people, both CAMHS and adult mental health services must have a ready dialogue to decide which service can most helpfully meet their mental health needs and ensure a smooth care pathway in the management of their mental disorder. Clear statements of boundaries by either service without such dialogue are not in the interests of the young people we serve.

Fortunately, the *National CAMHS Review* advised a National Advisory Council to oversee the progress of CAMHS throughout England, but this does not affect the other countries in the UK, so at least if things are not going well you know who to complain to.

Conclusion

Unprecedented resources have come into mental health services for children and adolescents in recent years. For children and families to benefit there must be an overarching coordination of the many initiatives, which need to be owned by all agencies working with them. Extra resources in CAMHS will benefit children, young people and their families only if those services are properly commissioned, organised, managed and targeted.

References

Audit Commission (1992) *Getting in on the Act. Provision for Pupils with Special Educational Needs: The National Picture*. HMSO.

Audit Commission (1999) *Children in Mind*. Audit Commission Publications.

Audit Commission & Healthcare Commission (2007) *Better Safe Than Sorry: Preventing Unintentional Injury to Children*. Audit Commission.

BMA Board of Science (2006) *Child and Adolescent Mental Health: A Guide for Healthcare Professionals*. British Medical Association.

BMA Board of Science (2007) *Breaking the Cycle of Children's Exposure to Tobacco Smoke*. British Medical Association.

CAMHS Evidence-Based Practice Unit (2007) *Choosing What's Best For You*. CAMHS Publications.

Crawley, H. (2005) *Eating Well At School: Nutritional and Practical Guidelines*. The Caroline Walker Trust.

Crawley, H. (2006) *Eating Well For Under-5s In Child Care: Practical and Nutritional Guidelines*. The Caroline Walker Trust.

Department for Children, Schools and Families & Department of Health (2008) *Children and Young People In Mind: The Final Report of the National CAMHS Review*. Department for Children, Schools and Families & Department of Health (http://www.dcsf.gov.uk/CAMHSreview/).

Department of Health (1990) *Joint Health and Social Services Council: The Care Programme Approach for People with a Mental Illness Referred to Specialist Psychiatric Services*. Department of Health.

Department of Health (1993) *Working Together for Better Health*. Department of Health.

Department of Health (1998) *Our Healthier Nation: A Contract for Health*. TSO (The Stationery Office).

Department of Health (1999) *Quality Protects Programme –2000/01. Transforming Children's Services*. Department of Health.

Department of Health (2001) *The Journey to Recovery – The Government's Vision for Mental Health Care*. TSO (The Stationery Office).

Department of Health (2004) *The National Service Framework for Mental Health – Five Years On*. Department of Health Publications.

Department of Health (2007) *Promoting Mental Health for Children Held in Secure Settings: A Framework for Commissioning Services*. Department of Health Publications.

Department of Health (2008) *Transition: Moving On Well*. TSO (The Stationery Office).

Department of Health & Department for Education and Skills (2004) *National Service Framework for Children, Young People and Maternity Services. The Mental Health and Psychological Well-being of Children and Young People*. Department of Health Publications.

Department of Health & Home Office (2003) *The Victoria Climbié Inquiry: Report of an Inquiry by Lord Laming* (http://publications.everychildmatters.gov.uk/eOrderingDownload/CM-5730PDF.pdf). Department of Health & Home Office.

Department of Health & Social Services Inspectorate (1991) *Children in the Public Care*. HMSO.

Department of Health and Social Security (1975) *Better Services for the Mentally Ill*. HMSO.

Fonagy, P., Target, M., Cottrell, D., et al (2002) *What Works for Whom – A Critical Review of Treatments for Children and Adolescents*. Guilford Press.

Garcia, I., Vasilou, C. & Penketh, K. (2007) *Listen Up! Person-Centred Approaches to Help Young People Experiencing Mental Health and Emotional Problems*. Mental Health Foundation.

HM Government (2004) *Every Child Matters*. Department for Education and Skills Publications.

HM Government (2008) *Information Sharing: Guidance for Practitioners and Managers*. Department for Children, Schools and Families Publications.

Kurtz, Z. (1992) *With Health in Mind: Mental Health Care for Children and Young People*. Action for Sick Children.

Kurtz, Z., Thornes, R. & Wolkind, S. (1994) *Services for the Mental Health of Children and Young People in England: A National Review*. Maudsley Hospital and South Thames (West) Regional Health Authority.

Lamb, C., Hall, D., Kelvin, R., et al (2008) *Working at the CAMHS/Adult Interface: Good Practice Guidance for the Provision of Psychiatric Services to Adolescents/Young Adults*. Royal College of Psychiatrists.

Mental Health Foundation (2002) *From Pregnancy to Early Childhood: Early Interventions to Enhance the Mental Health of Children and Families*. Mental Health Foundation.

NHS Health Advisory Service (1995) *Together We Stand: Commissioning, Role and Management of Child and Adolescent Mental Health Services*. HMSO.

UNICEF (2007) *An Overview of Child Well-being in Rich Countries: A Comprehensive Assessment of the Lives and Well-being of Children and Adolescents in the Economically Advanced Nations*. Innocenti Report Card 7. UNICEF.

Wolpert, M., Fuggle, P., Cottrell, D., et al (2006) *Drawing on the Evidence*. CAMHS Publications.

World Health Organization (2005) *Child and Adolescent Mental Health Policies and Plans*. WHO.

Wright, B., Williams, C. & Richardson, G. (2008) Services for children with learning disabilities. *Psychiatric Bulletin*, **32**, 81–84.

CHAPTER 3

CAMHS and the law

Ian Partridge, Greg Richardson and Mary Mitchell

'My nature is subdued
To what it works in, like the dyer's hand.'
Shakespeare, Sonnet 140

Introduction

The law clarifies responsibilities and legitimises interventions, providing a framework in which CAMHS may address the best interests of the young person and family. The central pieces of legislation relevant to CAMHS are the Children Act 1989, the Human Rights Act 1998, the Mental Health Act 1983 as amended in 2007, and the Mental Capacity Act 2005, although this has limited relevance to those under 16. The implications of these and related Acts to CAMHS practice are detailed for professionals (White *et al*, 2004; Harbour, 2008) and for parents (Family and Parenting Institute, 2007). The National Institute for Mental Health in England (NIMHE; 2009) has recently produced a helpful text, which navigates through the recent changes in legislation.

Children Act 1989

The Act represented a major rationalisation of the legal framework for dealing with children and identifies principles (Box 3.1) that are central to working with children and families. The welfare checklist (Box 3.2) provides a framework for planning for children and their families. As defined in the Act, a child is a minor until their 18th birthday. The Act also defines and upholds the principle of parental responsibility as:

'All the rights, duties, powers, responsibilities and authority which by law a parent of a child has in relation to the child and his property.'

The Act also provides guidance as to who holds parental responsibility, although the list has grown following subsequent acts (Adoption and Children Act 2002, Civil Partnership Act 2004). It goes on to identify principles that govern the courts and any court orders that relate to the care of children.

- The welfare of the child is paramount – Section 1(1).
- Delay must be reduced and avoided – Section 1(1).

Box 3.1 Principles of the Children Act 1989

Partnership
The importance of working together with children, families and other professionals. The notions of fairness, natural justice, openness, directness, honesty, empathy and support should generate interventions.

Paramountcy
Any involvement with and interventions into the lives of children and their families must begin and end with the principle that the welfare of the child (physical, psychological, developmental and emotional) is paramount.

Assessment of risk
If there are concerns regarding the welfare of children, the Local Authority has a duty (Section 4) to investigate. This has implications for CAMHS professionals who have concerns about children's welfare.

Significant harm
In terms of welfare and risks, the central concept is that of significant harm and the risk of significant harm. This arises from both acts of commission and acts of omission (Adcock & White, 1998).

Planning
The Act states that there is always a need for multidisciplinary and inter-agency cooperation and planning in working with children in need and at risk.

Communication
Identifiable networks of inter-agency communication, as well as communication with families, must be clarified.

- An order cannot be considered unless it is demonstrably better for the child than making no order at all.
- Account is taken of limiting legislation – Section 91(14).

The principles recognise that the child must be seen and understood in a developmental as well as a relational and family context. Interventions must be both realistic and pragmatic, with reasonable aims and expectations, always striving for the least restrictive alternative and the intervention that will do not only the most good but also the least harm.

Mental Health Act 1983

The Mental Health Act 1983 and the amendments in 2007 apply to children and young people; there is no minimum age for detention under the Act. The only age limitation is for guardianship, which applies to adults and young people over the age of 16. When young people require detention against their will the choice between using the Mental Health Act or the Children Act may not be an easy one, and usually only arises in relation to in-patient psychiatric care. The principle aim of the Children Act is to safeguard the child's welfare. The Mental Health Act safeguards the rights

---

Box 3.2 The welfare checklist

- The ascertainable wishes and feelings of the child, in light of age and understanding
- The child's physical, emotional and educational needs
- The likely effect on the child of any change in circumstances
- The child's age, gender, background and any other characteristics the court considers relevant
- Any harm the child has suffered or is likely to suffer
- How capable each of the child's parents, or any other person in relation to whom the court considers the question to be relevant, is of meeting the child's needs
- The range of powers available to the court under the Children Act in the proceedings in question

---

of people who require detention and compulsory treatment of a mental disorder by providing due process and rights of appeal. When a young person needs to be detained for their safety on account of behavioural disturbance rather than for the treatment of mental illness, consideration should be given to the use of a secure order (Section 25) of the Children Act 1989. In situations where consideration of these two legal frameworks is necessary, there must be clarity over the purpose of the intervention, and a decision as to whether the child's interests are best safeguarded by recognising their primary status as a child in need of protection, or as mentally ill and in need of in-patient treatment. Consideration should also be given to the least restrictive course of action.

Detention under the Mental Health Act 1983

In the vast majority of cases, the in-patient and community treatment of young people with mental disorders takes place on an informal basis, usually with the consent of both child and parents. The 2008 Code of Practice to the Mental Health Act 1983 as amended in 2007 (Department of Health, 2008) recognises the specific needs of children and recommends that the following should always be borne in mind when consideration is being given to the use of this legislation in the treatment of children and young people.

- Consideration of the best interests of the child or young person.
- Keeping the young person fully informed of their treatment.
- Taking into account their wishes (with due regard to age and understanding).
- Any intervention should be the least restrictive, least likely to expose them to stigmatisation, separation from family and interruption of their education.
- Providing access to education.

- The right of young people to dignity, privacy and confidentiality.
- The provision of facilities geared to their developmental needs.

In addition, when seeking the authority to detain and treat young people, the amended Mental Health Act 1983 recommends that at least one of the people involved in the Mental Health Act assessment of a person who is under 18 years old should be a clinician specialising in CAMHS, and where this is not possible, a CAMHS clinician should be consulted as soon as possible. In such an assessment the following will need consideration.

- Who has parental responsibility and what are their views?
- If parents are separated, with whom does the child live, is there a residence order and should contact be made with both families?
- What is the child's capacity for decision-making, offering consent to, or refusing, treatment?
- Local Authorities can under Section 33(3)(b) of the Children Act 1989 limit the extent to which parents may exercise their parental responsibility when a child is the subject of a care order.
- The 2008 Code of Practice introduces the concept of the 'zone of parental control' and provides guidance on the limits of parental power in treatment decisions when a young person is unable to make the decision (Department of Health, 2008). The more extreme the intervention, the more likely it is to fall outside the zone and the less likely it will be appropriate for the mental health professional to rely on the authority of a parent to treat a young person.

Section 131 of the Mental Health Act 1983, as amended by the 2007 Act, provides that a 16- or 17-year-old patient who has capacity to consent to being admitted to hospital for treatment of a mental disorder may give and withhold consent regardless of parental views. Such a young person therefore may be admitted even if a parent does not agree and, perhaps more importantly, may not be admitted against their will if parents seek to consent on their behalf. Where a 16- or 17-year-old lacks capacity to make such treatment decisions, the Mental Capacity Act may apply as it would to adults. However, if the treatment amounts to a deprivation of liberty as for example admission to a secure psychiatric unit, such action cannot go ahead under the Mental Capacity Act and any such admission should be assessed under the Mental Health Act 1983. Otherwise, common law principles may be considered, which permit a parent with parental responsibility to consent on behalf of the young person if the matter falls within the zone of parental control. If the intervention falls outside the zone and the young person does not fulfil criteria for detention under the Mental Health Act 1983, it may be necessary to seek authorisation from the court to proceed with treatment refused by the young person.

- If a young person under 18 is to be detained under the Mental Health Act, the hospital manager is now tasked by amendments to the Mental Health Act 1983 with providing appropriate facilities to ensure that the young person is placed in facilities geared to meeting their developmental needs. The definition of appropriate facilities is described in the Act, and includes guidance on segregation, staffing, routine and access to education.

- Careful consideration should be given to whether or not the child's needs could be met via an alternative placement (i.e. provision by the Social Services department or the education service).
- The 2008 Code of Practice advises that emergency treatment can and should be given if delay would be dangerous to the young person.

The sections of the Mental Health Act most often used within in-patient CAMHS are the following.

- Section 5.4 – whereby nursing staff are able to detain children wishing to self-discharge should they be concerned about their mental state, well-being and safety (this section expires after 4 hours).
- Section 5.2 – another interim section instigated by medical staff, which stays in force for 72 hours and should precede assessment for conversion to Section 2 or 3.
- Section 2 – expiring after 28 days, this allows for assessment within an in-patient setting.
- Section 3 – expiring after 6 months to allow treatment, but needs to be reviewed after 3 months.
- Section 117 – provides for a coordinating meeting before the discharge of any patient who has been detained under Section 3, and allows for multi-agency planning for care and treatment after discharge.

Mental Capacity Act 2005

The Mental Capacity Act 2005 applies to people aged 16 and over, and therefore has little impact on those under 16, who remain subject to the common law (Department for Constitutional Affairs, 2007). Most of the Act applies to 16- and 17-year-olds. An adult (18 years or over) and a young person (16–18 years) are presumed to have capacity unless:

'at the material time he is unable to make a decision for himself in relation to the matter because of an impairment of, or a disturbance in the functioning of the mind and brain.'

The doctor must establish first that there is such an impairment or disturbance, and second that it is sufficient to render the person incapable of making the particular decision. A person is unable to make the decision if they are unable to:

- understand the information relevant to the decision
- retain the information
- use or weigh the information as part of the process of making the decision
- communicate their decision.

Gillick competence

Young people under 16 years of age may make treatment decisions if the health professional decides that they have Gillick competence, which is defined as:

> 'sufficient understanding and intelligence to enable him or her to fully understand what is being proposed.' (*Gillick v. West Norfolk and Wisbech AHA [1986]*)

The concept of Gillick competence reflects the child's increasing development to maturity (Department of Health, 2008: p. 337). The doctor must assess that the young person is able to understand the risks and benefits of the intervention beyond immediate discomforts; for example, in some cases, a child's competence may fluctuate or while seeming to have the competence to make one decision a child may not necessarily have the competence to make another. The assessment must therefore be carefully considered with regard to each specific question. If the young person has the competence to make the particular treatment decision, they may give consent whatever their age. If the young person consents to treatment and is assessed by a healthcare professional as having Gillick competence then there is no need, legally, to obtain parental consent. However, it is good practice and preferable to gain both the consent of the young person and the parent when at all possible, and to involve all those close to the child in the decision-making process (Department of Health, 2001a).

Where a child with Gillick competence refuses treatment, the 2008 Code of Practice advises that the trend is to reflect greater autonomy for competent under-18s (Department of Health, 2008), so it may be unwise to rely on the consent of the person with parental responsibility and consideration should be given to whether or not the child meets criteria for detention under the Mental Health Act. Children who are not competent to make the decision about hospital treatment may be admitted with the consent of a parent with parental responsibility if the intervention is within the zone of parental control.

Assessing competence in young people

There are no formalised assessment procedures for the evaluation of competence in children. However, criteria from the practice guidelines for clinical psychologists (British Psychological Society, 2001) are consistent with guidelines from the BMA (2001) and have been updated by the General Medical Council (GMC; 2007). They provide a useful outline for assessing the competence of children and young persons relevant to all healthcare professionals (Boxes 3.3 & 3.4).

Human Rights Act 1998

The Human Rights Act seeks to ensure that laws, practices and procedures comply with the rights set out in the European Convention on Human

---

Box 3.3 Areas for assessment of capacity in children and young people

- Ability to understand choice and consequences of choice
- Willingness and ability to make choice
- Understanding of purpose, nature and effects of intervention
- Understanding of no intervention or alternative interventions, including attendant risks
- Freedom from pressure
- Reason for absence of parental consent

Rights (ECHR). The ECHR aims to protect human rights and fundamental freedoms, and to maintain and promote the ideals and values of a democratic society. The European Human Rights Act consists of 18 articles and 6 protocols, but not all of these are incorporated into UK law.

The introduction of the Human Rights Act will continue to have a major impact on the development of mental health law and practice, as it requires all public authorities (which include health and social care agencies) to act in a manner that is compatible with the ECHR. Individuals who have had their rights violated within mental health services can take legal action against the relevant authority. Many of the rights found in the ECHR have a direct impact on the provision of care for people with mental health problems. Those agencies and professionals involved in such care need to review their practices and procedures to ensure they lie within the ECHR (Sainsbury Centre for Mental Health, 2000). This has the potential for increasing good practice and ensuring respect for individual rights.

Consent

Articles 3 and 8 of the ECHR, 'freedom from torture and inhuman or degrading treatment or punishment' and 'the right to respect for private and family life, home and correspondence' respectively, have implications for ensuring consent of individuals is obtained before that individual undertakes medical treatment or psychological assessment, investigation or intervention (Hewson, 2000; Lilley et al, 2001). In Denmark (X v. Denmark (1983)), the court found experimental or non-consensual medical treatment to be in breach of Article 3. Absence of obtaining consent or acting in the best interests of an individual are in breach of Article 8 if the exceptions laid out in the article are not met. If informed consent is not obtained, or incapacity is not demonstrated and acting in the best interests of an individual is not indicated, then the healthcare professional in question would be in breach of Article 3 or 8 of the ECHR and could be charged as such in a UK court of law. Furthermore, it is vital for all healthcare professionals to be able to show that they have made methodical and continuous documentary records in both clinical and research work.

Box 3.4 Good practice in relation to consent and the assessment of capacity

Principles

- Although parental consent is not legally required if a child is assessed by a healthcare professional to be competent and the child consents to treatment, it is preferable to gain both child and parental consent.
- If the views of the parent differ from those of the child and this cannot be resolved through negotiation, the primary obligation is always the child's interests.
- Informed consent is a process, needing continual review.
- If a child is not considered to have capacity, clinical work should support active participation in decision-making by giving clear information and eliciting the child's views.

Standards of good practice

- Information should be provided at the appropriate developmental level of the child. The amount of information given should be appropriate to the length and nature of the intervention.
- Children should always be informed of the purpose of the work and the practical arrangements involved, even if their consent has not been obtained.
- Consent may need to be gained in a series of steps, in which case each stage should be recorded in the notes.
- When a child consents to treatment but the parent does not consent, then: record clearly the assessment of the child's competence, reasons why the parent has not provided consent and the agreement reached with the child concerning confidentiality; provide the child with written confirmation of the arrangements made; discuss the case in supervision or with senior colleagues and record this in the notes.
- The rare situation of a child assessed to have competence but refusing an intervention will best be resolved in a multidisciplinary setting. Supervision and consultation with other colleagues are essential. Overriding a competent child's wishes is justifiable only in circumstances where there is a significant threat to life or a threat of long-term significant harm and where the benefits of the intervention are relatively clear, for example when the withholding of antipsychotic medication in an early-onset psychosis could contribute to avoidable developmental damage. Legal advice or court approval may be necessary in these situations, especially when the parent refuses consent as well. For instance, if a young person with anorexia without capacity refuses food, nasogastric feeding will need to take place under Section 3 of the Mental Heath Act in order to protect the rights of the child to appeal and due process, and to ensure the welfare of the child.
- The more complex and problematic decisions should always be made with multidisciplinary input.
- Consent is required for sharing or obtaining information from other professionals or agencies. Again, if the child's best interests override consent, then this should be documented.
- Regular supervision and peer review are recommended.

Definition

Consent is defined in the Mental Health Act 1983 Code of Practice (Department of Health & Welsh Office, 1999: para. 15.13) as:

> 'The voluntary and continuing permission of the patient to receive a particular treatment, based on an adequate knowledge of the purpose, nature, likely effects and risks of that treatment including the likelihood of its success and any alternatives to it. Permission given under any unfair or undue pressure is not consent.'

For consent to be valid, four components are required.

- Adequate information needs to be provided to the individual.
- The individual must have capacity to give consent.
- There must be an absence of coercion.
- Available alternatives to the intervention offered need to be outlined.

The subject of consent to treatment for mental illness is a complex issue when working with children and young people, as it requires the professional to consider the consent of parents as well as their children. The introduction of the Human Rights Act also has some important implications in this area for healthcare professionals. However, the first test is whether the young person has the capacity to consent:

> 'Only if they are able to understand, retain, use and weigh this information, and communicate their decision to others can they consent to that investigation or treatment.' (General Medical Council, 2007)

Fortunately, guidance is provided for all clinicians by the Department of Health (2001b) and, for doctors, by the GMC (2008).

Confidentiality

Article 8 of the ECHR, 'the right to respect for private and family life, home and correspondence', has clear implications on confidentiality of information acquired through professional practice or research (Gostin, 2000; Lilley *et al*, 2001). This implies a responsibility for the protection of the privacy of individuals or organisations about whom information is collected or held. Part of the wide interpretation of Article 8 includes cases (e.g. *MS v. Sweden (1997)*, and *Z v. Finland (1998)*) where the court found that an individual's right to privacy (under Article 8) was breached through the lack of protection of medical notes and other data. This has clear implications and relevance for healthcare records. A healthcare professional who does not maintain confidentiality without the individual's consent, or who breaks confidentiality without just cause, will be in breach of Article 8 of the ECHR and could face charges brought in a UK court. The duty owed to children and young people regarding confidentiality is the same as for adults, and should only be breached if there is a risk of significant harm and a 'need to know' basis for disclosure. The young person is entitled to an opportunity to disclose such information themselves and to be involved in the decision to share information without their consent.

Safeguarding children

All agencies working with CAMHS have a responsibility to safeguard children and to understand the legal framework in which those responsibilities operate. Child and adolescent mental health services are required to work at the interface of clinical practice and children's safety in both a proactive and a reactive manner. This requires balancing responsibilities for the therapeutic management of children and their families with those of safeguarding children. The complexities in maintaining this balance are best addressed by reference to the welfare of the child being at all times paramount. Assessment of the best interests of the child should always take place within a multidisciplinary and multi-agency context (HM Government, 2004).

Through their work, CAMHS have a role in informing and developing effective methods of safeguarding children (Brophy, 2001). Both the Children Acts 1989 and 2004, and other guidance (Home Office et al, 1991; Department of Health et al, 1994, 1999; Department of Health & Welsh Office, 1995) restated the need for disciplines and agencies to work together in a network of communication and liaison to ensure the welfare of the child remains paramount.

Suspicion, and disclosure, of abuse or neglect

The local area safeguarding children committee will have clear guidelines for the management of child abuse and neglect, of which all CAMHS staff should be aware. Within CAMHS, there should be clear lines of communication, responsibility and accountability for staff faced with concerns about safeguarding children. All staff should be aware of the management of confidentiality, as differing criteria exist for different disciplines. The overriding duty to the child's welfare means that, within CAMHS, the guiding principle is limited confidentiality. Significant harm or the risk of significant harm necessitates the activation of procedures designed to safeguard the welfare of the child, regardless of the fashion in which information was obtained.

Linked to this is the responsibility of managing the situation in such a fashion as to minimise any additional stress and distress caused to the child and family. The principles that apply are listed in Box 3.5.

In general, it is not the role of CAMHS professionals to undertake child protection investigations unless they are asked to perform a specific assessment following the instigation of child protection procedures.

Inter-agency cooperation

The importance of inter-agency cooperation can be seen in the number of guidelines and publications with 'working together' in the title. Practical steps must be taken by CAMHS to operationalise this cooperation beyond attendance at occasional case conferences. The tiered system gives a clear

---

Box 3.5 Principles of safeguarding children

- The safeguarding of children is supported with established guidelines familiar to all members of staff working with children
- Senior staff are consulted and informed
- Information is presented to and discussed with the relevant agencies (e.g. Social Services, police)
- The child is kept fully and clearly informed of what is happening
- The family are informed as soon as is safe for the child
- The child is never put in more danger by the intervention
- Clear, detailed and, where possible, contemporaneous notes are kept
- Attendance at any subsequent inter-agency meeting is prioritised

---

framework for doing so and offers a mechanism whereby CAMHS can contribute fully and effectively to safeguarding children.

Tier 1

Providing support to Tier 1 workers is a vital part of CAMHS function, and never more so than when safeguarding children. Some Tier 1 workers (e.g. social workers) have primary responsibility for safeguarding children in terms of investigation and ensuring the child's safety and well-being. Advice, consultation and support from a CAMHS professional regarding psychological impact and sequelae, and the placing of child abuse within a systemic and developmental context, can enable this process to be more effective. A wider supervisory and advisory function may exist in work with other Tier 1 professionals.

Work in child abuse is emotionally draining and can have an impact upon individual professionals and professional networks, as well as the children and their families. The CAMHS professional may be able to offer support and understanding to such professionals, as well as a sense of detachment from the decision-making process.

Tier 2

Child and adolescent mental health service workers operating individually at Tier 2 may be involved in working with children and families where safeguarding children is of direct importance or indirect concern. In such work, multi-agency liaison and effective communication networks must exist, so that each agency understands its role and the questions it has to address. Knowing who's who in Social Services and the police, as well as developing relationships with these agencies, enables effective safeguarding of children. Being aware of guidelines, responsibilities and what is expected of various agencies and professionals ensures that work can be performed without recourse to panic; it also offers a calmer background for both child and family.

Tier 2 professionals may also be involved in post-investigation therapeutic work with children and families. The issue of therapeutic work during investigation and possible prosecution can be problematic; however, the clinical needs of children in terms of their emotional, psychological and physical well-being must be weighed carefully in terms of the responsibility to prioritise the welfare of the child.

Tier 3

Child and adolescent mental health services may develop particular Tier 3 services to work in safeguarding children on a reactive and preventive level. Examples include risk assessment teams, therapeutic group work, family therapy and parent–child relationship groups. In all these areas, liaison with other agencies must be clearly established to avoid isolated working and to establish their task in the management of the situation. Such specialist teams may also have an input to inter-agency training initiatives.

Tier 4

Specialist services such as in-patient units may provide a setting wherein disclosure of, or awareness of, child abuse occurs. The principles outlined above also apply here. It may be that children who develop serious mental health problems have experienced some form of neglect or abuse that is pertinent to their present condition and which may affect planning for them. The structural isolation of an in-patient unit must not detract from multidisciplinary and multi-agency planning and working for the young person's welfare.

References

Adcock, M. & White, R. (1998) *Significant Harm*. Significant Publications.

British Medical Association (2001) *Report of the Consent Working Party: Incorporating Consent Tool Kit*. BMA.

British Psychological Society (2001) *SIG Position Paper: Practice Guidance on Consent for Clinical Psychologists Working with Children and Young People*. BPS.

Brophy, J. (2001) *Child Psychiatry and Child Protection Litigation*. Gaskell.

Department for Constitutional Affairs (2007) *Mental Capacity Act 2005 Code of Practice*. TSO (The Stationery Office).

Department of Health (2001a) *Seeking Consent: Working With Children*. TSO (The Stationery Office).

Department of Health (2001b) *Reference Guide to Consent for Examination or Treatment*. TSO (The Stationery Office).

Department of Health (2008) *Mental Health Act 1983: Revised Code of Practice. Summary of Changes from Current Code*. TSO (The Stationery Office).

Department of Health & Welsh Office (1995) *Child Protection: Clarification of Arrangements Between the NHS and Other Agencies*. HMSO.

Department of Health & Welsh Office (1999) *Mental Health Act 1983 Code of Practice*. TSO (The Stationery Office).

Department of Health, British Medical Association & Conference of Medical Royal Colleges (1994) *Child Protection. Medical Responsibilities: Guidance for Doctors Working with Child Protection Agencies*. HMSO.

Department of Health, Home Office & Department for Education and Employment (1999) *Working Together to Safeguard Children*. TSO (The Stationery Office).

Family and Parenting Institute (2007) *Is It Legal? A Parents' Guide to the Law*. Family and Parenting Institute.

General Medical Council (2007) *0–18 Years: Guidance for All Doctors*. GMC.

General Medical Council (2008) *Consent: Patients and Doctors Making Decisions Together*. GMC.

Gillick v. West Norfolk and Wisbech AHA [1986] AC 112.

Gostin, L. O. (2000) Human rights of persons with mental disabilities: the European Convention of Human Rights. *International Journal of Law and Psychiatry*, **23**, 125–159.

Harbour, A. (2008) *Children with Mental Disorder and the Law*. Jessica Kingsley.

Hewson, B. (2000) Why the Human Rights Act matters to doctors. *BMJ*, **321**, 780–781.

HM Government (2004) *Every Child Matters: Change for Children*. Department for Education and Skills Publications.

Home Office, Department of Health, Department of Education and Science & Welsh Office (1991) *Working Together under the Children Act 1989: A Guide to Arrangements for Inter-Agency Cooperation for the Protection of Children from Abuse*. HMSO.

Lilley, R., Lambden, P. & Newdick, C. (2001) *Understanding the Human Rights Act: A Tool Kit for the Health Service*. Radcliffe Medical Press.

MS v. Sweden (1997) 3 BHRC 248.

National Institute for Mental Health in England (2009) *The Legal Aspects of the Care and Treatment of Children and Young People with Mental Disorder: A Guide for Professionals*. NIMHE.

Sainsbury Centre for Mental Health (2000) *An Executive Briefing on the Implications of the Human Rights Act 1998 for Mental Health Services*. Sainsbury Centre for Mental Health.

White, R., Harbour, A. & Williams, R. (2004) *Safeguards for Young Minds: Young People and Protective Legislation*. Gaskell.

X v. Denmark (1983) 32 DR 282.

Z v. Finland (1998) 25 EHRR 371.

CHAPTER 4

Structure, organisation and management of CAMHS

Ian Partridge and Greg Richardson

'Here is Edward Bear, coming downstairs now, bump, bump, bump, on the back of his head, behind Christopher Robin. It is, as far as he knows, the only way of coming downstairs, but sometimes he feels that there really is another way, if only he could stop bumping for a moment and think of it. And then he feels that perhaps there isn't.'

A. A. Milne, *Winnie the Pooh*

Introduction

The starting point of the management structure of CAMHS must be the young person and family – not the requirements of the institution. We are still learning about what suits young people and families best, but a service based on the principles described in *Together We Stand* (NHS Health Advisory Service, 1995) appears to go some way to meeting them. For the service to be geared to meeting the needs of the local community and its partner agencies, it must be clearly structured and efficiently managed (Box 4.1). It must understand the reality of commissioning priorities, staffing and retention levels, and shifts in national, regional or local initiatives, and incorporate them into the managerial framework so that service provision to the child and family is systemically informed by what is, rather than what we may wish in an ideal world should be. The CAMHS review has provided some clear principles about how CAMHS should develop to meet the broader mental health needs of all those at risk of mental health problems (Department for Children, Schools and Families & Department of Health, 2008).

A lack of attention to basic managerial principles often undermines the service provided, creating discord among, as well as pressure upon, individual professionals and teams. The resultant dysfunction can lead to inadequate service provision and low morale. Equally, a service that is perceived to be poorly organised and idiosyncratic is not going to attract investment.

Management in tiers

The tiered model starts with the young person and family, whose first contact with mental health services will be at Tier 1. Child and adolescent

---

Box 4.1 Foundations for effective CAMHS

- A 'critical mass' of multidisciplinary staff
- Coordination and integration of professions and teams
- Organisation within the tiered framework
- The use of the individual and professional skills of all service members to their full potential
- Clear lines of accountability, responsibility and supervision
- A training and development programme for all disciplines
- Prioritisation and management of workload
- Clear operational policies
- Adequate administrative support
- Overt inter-agency networks of communication
- An agreed strategy
- An interested and supportive management structure
- A designated, consistent budget
- Clinical governance

---

mental health services must be structured around them to ensure their pathway of care through the service is as smooth as possible; CAMHS must therefore provide mental health input to young people through those with whom they have contact in their everyday lives. There is no reason why all CAMHS disciplines, with training and experience, cannot and indeed should not be involved in liaison and consultation with Tier 1 staff. Developing contacts, relationships and joint working with outside agencies will ensure that CAMHS are understood and used effectively by those providing a direct service to children and families.

At Tier 2, CAMHS must be organised for individual professionals to work with children and families, as this is a large percentage of the work undertaken by any CAMHS. They will require, in addition to the principles listed in Box 4.1, an awareness of the functioning and specialist skills of other disciplines inside and outside CAMHS, and the operational practices of partner agencies, so that they can involve other disciplines and agencies as required by the children they see.

Tier 3 specialist teams provide an opportunity for CAMHS members to work together with a specific focus and to develop their skills in specific complex areas. Tier 3 teams should offer training opportunities for all disciplines and model good interdisciplinary working. They require coordinators to perform the everyday administrative tasks of the team, to ensure work allocated to the team is appropriately managed and to provide a focal point for other members of the CAMHS.

Most CAMHS will not have a Tier 4 function, and staff working at Tier 4 have specialist skills and often require their own discrete management structure.

A multidisciplinary service

To work effectively at all tiers, a range of disciplines, skills and perspectives are required, so that children are offered a care package geared to their individual needs. A multidisciplinary CAMHS must incorporate the skills necessary to address the clinical management of the wide and complex clinical problems presented. Each discipline and all professionals have a responsibility to work in and provide support across all tiers. The effective working of each tier and the free movement of staff to work and provide support in each tier are part of the functioning of a CAMHS as a whole. Within the service, each discipline will have its hierarchical and supervisory structure supporting the autonomous effectiveness of each profession.

Administrative staff are vital to the smooth and efficient running of any organisation. In addition to compiling and maintaining records for all aspects of the service, they may also take responsibility for the collection of statistical data that may be used for research and audit. These staff usually also work with patients and carers on the telephone and in the building, as well as with the many professionals involved with patient care. Administrative staff are the direct link with the public and other agencies, and are often the first point of contact for both. To ensure the right skill mix, it is necessary to invest and train the staff not only in appropriate clerical and administrative skills, but also in skills of diplomacy for this demanding and responsible area of work. The secretariat is often the service engine room, whose functioning is vital to the running of the ship. It should be recognised as such, and at times of financial hardship, if regarded as an expendable ancillary service, such short-sightedness will bring the service to a juddering halt.

Management of the service

The professions and specialist teams within CAMHS generate many management roles. These roles must be recognised and differentiated, members of CAMHS taking on responsibility for different roles at different times, for example coordinator of a Tier 3 team as well as professional supervisor of a less experienced member of the same discipline and possibly the professional lead.

All meetings and teams within the service will require a chair or coordinator who ensures that the meeting or team deals with the business in hand (e.g. the management of referrals or professional supervision) and that action is taken on decisions. Staff meetings, which are geared to under-standing the work of the service, as opposed to decision-making meetings, may require a facilitator, who may be another staff member or someone from outside the service.

Within each profession there are hierarchies and the senior members have responsibility for the professional supervision and management of those more junior (e.g. senior doctors ensuring there is a duty rota of junior doctors).

The site on which the CAMHS is based will also require management, so that the accommodation and working environment of all staff members are attended to. The staff member who takes on this responsibility must be able to network well in the rest of the host organisation and have considerable skills in managing people.

The CAMHS management team

Overarching responsibility for the structure, organisation and operation of CAMHS is the task of the CAMHS manager and their management team. This team should consist of the senior members of all the professions working in the service and relevant members of the host organisation's management, so that they may address the tasks listed in Box 4.2. The CAMHS manager will be the 'chief executive' for this meeting and takes responsibility for ensuring that decisions made by the CAMHS management team are put in place. They are the link between CAMHS and the host provider organisation, and both must hold them in high regard. They require considerable management and negotiating skills while maintaining a close grasp of what is realistically possible.

The achievement of the management tasks will require regular meetings, possibly monthly, to discuss clinical governance and financial matters as well as performance. The annual budget for CAMHS should be clearly differentiated from other budgets in the trust. The budget will then require monitoring and managing (Gale, 1996). It may also be useful to have the budget further subdivided for different parts of CAMHS (e.g. the Tier 4 service and the community CAMHS). The budget will also be divided under separate headings, such as staff costs, travel and overheads. A member of the host organisation's finance staff on the management group can be very helpful in understanding the financial situation. Child and adolescent mental health services that offer a specialist service such as Tier 4 provision,

---

Box 4.2 Tasks of the CAMHS management team

- Monitoring the distribution of workload and service delivery
- Ensuring clinical governance
- Monitoring progress of the service against the strategy
- Understanding, monitoring and containment of the service budget
- Developing business plans to enhance the service
- Ensuring partner agencies are involved in the operation of CAMHS
- Ensuring the operational policy for the service is up to date
- Ensuring all disciplines within CAMHS are represented
- Bringing serious opportunities or threats to the notice of the host organisation
- Informing and supporting the CAMHS manager in their management role

may have the potential to generate income for the host organisation, which may be a useful lever to gain more resources for CAMHS and certainly to support the Tier 4 service. Close monitoring at year-end (January–March) may reveal an under-spend which may enable the purchase of capital items before 31 March.

Management within the wider host organisation

The CAMHS management team may be a clinical directorate in its own right, or a subgroup of a larger directorate. There has been considerable discussion as to whether CAMHS are best placed within the management of child health services or mental health services. Child and adolescent mental health services can be well managed and understood in both settings and such services often wish to stay where they are. Equally, CAMHS can be poorly understood and badly managed in both settings. The lesson seems to be to develop relationships with the existing management structure rather than leave it in hope of finding a more understanding master. Child and adolescent mental health services are managed within the burgeoning variety of trusts that are now developing: they may be part of a community and mental health trust, a mental health foundation trust, a whole-district trust (in Wales only now), a primary care trust or a social care trust. They all have their advantages and disadvantages.

Trusts are organised upon a continuum from general management to clinical directorates and the CAMHS management group must ensure it is fitted firmly into whichever organisational structure is in place. There is no reason why members of the CAMHS management group cannot take on wider management responsibilities (e.g. the nurse manager being on the trust board or the consultant psychiatrist being the clinical director of child health), but the CAMHS manager must remain firmly focused on that task.

A CAMHS is only as strong as its weakest link. A service that does not integrate its component parts into a cohesive whole will find itself in danger of fragmentation at times of pressure, retrenching to a position of low staff morale and complaints of lack of resources. A well-managed service has within it the recognition and support of all members of the team and will be fit for purpose in obtaining and using resources effectively.

References

Department for Children, Schools and Families & Department of Health (2008) *Children and Young People In Mind: The Final Report of the National CAMHS Review*. Department for Children, Schools and Families & Department of Health (http://www.dcsf.gov.uk/CAMHSreview).

Gale, R. (1996) Managing a budget. In *Textbook of Management for Doctors* (ed. T. White), pp. 211–220. Churchill Livingstone.

NHS Health Advisory Service (1995) *Together We Stand: Commissioning, Role and Management of Child and Adolescent Mental Health Services*. HMSO.

CHAPTER 5

Evidence-based practice

Jonathan Barrett, Juliette Kennedy and Ian Partridge

'The good educationalist works from within the material drawing it out, he does not impose the pattern he has chosen on "ungrateful material".'

    Cornelius Cardew

Introduction

Evidence-based practice in CAMHS is epitomised by the conscientious, explicit and judicious use of current best evidence in decision-making about the care of young people and families (Sackett *et al*, 1997). Evidence-based practice therefore strives to:

- improve decision-making
- encourage cost-effective use of limited resources
- enhance knowledge among CAMHS practitioners
- assist in communication with families and facilitate collaborative, informed decision-making.

The underlying philosophy of evidence-based practice is that therapeutic interventions should be rational, measurable and observed to benefit their recipient (Laugharne, 1999). This leads to an attempt to standardise the way that all healthcare workers make clinical decisions, with a strong emphasis on using the best evidence available from research.

> 'The aim is to see that Research and Development becomes an integral part of healthcare, so that managers and practitioners find it natural to rely on the results of research in their day to day decision making. ... Strongly held views, based on belief rather than sound information, still exert too much influence in healthcare. In some instances knowledge is available but is not being used, in other situations additional knowledge needs to be generated from reliable sources.' (Peckham, 1991)

In this statement the government set an agenda that obliges all healthcare professionals to use evidence-based approaches to their clinical decision-making. *A First Class Service* (Department of Health, 1998) specifies that a quality organisation will ensure that evidence-based practice is in day-to-day use, with the infrastructure to support it. Evidence-based practice has been driven by the need for accountability to commissioners, families and those funding services. *Standards for Better Health* (Department of Health, 2006) states that healthcare organisations ensure that they conform to NICE technology appraisals and, where it is available, take into account nationally agreed guidance when planning and delivering treatment and care. Inertia can be induced when practitioners are required to work differently, which might present a barrier to the implementation of evidence-based practice. There are attendant risks of evidence-based nihilism, if professionals seek 'perfect' rather than the best-available evidence (Ramchandani *et al*, 2001). Research is provisional by nature, and will only provide definitive answers to specific populations.

Access to evidence

Research evidence requires interpretation (Fig. 5.1). In order to find an answer to many clinical dilemmas, evidence should be reviewed and interpreted by the practising clinician. The National Institute for Health and Clinical Excellence have issued some evidence-based guidelines as directives for clinical practice, in order to try to reduce the inevitable time lag between some clinicians determining and developing best practice, and everyone else catching up (Box 5.1); in addition, the Social Care Institute for Excellence (SCIE; www.scie.org.uk/children/index.asp) have published research briefings and guidance relevant to CAMHS (e.g. Social Care Institute for Excellence, 2005), as has the National Initiative for Autism: Screening and Assessment (NIASA) (e.g. Le Couteur & NIASA Working Group, 2003). Evidence comes primarily from scientific research; but also from reasoning from basic physiology, pathology, psychology or clinical intuition (Evidence-Based Medicine Working Group, 1992). Research evidence must be combined with clinical expertise, along with the views of the young person and their family to arrive at a sound clinical decision

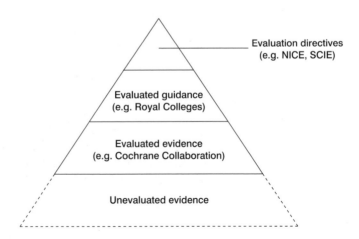

Fig. 5.1 Access to research evidence. NICE, National Institute for Health and Clinical Excellence; SCIE, Social Care Institute for Excellence.

Box 5.1 Guidance relevant to CAMHS

- Psychosis (National Collaborating Centre for Mental Health, 2009), adult specific
- Anxiety (National Institute for Health and Clinical Excellence, 2004), adult specific
- Eating disorders (National Collaborating Centre for Mental Health, 2004*a*), 8 years and upwards
- Self-harm (National Collaborating Centre for Mental Health, 2004*b*), section on children and young people
- Substance misuse (National Collaborating Centre for Mental Health, 2007), all ages
- Post-traumatic stress disorder (National Collaborating Centre for Mental Health, 2005*a*), children and adults
- Obsessive–compulsive disorder (National Collaborating Centre for Mental Health, 2005*b*), 8 years and upwards
- Children and young people with cancer (National Collaborating Centre for Cancer, 2005)
- Depressive disorder (National Collaborating Centre for Mental Health, 2005*c*), children and young people
- Bipolar disorder (National Collaborating Centre for Mental Health, 2006), all ages
- Attention-deficit hyperactivity disorder (National Collaborating Centre for Mental Health, 2008)
- Conduct disorders (National Institute for Health and Clinical Excellence, 2006)
- Chronic fatigue syndrome (Turnbull *et al*, 2007)
- Interventions to reduce substance misuse among vulnerable young people (National Institute for Health and Clinical Excellence, 2007*a*)
- School-based interventions on alcohol (National Institute for Health and Clinical Excellence, 2007*b*)
- Structural neuroimaging in first-episode psychosis (National Institute for Health and Clinical Excellence, 2008*a*), all ages
- Social and emotional well-being in primary education (National Institute for Health and Clinical Excellence, 2008*b*)
- Guidance on assessment and screening for autism in children has been published by the National Autistic Society (Le Couteur & NIASA Working Group, 2003) and by the Social Care Institute for Excellence (2005).

(Box 5.2). The dichotomy between clinical intuition and an evidence-based approach is false (Greenhalgh, 2002), and placing a higher value on evidence gained from RCTs can divert attention from other studies that have much to offer clinical practice. Although a trial might be of good quality, using robust methodology, and the logic behind it irrefutable, a discerning attitude is required to apply it ethically to individuals.

Clinical practice

Views about evidence-based practice can become polarised; critics may caricature its enthusiasts as research evangelists who fail to appreciate the

---

Box 5.2 The functions of research

- Generating new knowledge
- Providing 'generalisable' results (i.e. that can be applied to a wider population of similar patients)
- Challenging current practice
- Informing policy and service delivery

Adapted from Bury & Mead, 1998

---

complexity of everyday practice, and overlook the wisdom of experienced clinicians. Advocates of evidence-based practice might view its opponents as 'Luddites' who have overvalued ideas about their clinical acumen (Geddes & Harrison, 1997). Practitioners cannot rely solely on clinical judgement and experience, which may be influenced by assumptions and anecdotes. Clinical decision-making is informed by the following factors (Graham, 2000):

- the best available external clinical evidence from systematic research that is relevant to the child and family's problem;
- individual clinical expertise (i.e. the skills and judgement clinicians acquire from the experience of seeing patients), and in particular the skills in diagnosis and in understanding the context in which the family's problem has occurred;
- an appreciation of the child and family's preferences and rights when making decisions about their care.

Good clinicians will use each of these components in an integrated way. One alone is not enough (Fig. 5.2). Without clinical expertise, practice risks becoming tyrannised by external evidence, as even excellent external evidence may not be relevant for the individual patient (Sackett et al, 1997). Patient preference may override research evidence in some cases, for example if the family declines to engage in family therapy, despite this intervention being supported by the best research evidence for their problem. The service would then need to consider alternative options, taking into account any other available external evidence. The importance of informing families about evidence-based approaches has been discussed by Szatmari (1999); the challenge of how to impart this knowledge to young people and their families has been taken up by the CAMHS Evidence-Based Practice Unit in their publication *Choosing What's Best For You* (Wolpert et al, 2007).

'The sharp distinction between external evidence and clinical expertise can have the serious disadvantage of conveying a message that clinical experience does not produce evidence. In common terms the average child and adolescent mental health worker is likely to define "evidence" broadly, as any information

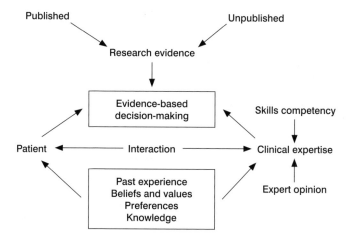

Fig. 5.2 Sources of information needed for clinical decision-making. Reproduced with permission from Bury & Mead, 1998, © Elsevier.

useful in making a clinical decision. Most clinicians would think of several relevant clinical experiences with similar patients as reasonably strong evidence.' (Graham, 2000)

There is a need to integrate all available information in clinical decision-making (Box 5.3); data obtained from a clinical assessment should be combined with information derived from generalisable research to form a theory about a particular young person in a particular family. The theory can then be tested, by checking with other sources of information or by trying an intervention and seeing if the outcome is consistent with the theory. If the theory is correct, the intervention will ameliorate the problem (Graham, 2000). Clinical expertise is the essential tool for the efficient gathering of case evidence; it is necessary in integrating case

---

Box 5.3 Evidence-based decision-making

- Formulate a clear clinical question from the patient's problem
- Search the literature for relevant articles (using MEDLINE and other databases)
- Critically appraise the evidence for its validity and usefulness
- Implement useful findings in clinical practice
- Evaluate, via clinical audit, the impact of the change in practice[a]

Reproduced from Rosenberg & Donald, 1995
[a]Bury & Mead, 1998

evidence with external evidence from research, applying that which is relevant to the problem in hand, engaging the family and integrating their views and preferences. Only then can an effective management plan be formulated.

Clinical questions are produced from the clinical dilemmas that arise when constructing management plans for patients or when attempting to improve an element of the service. A common question might be: 'For this young person with anxiety what are the possible effects of cognitive–behavioural therapy versus relaxation training and therefore which therapy should be offered?'

Increasingly, the public are informing themselves, particularly through the internet, of the evidence available from research. They may be basing their choices about their own and their family's healthcare on this information (Wright et al, 1999; Powell & Clarke, 2006). Professionals need to be aware of the latest research, but importantly they need to develop a facility for both critical selection and appraisal. Critical appraisal is a complex skill that requires practice. Clinicians occasionally feel oppressed by these challenges in the face of the time constraints of clinical practice: evidence-based resources can assist the browbeaten clinician.

Evidence-based resources

There is increasing interest in evidence-based resources (Guyatt et al, 2000), where experts in critical appraisal produce summaries of important new studies they have analysed, which can be quickly read by others. *Evidence-Based Mental Health* (ebmh.bmj.com/), the FOCUS initiative of the Royal College of Psychiatrists (www.rcpsych.ac.uk/clinicalservicestandards/focus.aspx) and MORE (McMaster Online Rating of Evidence; http://hiru.mcmaster.ca/more/), produce evidence-based briefings in a timely and manageable way for clinicians who might otherwise be overwhelmed by the evidence base – the biomedical evidence base alone doubles every 10 years. The phenomenon of information overload is not isolated to healthcare; in the last three decades of the 20th century humans produced more information than in the previous 5000 years (Wigington, 2008). Useful summaries such as *Drawing on the Evidence* (Wolpert et al, 2006), precis the evidence base and highlight the gaps in knowledge as well as the key findings. The CAMHS Evidence-Based Practice Unit has also produced *Knowing Where to Look* (Lavis, 2008), which provides a signpost for CAMHS clinicians in locating and appraising appropriate evidence to support their practice.

Other options include adapting national guidelines for local implementation where these are available (Box 5.1), or a member of the service looking at the primary studies and any systematic reviews (Box 5.4) and producing guidelines or protocols for all team members to use at a local level.

Box 5.4 Article selection guide

Treatment
- Was the assignment of patients to treatment randomised?
- Were all the patients who entered the trial accounted for at the end?

Diagnosis
- Was there an independent, masked comparison with a control group?
- Did the patient sample include an appropriate spectrum of the sort of patients to whom the diagnostic test will be applied in clinical practice?

Harm
- Were there clearly identified comparison groups that were similar with respect to important determinants of outcome (other than the one of interest)?
- Were the outcomes and exposures measured in the same way in the groups being compared?

Prognosis
- Was there a representative patient sample at a well-defined point in the course of the disorder?
- Was follow-up sufficiently long and complete?

From Oxman *et al*, 1993

Clinical effectiveness and cost-effectiveness

Clinical effectiveness can be understood in the following terms:

> 'the extent to which specific clinical interventions, when deployed in the field for a particular individual, group or population, do what they are intended to do. i.e. Maintain and improve health and secure the greatest possible health gain from the available resources. An intervention must be both clinically effective and cost effective and be shown to produce those benefits in practice.' (Chambers, 1998)

Promoting Action on Clinical Effectiveness (PACE) is an initiative to develop evidence-based practice as a routine way of working for health services. It has described the successful outcomes when clinical effectiveness is linked to local needs and priorities as long as clinicians, managers, policy-makers and patients are all involved in the process (Chambers, 1998). Effectiveness is an integral consideration when commissioning services, forming part of the needs assessment and planning process, to ensure that a quality service is ultimately delivered (Smith *et al*, 2006).

Consideration must also be taken of the cost-effectiveness of decision-making 'to maximise the benefit to patients, given the constraints of scarce resources' (Pettite, 1994). Cost is now a part of every treatment decision, and cost-effective decision-making is part of the rationing debate. There is a paradox here in that cost-effectiveness is concerned with relative benefits for populations of patients, while evidence-based practice is concerned with absolute benefit to the individual.

Audit forms the last stage in the process. Clinical audit helps the team reach a standard of working as close to best practice as possible.

Evidence-based practice and CAMHS

How 'evidence' is defined has major implications for the provision of CAMHS. A narrow view, for example that only RCTs should be considered when planning treatment interventions, may suit surgical and perhaps medical teams; however, RCTs can be limited in helping child mental health workers make decisions about interventions for young people. There are three principal reasons for this (Graham, 2000).

1   Systemic thinking often considers the young person's symptoms as secondary to, or in the context of, a predicament they are experiencing. Randomised controlled trials focus on comparing groups of individuals who have the same symptom cluster (diagnosis) and usually ignore their predicaments. It makes little sense to focus on symptoms and make no reference to context when the symptoms are clearly secondary and would often resolve spontaneously if the predicament were attended to.

2   Ninety-five per cent of children attending CAMHS have more than one diagnosis (Audit Commission, 1999), yet the majority of RCTs are done to establish an intervention to improve the outcome of a single disorder. The presence of comorbidity is likely to significantly affect both intervention and outcome for the young person.

3   Criteria for entry into the majority of RCTs generally demand that individuals meet either ICD–10 or DSM–IV research criteria for diagnosis of the disorder under study. Yet many young people who are suffering and in need of help from CAMHS do not achieve this level of diagnosis. Therefore, the degree to which the results of the RCT are generalisable to this clinical population is doubtful.

Different disorders respond to different therapies (Wolpert *et al*, 2006). Consequently, CAMHS require members with expertise in behavioural therapy, CBT, family therapy, individual psychodynamic psychotherapy and group therapy. Any gap in available skills will prevent the team practising in an evidence-based way when faced with a clinical problem for which evidence of efficacy for a specific therapy exists.

In general, when either might be applied, the evidence for the effectiveness of behavioural therapies is greater than that for non-behavioural therapies (Fonagy *et al*, 2002). This may reflect, however, that more behavioural therapies have been evaluated (Graham, 2000). Clearly, unevaluated therapies cannot be considered ineffective; 'absence of evidence is not evidence of absence', an aphorism often attributed to the astronomer Carl Sagan, is apposite.

Issues in practice

Treatment

How does any member of CAMHS decide whom to treat? Should a child with asthma take precedence when there is a good evidence base that family therapy will reduce the incidence and severity of asthma attacks (Lask & Matthew, 1979), but the child has a low level of emotional disturbance? Or should work be directed to an adolescent with conduct disorder, who will have massive psychological disturbance, in the care of the Local Authority, but for whom there is no recognised curative intervention? The practice of evidence-based medicine dictates the former, but the need to support other agencies working with very difficult young people dictates the latter. A CAMHS, therefore, has to think very carefully about how it prioritises its workload and to have clear operational policies stating why it has those priorities, so that other agencies, professionals and management structures understand them. Many outcomes of CAMHS interventions are not easily quantifiable, which makes the implementation of evidence-based practice challenging. Exclusive reliance on research outcomes can be to the detriment of young people and families if the view is taken that interventions without substantial evidence are also without substantial value.

Prevention

How do CAMHS professionals influence risk factors such as poverty, intellectual disability or bullying for the development of conditions when those risk factors are in operation before any referral and are often impervious to CAMHS intervention?

Professionals working in CAMHS are mainly involved in secondary and tertiary prevention through their clinical work. However, they may also be involved in primary prevention either through seeking to influence government policy (e.g. in education, employment policy) or local policy (e.g. housing), but these are political activities not defined by the professional role. Child and adolescent mental health service professionals may be involved in teaching or training outside the team with other agencies, whether statutory (e.g. Social Services, education), voluntary or academic (e.g. university), or on an *ad hoc* basis as a result of local requests from statutory organisations or self-help groups. All of these heighten awareness of mental health issues and psychiatric disorders.

More directly, CAMHS professionals may provide consultation to a range of Tier 1 professionals who are seeing young people at risk of developing mental disorders. In addition, they may develop, or be part of, multidisciplinary groups arranging early intervention programmes for vulnerable children such as an 'early bird' intervention programme in preschool children with autism or early intervention programmes for children at risk of conduct disorder (Little & Mount, 1999).

Outcomes

To whom are CAMHS professionals answerable in terms of the outcomes of their work – the children, their parents, their schools, their neighbours, their social workers, the police or the courts? They will all have their own expectations and it is unlikely they will all be the same. The welfare principle puts the child at the head of a CAMHS priority list. However, CAMHS have to work with the parents in most cases, so it is important not to alienate them. This is also true of schools, but CAMHS are not answerable to them. Only when considerations of abuse arise do responsibilities to the child through other agencies override those of the parents. Child and adolescent mental health services are required to work with other agencies but cannot let them dictate what should be the outcome of their work, otherwise CAMHS become primarily agents of state control.

Conclusion

Evidence-based practice underpins contemporary CAMHS as a scientific endeavour. Evidence-based healthcare can promote team working by providing a common framework for problem-solving and understanding between team members from different professional backgrounds. It may also contribute to removing hierarchical distinctions that are based on seniority, as any member of the team can perform a search and critical appraisal and then be in a position to advise others. The application of scientific evidence can justify our work with young people and families, and has the potential to improve vastly the quality of service provided by CAMHS over time.

e-Resources

CAMHS Outcome Research Consortium (http://www.corc.uk.net/).
Centre for Evidence-Based Medicine (http://www.cebm.net/).
Centre for Reviews and Dissemination (http://www.york.ac.uk/inst/crd/).
Child and Adolescent Mental Health Services Evidence-Based Practice Unit (CAMHS EBPU) (http://www.annafreudcentre.org/ebpu/).
Cochrane Collaboration (http://www.cochrane.org/).
National Institute for Health and Clinical Excellence (NICE) (http://www.nice.org.uk).
Social Care Institute for Excellence (SCIE) (http://www.scie.org.uk).

References

Audit Commission (1999) *Children in Mind*. Audit Commission Publications.
Bury, T. & Mead, J. (1998) *Evidence-Based Healthcare: A Practical Guide for Therapists*. Heinemann.
Chambers, R. (1998) *Clinical Effectiveness Made Easy. First Thoughts on Clinical Governance*. Radcliffe Medical Press.
Department of Health (1998) *A First Class Service: Quality in the New NHS*. TSO (The Stationery Office).
Department of Health (2006) *Standards for Better Health*. TSO (The Stationery Office).

Evidence-Based Medicine Working Group (1992) Evidence-based medicine. A new approach to teaching the practice of medicine. *JAMA*, **268**, 2420–2425.

Fonagy, P., Target, M., Cottrell, D., *et al* (2002) *What Works for Whom – A Critical Review of Treatments for Children and Adolescents*. Guilford Press.

Geddes, J. & Harrison, P. J. (1997) Closing the gap between research and practice. *British Journal of Psychiatry*, **171**, 220–225.

Graham, P. (2000) Treatment interventions and findings from research: bridging the chasm in child psychiatry. *British Journal of Psychiatry*, **176**, 414–419.

Greenhalgh, T. (2002) Uneasy bedfellows? Reconciling intuition and evidence-based practice. *British Journal of General Practice*, **52**, 395–400.

Guyatt, G. H., Meade, M. O., Jaeschke, R. J., *et al* (2000) Practitioners of evidence based care. *BMJ*, **320**, 954–955.

Lask, B. & Matthew, D. (1979) Childhood asthma – a controlled trial of family psychotherapy. *Archives of Disease in Childhood*, **54**, 116–119.

Laugharne, R. (1999) Evidence-based medicine, user involvement and the post-modern paradigm. *Psychiatric Bulletin*, **23**, 641–643.

Lavis, P. (2008) *Knowing Where to Look: How to Find the Evidence You Need*. CAMHS Evidence Based Practice Unit.

Le Couteur, A. & NIASA Working Group (2003) *National Autism Plan for Children*. National Autistic Society.

Little, M. & Mount, K. (1999) *Prevention and Early Intervention with Children in Need*. Action for Young People.

National Collaborating Centre for Cancer (2005) *Improving Outcomes in Children and Young People with Cancer*. National Institute for Health and Clinical Excellence.

National Collaborating Centre for Mental Health (2004a) *Eating Disorders. Core Interventions in the Treatment and Management of Anorexia Nervosa, Bulimia Nervosa and Related Eating Disorders. Clinical Guideline CG9*. Gaskell & British Psychological Society

National Collaborating Centre for Mental Health (2004b) *Self-Harm: The Short-Term Physical and Psychological Management and Secondary Prevention of Self-Harm in Primary and Secondary Care*. British Psychological Society & Royal College of Psychiatrists.

National Collaborating Centre for Mental Health (2005a) *Post-traumatic Stress Disorder: The Management of PTSD in Adults and Children in Primary and Secondary Care. Clinical Guideline CG26*. National Institute for Health and Clinical Excellence.

National Collaborating Centre for Mental Health (2005b) *Obsessive Compulsive Disorder: Core Interventions in the Treatment of Obsessive Compulsive Disorder and Body Dysmorphic Disorder. Clinical Guideline CG31*. National Institute for Health and Clinical Excellence.

National Collaborating Centre for Mental Health (2005c) *Depression in Children and Young People: Identification and Management in Primary, Community and Secondary Care. Clinical Guideline CG28*. British Psychological Society & Royal College of Psychiatrists.

National Collaborating Centre for Mental Health (2006) *Bipolar Disorder: The Management of Bipolar Disorder in Adults, Children and Adolescents, in Primary and Secondary Care. Clinical Guideline CG38*. British Psychological Society & Gaskell.

National Collaborating Centre for Mental Health (2007) *Drug Misuse: Psychosocial Interventions. Clinical Guideline CG51*. National Institute for Health and Clinical Excellence.

National Collaborating Centre for Mental Health (2008) *Attention Deficit Hyperactivity Disorder: Diagnosis and Management of ADHD in Children, Young People and Adults. Clinical Guideline CG72*. British Psychological Society & Royal College of Psychiatrists.

National Collaborating Centre for Mental Health (2009) *Schizophrenia: Core Interventions in the Treatment and Management of Schizophrenia in Primary and Secondary Care (update). Clinical Guideline CG82*. National Institute for Health and Clinical Excellence.

National Institute for Health and Clinical Excellence (2004) *Anxiety: Management of Anxiety (Panic Disorder, with or without Agoraphobia, and Generalised Anxiety Disorder) in Adults in Primary, Secondary and Community Care. Clinical Guideline CG22*. NICE.

National Institute for Health and Clinical Excellence (2006) *Parent-Training/Education Programmes in the Management of Children with Conduct Disorders*. NICE.

National Institute for Health and Clinical Excellence (2007a) *Community-based Interventions to Reduce Substance Misuse among Vulnerable and Disadvantaged Children and Young People.* NICE.

National Institute for Health and Clinical Excellence (2007b) *Interventions in Schools to Prevent and Reduce Alcohol Use among Children and Young People.* NICE.

National Institute for Health and Clinical Excellence (2008a) *Structural Neuroimaging in First-Episode Psychosis.* NICE.

National Institute for Health and Clinical Excellence (2008b) *Promoting Children's Social and Emotional Wellbeing in Primary Education.* NICE.

Oxman, A., Sackett, D. L. & Guyatt, G. H. (1993) Users' guides to the medical literature. 1: How to get started. The Evidence-Based Medicine Working Group. *JAMA,* **270,** 2093–2095.

Peckham, M. (1991) *Research for Health: A Research and Development Strategy for the NHS.* Department of Health.

Pettite, D. B. (1994) *Meta-Analysis, Decision Analysis and Cost Effectiveness Analysis.* Oxford University Press.

Powell, J. & Clarke, A. (2006) Internet Information-seeking in mental health. *British Journal of Psychiatry,* **189,** 273–277.

Ramchandani, P., Joughin, C. & Zwi, M. (2001) Evidence-based child and adolescent mental health services: oxymoron or brave new dawn? *Child Psychology and Psychiatry Review,* **6,** 59–64.

Rosenberg, W. & Donald, A. (1995) Evidence-based medicine: an approach to clinical problem solving. *BMJ,* **310,** 1122–1125.

Sackett, D., Rosenberg, W. M. C., Gray, J. A. M., *et al* (1997) *Evidence-Based Medicine. How to Practice and Teach E.B.M.* Churchill Livingstone.

Smith, J., Lewis, R. & Harrison, T. (2006) *Making Commissioning Effective in the Reformed NHS in England.* Health Policy Forum.

Social Care Institute for Excellence (2005) *Therapies and Approaches for Helping Children and Adolescents who Deliberately Self-harm (DSH).* SCIE (http://www.scie.org.uk/publications/briefings/files/briefing17.pdf).

Szatmari, P. (1999) Evidence-based child psychiatry and the two solitudes. *Evidence-Based Mental Health,* **2,** 6–7.

Turnbull, N., Shaw, E. J., Baker, R., *et al* (2007) *Chronic Fatigue Syndrome/Myalgic Encephalomyelitis (or Encephalopathy): Diagnosis and Management of Chronic Fatigue Syndrome/Myalgic Encephalomyelitis (or Encephalopathy) in Adults and Children.* Royal College of General Practitioners.

Wigington, P. (2008) Clear messages for effective communication. *Journal of Environmental Health,* **70,** 71–73.

Wolpert, M., Fuggle, P., Cottrell, D., *et al* (2006) *Drawing on the Evidence* (2nd edn). CAMHS Publications.

Wolpert, M., Goodman, R., Raby, C., *et al* (2007) *Choosing What's Best For You.* CAMHS Publications.

Wright, B., Williams, C. & Partridge, I. (1999) Management advice for children with chronic fatigue syndrome: a systematic study of information from the internet. *Irish Journal of Psychological Medicine,* **16,** 67–71.

CHAPTER 6

Clinical governance

Greg Richardson

'My own rules are very simple. Don't hurt nobody. Be nice to people.'
Sammy Davis Jr

Definition

'Clinical governance is the system through which NHS organisations [and independent health providers] are accountable for continuously improving the quality of their services and safeguarding high standards of care, by creating an environment in which clinical excellence will flourish.' (Department of Health, 2003)

Clinical governance is a way of integrating financial control, service performance and clinical quality into the management of health services (Scally & Donaldson, 1998), and provides:

'an organising principle, a state of mind, the day-by-day, flesh-and-blood embodiment of how we practise – acting together across the traditional boundaries of our different roles and responsibilities; concentrating our will to care, the skills we have acquired, and the resources at our disposal – in order to give our patients – all of them, whatever their means, wherever they are – the best and safest care that a good health service can deliver.' (Donaldson, 2003).

It became an integral part of the health service with the publication of *A First Class Service* (Department of Health, 1998), which described the methods by which the quality of services would be set, delivered and monitored with the publication of *Providing Assurance on Clinical Governance* (Department of Health, 2005).

Objectives

The objective of clinical governance is to provide clinical excellence to those served by the health services. In CAMHS, this may be achieved by:

- focusing on the quality of services;
- placing the patient and family at the centre of work with them through an informed therapeutic alliance;
- safeguarding high standards of service delivery;

- creating an environment in which excellence in clinical care and awareness of current evidence will flourish;
- using failures and exemplars to improve the quality of care;
- providing an organisational culture that encourages clear role definition within supportive teams and that discourages control by blaming;
- protecting patients and their families from harmful interventions or side-effects of treatments;
- effective regulation of mental health professionals.

Clinical governance processes[1]

Patient experience

Clinical practice means incorporating user and carer views into the management plan of every child. Although choice has become a front-runner in the NHS, most young people and families wish to have a service local and relevant to them, therefore such a service must be able to incorporate them in the most effective management package. Child and adolescent mental health services are perhaps ahead in the choice agenda, for they have to negotiate treatment as part of the treatment, and interventions are only really effective if there is a therapeutic alliance.

Patient and public involvement

User involvement is a complex area in child and adolescent mental health as children, parents, teachers, advocacy groups and social agencies often have conflicting views about what is an effective and helpful service and which of them is the user. Formal reviews of users' views of a particular part of the service such as those described in Chapter 9 can be part of an active audit programme.

Clinical audit

Mental health professionals need time out to review what they are doing to children, families and fellow professionals. Both community and in-patient teams require at least a half day every 6–12 months in which to take a more detached view of their work and to review service provision. Only when the nose is taken from the grindstone is it recognised that the nose is perhaps not the correct organ to be using and that the grindstone is not the most useful tool in these circumstances. All CAMHS should have an active multidisciplinary audit programme (Hardman & Joughin, 1998) that encompasses observational studies of how the service functions. This can lead on to the establishment of protocols and standards, which will

---

1. Taken from *Providing Assurance on Clinical Governance: A Practical Guide* (Department of Health, 2005).

then require regular monitoring. Initially, these projects may be internally generated, but with input from involved agencies such as primary care organisations and user groups, outside interests can be incorporated into the annual audit cycle. Evaluations of service and user perspectives also provide audit material, and so affect service delivery.

Risk management

Risks arise from individuals be they designated patients, parents, carers, fellow professionals or mental health staff as well as from the environments in which they work. Methods of recognising, estimating and managing those risks are part of everyday work and require increasing formalisation if services are not to be found deficient (Carson, 1990). Some risks are managed by statutory provision such as Criminal Records Bureau (CRB) checks and health and safety legislation, but others have to be assessed regularly to ensure the safest setting for the young person and those looking after them. The safety of children in the waiting area, the protection of lone workers, the facility for speedy communication and the safety of adolescents who self-harm are examples of topics that need to be addressed. If necessary, protocols should be developed for certain high-risk groups. Risk-averse organisations quickly become stifling institutions, so risk has to be actively assessed and managed to ensure a therapeutic experience for the patient and family. The risk management strategy should contain a process for learning from serious incidents to ensure that such incidents are monitored and investigated, that recommendations are implemented, and that the changes required to prevent such an incident occurring again are monitored as part of the audit process.

Clinical incident reporting

Schemes for the reporting of adverse incidents, both major and minor, should investigate the way the organisational system is letting down the staff working in them, as everyone makes mistakes and random blame encourages defensive and bureaucratic practice. However, in the wider health service, there is often a perception that there is only ever interest when something goes wrong and that interest is investigative, not supportive, always looking for someone to blame.

Complaints

All health organisations have processes for dealing with complaints that must meet certain time targets. Child and adolescent mental health service professionals usually have particular skills in dealing with complaints as their stock in trade is the management of difficult situations in which there are highly aroused emotions. A CAMHS professional can often prevent a dissatisfaction with the service from becoming a complaint, as long as they take action on that which is being complained about and review with other members of the CAMHS the implications of the dissatisfaction.

Clinical effectiveness

What Works for Whom was published in 2002 (Fonagy *et al*) and has been updated (Wolpert *et al*, 2006). The National Institute for Health and Clinical Excellence has also published guidelines for disorders relevant to CAMHS (e.g. depression, ADHD; National Collaborating Centre for Mental Health, 2005, 2008)), but many requests for treatment do not fit neatly into crisp diagnosis-based care pathways. Structuring and managing treatment options is the subject of Chapter 14.

Clinical pathways and guidelines

The first part of engagement with any young person and family after the initial assessment has been made will be to describe to them a clinical pathway along which the CAMHS professional is going to accompany them and provide some of the therapeutic input. For some disorders, such as ADHD, eating disorders and self-harm, NICE has produced clear care pathways (National Collaborating Centre for Mental Health, 2004*a*,*b*, 2005, 2008).

Staffing and staff management

Child and adolescent mental health service working should be based on professional and individual role clarity, role confidence, role legitimacy, ownership of responsibility, commitment to children and families, collaborative agencies and colleagues, organisational clarity, high-level communication skills and, if possible, humour. Staff will feel valued and supported if there is a strong team ethos. All the very best efforts are wasted if they are not coordinated to a directed end. As every CAMHS requires a manager, so every Tier 3 team requires a member to take responsibility for coordinating the efforts of that team so that it works efficiently. Their role should be defined in the operational policy. Good management encourages all of the above requirements for clinical governance while giving a sense of belonging and worth to the service. Each profession has regulatory mechanisms (General Medical Council, 2006). Service members should be close to each other's practice and use supervision, consultation and joint working to maintain professional standards.

Education and training

Doctors generally have better access to training activities than other disciplines that tend to be poorly supported financially for their training. There is therefore a need for all CAMHS members to be involved in the training of others in CAMHS so that it can be done as locally as possible. Conference attendance on an occasional basis keeps isolationism at bay. All training must be discussed annually with every staff member and development needs addressed as part of annual appraisal. Access to the internet should be available in all services but should not replace libraries where journals and reference texts can be referred to. Chapter 7 addresses training matters.

Continuing professional development

All CAMHS members need to be involved in an active process of continuing professional development (CPD), which ensures they keep themselves up to date (Royal College of Psychiatrists, 2001, 2009). Personal development plans based on yearly appraisals and CPD needs are an absolute essential and integral to the employment of health service staff. Accreditation is just over the horizon for doctors. Research and audit activities encourage service members' inquisitiveness about their practice.

Mortality and morbidity reviews

Mortality is not unknown in CAMHS and is monitored through the National Confidential Inquiry into Suicide and Homicide by People with Mental Illness (www.medicine.manchester.ac.uk/psychiatry/research/suicide/prevention/nci/), and any death of a person involved with CAMHS should precipitate a serious untoward incident enquiry. Child and adolescent mental health services have not been good at monitoring the progress of and outcomes for patients and families, but should routinely use recognised measures to assess incapacity and progress.

Clinical performance indicators

A CAMHS operational policy should integrate national and local requirements into its compliance with the local CAMHS strategy. Increasingly, standards are being set nationally (Royal College of Psychiatrists' Research and Training Unit, 2005). The benchmarking of in-patient services has reached a high level of sophistication with the Quality Network for In-patient CAMHS (QNIC) established in 2001. Currently, nearly 90% of in-patient units are members of QNIC and the annual report clarifies where units are meeting national standards and where they are failing (College Centre for Quality Improvement, 2006). Subsequently, a similar benchmarking organisation, the Quality Network for Multi-Agency CAMHS (QINMAC) has been established (www.rcpsych.ac.uk/crtu/centreforqualityimprovement/qinmaccamhs.aspx).

Measurement of outcomes

The measurement of outcomes in CAMHS has primarily occurred in research studies that have helped with clinical effectiveness. It is now incumbent on CAMHS that if they wish to have the resources to function effectively, they prove their effectiveness through outcome measures, many of which have now been used both in research and clinical practice. The use of rating scales at the commencement of treatment and during the course of treatment should now be routine.

Requirements

In order for the processes mentioned earlier to run effectively there are certain requirements.

Good information technology

Information in the health services has traditionally focused on face-to-face contact with patients or on meeting waiting list targets. However, as 'Payment by Results' (Department of Health, 2009) has been investigated for mental health services, the relevance of such a system has been called into question as it does not meet the needs of a service working with families, carers and other agencies rather than individual patients, although some ill-informed commissioners still try to purchase CAMHS on such terms. Performing a considerable amount of consultation, educational and supportive work at Tier 1 or involving Tier 3 teams dealing with different client groups does not fit current health information technology systems. The need for service-driven information systems geared to team working and Tier 1 support requires intensive work with information technology departments and has still not been addressed.

A developing service

Child and adolescent mental health services that take clinical governance seriously will be developing all the time, informed by research evidence, national and local requirements, the results of audit processes, the risk management strategy and as a result of consumer surveys. New developments such as primary mental health workers or a new Tier 3 team, as well as new resources, require monitoring to ensure that they are meeting their objectives in an efficient manner. Service development does not imply adding on new services to old, but giving up old methods of practice as new ones are shown to be more useful or expedient. Innovation in CAMHS requires the development and encouragement of empowerment and facilitation skills. Having different professionals taking on coordinating and management roles in different parts of the service and in different Tier 3 teams encourages innovative and developmental thinking.

Annual reports

All trust medical directors have to produce an annual clinical governance report. Child and adolescent mental health services within the trust are required to contribute to this as an integral part of performance management within the trust. This is an ideal opportunity to show that CAMHS are taking the quality of their services seriously and developing them accordingly.

References

Carson, D. (1990) *Risk Taking in Mental Disorder: Analyses, Policies and Practical Strategies.* SLE Publications.

College Centre for Quality Improvement (2006) *QNIC The Quality Network for In-Patient CAMHS Annual Report Review Cycle 5: 2005–2006.* Royal College of Psychiatrists.

Department of Health (1998) *A First Class Service: Quality in the New NHS.* TSO (The Stationery Office).

Department of Health (2003) Clinical governance. (http://www.dh.gov.uk/en/Publichealth/Patientsafety/Clinicalgovernance/index.htm). Department of Health

Department of Health (2005) *Providing Assurance on Clinical Governance: A Practical Guide.* Department of Health.

Department of Health (2009) Developing Payment by Results for mental health. Department of Health (http;//www.dh.gov.uk/en/Managingyourorganisation/financeandplanning/NHSmanagementcosts/index.htm).

Donaldson, L. (2003) CMO quotes – clinical governance and quality. Department of Health (http://www.dh.gov.uk/en/aboutus/MinistersandDepartmentLeaders/ChiefMedicalOfficer/CMOpublications/QuoteUnquote/DH_4102558).

Fonagy, P., Target, M., Cottrell, D., *et al* (2002) *What Works for Whom – A Critical Review of Treatments for Children and Adolescents.* Guilford Press.

General Medical Council (2006) Good medical practice. GMC.

Hardman, E. & Joughin, C. (1998) *FOCUS on Clinical Audit in Child and Adolescent Mental Health Services.* Gaskell.

National Collaborating Centre for Mental Health (2004a) *Eating Disorders. Core Interventions in the Treatment and Management of Anorexia Nervosa, Bulimia Nervosa and Related Eating Disorders. Clinical Guideline CG9.* British Psychological Society & Royal College of Psychiatrists.

National Collaborating Centre for Mental Health (2004b) *Self-Harm: The Short-Term Physical and Psychological Management and Secondary Prevention of Self-Harm in Primary and Secondary Care. Clinical Guideline CG16.* British Psychological Society & Royal College of Psychiatrists.

National Collaborating Centre for Mental Health (2005) *Depression in Children and Young People. Identification and Management in Primary, Community and Secondary Care. Clinical Guideline CG28.* National Institute for Health and Clinical Excellence

National Collaborating Centre for Mental Health (2008) *Attention Deficit Hyperactivity Disorder: Diagnosis and Management of ADHD in Children, Young People and Adults.* British Psychological Society & Royal College of Psychiatrists.

Royal College of Psychiatrists (2001) *Good Psychiatric Practice: CPD. Council Report CR90.* Royal College of Psychiatrists.

Royal College of Psychiatrists (2009) *Good Psychiatric Practice (Third Edition). College Report CR154.* Royal College of Psychiatrists

Royal College of Psychiatrists' College Research and Training Unit (2005) *Clinical Governance in Mental Health and Learning Disability Services: A Practical Guide.* Gaskell.

Scally, G. & Donaldson, L. J. (1998) Clinical governance and the drive for quality improvement in the new NHS in England. *BMJ,* **317,** 61–65.

Wolpert, M., Fuggle, P., Cottrell, D., *et al* (2006) *Drawing on the Evidence.* CAMHS Publications.

CHAPTER 7

Education, supervision and workforce development

Margaret Bamforth, Sophie Roberts, Sarah Bryan and Nick Jones

---

education n. that which discloses to the wise and disguises from the foolish their lack of understanding.

Ambrose Gwinett Bierce (1842–1914)

Introduction

Increased medical advances and a better-informed and more demanding public have put pressure on clinicians both to perform and to show themselves to perform at higher standards than ever before. National standards have been set through National Service Frameworks (NSFs) and by NICE. It is impossible to consider the future direction of education, training and workforce development within CAMHS without reference to two policy documents, the *National Service Framework for Children, Young People and Maternity Services* (Department of Health, 2004a) and *Every Child Matters* (HM Government, 2004). Further initiatives for health service staff include *Agenda for Change* (Department of Health, 2008) and *The NHS Knowledge and Skills Framework* (Department of Health, 2004b).

The delivery of education and training has changed. Competence and capability as educational outcomes are now valued over qualifications. Practice is linked more closely with education and training, and the competencies required for safe practice are identified through competency frameworks, such as the *NHS Knowledge and Skills Framework* and postgraduate medical curricula (Child and Adolescent Faculty Further Education and Curriculum Committee, 2008; Royal College of Psychiatrists, 2008). This change has been led by educationalists, clinicians and managers, and is evident in the design of some of the courses that have been developed to address the training gaps highlighted by the requirements of the NSF. The requirement for a capable workforce and the consideration of patient safety as paramount has led to the implementation of workplace-based training and assessment.

Challenges for CAMHS

The children's NSF set challenges for CAMHS, especially to provide services for children with severe learning disabilities, young people aged

16 and 17 years, and to manage emergencies presenting outside normal working hours. Guidance from NICE has presented challenges related to interventions, for example the need to provide CBT for young people with depression (National Collaborating Centre for Mental Health, 2005). The expansion of the workforce in all tiers has put pressure on managers and commissioners to ensure that the workforce has the knowledge, skills and attitudes to work effectively with their client group. This has been aided by the development of competency-based frameworks that aim to increase the capability and effectiveness of the workforce through the *Common Core of Skills and Knowledge for the Children's Workforce* (Department for Education and Skills, 2005), *Ten Essential Shared Capabilities* (Department of Health *et al*, 2004) and the National Occupational Standards (Care Services Improvement Partnership & National Institute for Mental Health in England, 2007).

The Care Services Improvement Partnership (CSIP) identified the following findings relating to the specialist CAMHS workforce (Edwards *et al*, 2007).

- Current provision of training does not systematically reflect national guidelines.
- There is a lack of strategic direction in workforce planning and a need to relate this to service development.
- A recent increase in expectations of services delivered by CAMHS has resulted in a corresponding increase in training needs.
- Experiences of training are variable owing to unclear career pathways for new staff who enter CAMHS and this highlights the requirement for a basic generic level of training.
- Specialist services are hampered by resource constraints that limit the availability and accessibility of training for practitioners who work in CAMHS.
- There is a requirement for a more flexible and practice-based approach towards the delivery of training.
- Training should have beneficial impacts for the children and young people who use the service that the staff work within.
- Continuing supervision is required to ensure the impact of training is maximised.
- Commissioning is essential to ensure that the workforce that delivers CAMHS is adequately resourced and trained to provide the services that are expected of it.

The availability of training is limited and accessibility can be a problem, often owing to lack of resources in both funding and the ability to 'back-fill' the time that training takes from the service.

The CSIP does not address professionals in Tier 1, but this workforce has significant training needs in early identification, intervention and signposting to services children require. Only with appropriate training will they be effective in addressing both emotional health and well-being, as well as more significant mental health problems of children and young people. Tier 1 looks to CAMHS to provide training or to work in collaboration in raising awareness across all agencies, in particular education services. The CAMHS workforce is also now working more commonly across tiers, with workers being involved in youth offending teams, looked-after children's teams or paediatric liaison teams. These arrangements generate their own demand for training in these specialist areas.

The introduction of New Ways of Working (Department of Health, 2005) presents a further set of challenges that require individual workers to be more flexible and possibly work in different ways in different roles. This generates additional training needs. An example is the New Ways of Working project to expand services for children with learning disabilities, which is being implemented in the North West of England (Morris, 2007). The provision of training and staff development is an integral part of this project, which aims to have all staff in community CAMHS able to manage children with a combination of learning disabilities and mental health problems.

Learning climate and methods of training

Critten (1993) described the conditions necessary for effective learning and suggested the establishment of a 'learning company' as an organisation able to create a climate in which individual members are encouraged to learn and fulfil their potential. Progressive CAMHS will create an atmosphere where learning and working are synonymous, promoting both collective and self-direction in order to meet the continuing process of care transformation. Training should be seen as a continuous process of reviewing and developing care in the light of evaluation. Fluctuations in training provision are a reaction due to change, as opposed to continual training, which is instrumental to change.

Child and adolescent mental health services have always been aware of the need to 'grow their own'. In other words, because of the lack of career pathways and formal qualifications, services have recruited clinicians with a range of skills and professional backgrounds. Learning has occurred through an apprenticeship model and through situated learning (Lave & Wenger, 1991). With the move to competency-based training, it is important not to lose these traditions.

Postgraduate medical training has embraced the competency-based model. This is largely because it allows standards of practice at different levels of training to be identified and assessed. Competencies are identified and incorporated into competency-based curricula. A large proportion of assessment takes place in the workplace. This allows assessment of what the trainee actually 'does' – it therefore assesses performance. The different levels of competency are demonstrated in Miller's triangle (Miller, 1990) (Fig. 7.1).

It is crucial to attempt to understand the meaning of competence: is competence simply the sum of a number of task-orientated skills, or is it

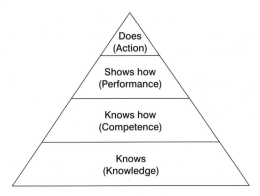

Fig. 7.1 Triangle of clinical competence. Reproduced from Miller (1990).

the ability to integrate competencies and apply them in a way that meets the needs of those being served (Leung, 2002; Rethans *et al*, 2002)?

Another important aim of education and training is to produce experienced learners. The future workforce will need to be more flexible and mobile. It is essential that the workforce is made up of practitioners who are adaptable and develop metacognitive skills (learning how to learn), so that they can more effectively meet service demands. Ways of learning are also becoming more flexible. As well as more learning taking place in the workplace, additional training is being provided through e-learning. All excellent practice will require the practitioner to use reflection as a means to develop and improve skills. Facilitating and enabling reflection to take place can be built into practice using portfolios incorporating reflective statements, and is an essential component of supervision.

Supervision

Supervision can be defined as:

> 'a formal process of professional support and learning which enables individual practitioners to develop knowledge and competence, assume responsibility for their own practice and enhance safe working practices in complex clinical situations. It should enable reflection of practice with the support of a skilled supervisor' (Department of Health, 1993).

All professional organisations recommend regular supervision, although there is scant evidence for its effectiveness (Wheeler & Richards, 2007). There are many models of supervision, including the functions model (Kadushin, 1992), the process model (Hawkins & Shohet, 2000), the systems approach (Holloway, 1995) and the developmental approach (Stoltenberg & Delworth, 1987). The consensus seems to be that a blend of supervision methods should be employed, geared to the needs of the supervisee (Falender & Shafranske, 2004).

Within CAMHS, supervision usually occurs in professional groups, and teams need to develop protocols that reflect the different recommendations of professional bodies regarding frequency, which often depends on seniority (Box 7.1). Standards should be developed within teams to protect relatively junior CAMHS clinicians who may not have established national agreements.

Strategy and workforce redesign

The challenges outlined previously cannot be met by a piecemeal approach to training and education. There must be a strategic approach from managers of services, commissioners and providers of higher education. Workforce redesign has to be used in the most effective way. A workforce redesign tool can facilitate the development of a comprehensive training-needs analysis. Such a tool has been developed, in collaboration between the National CAMHS Support Service and the Health and Social Care Advisory Service (Nixon & Anderson, 2006).

Box 7.1 Recommendations for supervision in CAMHS

- All clinical staff should receive supervision; the frequency of this should depend on experience and needs.
- A recommended level would be at least monthly supervision for more experienced staff.
- All clinical staff should receive managerial and clinical supervision, which might be at separate times or might be incorporated into the same session.
- Staff should agree with their supervisor which areas are to be discussed and how the supervision is to be recorded (including recording discussions in clinical notes). The issue of recording sensitive/child protection issues in supervision and how these should be recorded will be explored.
- Not all supervision needs to be 1:1. Small group supervision can be useful.
- All staff should have access to discipline-specific supervision if they feel it is appropriate and/or helpful. It may be necessary for some staff to set up mutual arrangements with other professionals outside the locality.
- Supervisors should have access to appropriate training in supervision skills.
- Supervisors should have access to supervision about the supervision they provide.
- *Ad hoc* clinical supervision can be difficult for supervisor and supervisee in terms of accountability and record-keeping. This is not recommended, although there are times when it is clinically appropriate to seek guidance/advice from a specific member of the team with specific skills/experience. It is good practice for this to be done in an appropriate place with agreements about what is to be recorded.

In developing a training and education strategy the following must be borne in mind.

- Workforce development has to be considered within a competency framework.
- CAMHS must be part of an integrated children's workforce. This includes generic mental health competencies as part of a strategy to deliver training at Tier 1.
- The workforce may require redesign to be fit for purpose; service delivery models need to be considered and mapped to workforce requirements. Historically the workforce has developed on a demand-led basis.
- Retention and recruitment needs to be considered in the light of finite investment and the requirement to develop a workforce capable of delivering the children's NSF (e.g. developing learning disability competencies).
- All of the above will determine what training needs to be developed. Training needs analysis should identify how training will be sustained and what needs to be delivered on what footprint. More courses need to be workplace-based and this should be evaluated.
- Leadership is needed to change practice as a result of training.
- Multidisciplinary and joint agency-based training should be considered.
- Effective appraisal and CPD programmes need to inform the business planning cycle.
- Methods of good practice dissemination and the cascading of training within services must be introduced.
- Outcome measures and audit should be used to identify training gaps.

For service managers, the use of appraisal methods and personal development plans are essential if skills are to be updated and maintained. Annual review of development plans and a service training needs analysis should reflect the need for joint training and be budgeted accordingly. There is often an inequity of training opportunities and training budgets within CAMHS. A way of managing this is to agree a principle of service training needs and to prioritise them in the training budget. The pooling of training budgets can be a challenge for individual disciplines but is a positive step towards shared learning.

Clinical governance and evidence-based practice

The implementation of evidence-based practice and clinical governance are covered in Chapters 5 and 6 respectively; however, their critical role in successful workforce development warrants some discussion here. Clinical governance is essential to the setting, delivery and monitoring of standards for achieving excellence in healthcare delivery. Although professional self-regulation provides clinicians with the opportunity to set standards, *First Class Service* (Department of Health, 1998) recognised that only lifelong learning would provide NHS staff with the prerequisites to offer contemporary, high-quality and effective care to patients. Clinicians should receive feedback on their performance that will inform supervision and support the development of high-quality practice, especially with regard to competent assessment and the delivery of treatment plans.

Aspiring to excellence is the aim of all services in the NHS, and feedback on service provision and delivery is also essential. The following organisations, listed below, all provide quality control and benchmarking processes, which informs subsequent training and education.

The CAMHS Outcomes Research Consortium (CORC) is a collaboration between CAMHS across the UK. The aims of CORC are the following.

- To develop and support the dissemination of a model of routine evaluation of outcome that can be used across a range of services.
- To help put in place systems to allow the data obtained to inform service providers, commissioners and users, and other relevant stakeholders within all member sites.
- To collate the data from all members who are anonymised, in order that this can be analysed centrally and the results shared with each service area.
- To collaborate in using outcome information to inform and develop good practice.

The current core outcome measures are the Strengths and Difficulties Questionnaire (SDQ) for the parent and child perspective (Goodman, 1997), Commission for Health Improvement Experience of Service Questionnaire (CHI–ESQ) for the parent and child feedback on the service (Commission for Health Improvement, 2002), and the Children's Global Assessment Scale (CGAS; Schaffer *et al*, 1983). In addition, more specific measures are being piloted which can supplement the routine measures. These measures are taken at two points: at the child's first appointment and around 6 months or at discharge if sooner.

The QNIC was pioneered in 2001 by the Royal College of Psychiatrists Research and Training Unit to establish benchmark standards for in-patient services and to monitor services against the benchmarks (www.rcpsych. ac.uk/crtu/centreforqualityimprovement/qnic.aspx). It has a membership of 85% of in-patient units in the UK and produces an annual report on how in-patient units are functioning against the standards (Davies & Thompson, 2008).

The QINMAC was established in 2005 and strives to facilitate quality improvement and development in community CAMHS through a supportive self- and peer-review network (www.rcpsych.ac.uk/crtu/ centreforqualityimprovement/qinmaccamhs.aspx). This professionally led network is designed to enable communication and the sharing of best practice between services. Part of QINMAC's focus is on the extent to which community CAMHS work with other services and agencies to deliver high standards of care for children, young people and their families. The standards were developed following extensive review of relevant policy and existing standards from the Healthcare Commission and the NSF for children (Department of Health, 2004a). The service standards were discussed in workshops involving professionals, parents, carers and young people (Dugmore et al, 2008). There was also a consultation exercise with key stakeholders.

Multidisciplinary and multi-agency training

Every Child Matters (HM Government, 2004) sets out clearly the policy direction towards an integrated children's workforce. Key competencies and capabilities for every worker dealing with children have been identified. The interplay between specialist and generic skills has long been regarded as an essential strength of multidisciplinary CAMHS. All disciplines within CAMHS will have undertaken professional training. Post-qualification 'specialist' training is usually undertaken, specific to working with young persons and their families, to develop skills and interests. Successful CAMHS will contain a strong element of interdisciplinary working. The strength of this working lies in its access to a wide range of skills.

All Local Authorities in partnership with health, education and voluntary agencies have in place multi-agency strategies and joint action plans for children's services. It appears logical that services working together require joint training for their professionals. In many areas this has resulted in multi-agency CAMHS training strategies being established with the intention of integrating training opportunities for staff across organisations.

Training for managers and commissioners

Delivering high-quality services is a complex task when there are different agencies involved, complex systems of service delivery, and differing cultures and values. It is therefore vital that managers and commissioners learn about such work through development programmes. Their training needs can be overlooked and the training of clinicians prioritised, but this is counterproductive as services and therefore service users benefit greatly from competent management and commissioning.

Leadership development

If services are to develop and become more accessible, effective and sensitive to feedback from the families that use them then it is essential that CAMHS practitioners have access to leadership programmes. Leaders are needed at all levels of an organisation to facilitate change, to champion evidence-based practice, to implement innovative service delivery and to support greater involvement of service users. The NHS has an established leadership programme (NHS Institution for Innovation and Improvement, 2006) which can support the development of leadership skills.

CAMHS as providers of training

Child and adolescent mental health service professionals have a role in providing training. This training may be in a formal setting such as a workshop or seminar, but is just as likely to occur informally through surgeries, consultations or direct clinical supervision. Whatever the venue, it is important the 'teacher' feels adequately prepared and skilled to teach the session. The training needs of the trainers should not be overlooked, and opportunity should be given for trainers to practise and to be given structured feedback on their performance. This can be achieved by a system of mentoring by the more experienced members of staff and by calling upon the expertise of the local university or higher-education departments for advice and support. In addition, if the team offers training regularly, they may consider producing a feedback/evaluation form for use at later supervision sessions.

Links with further education establishments

Clinical governance, NSFs, NICE, health improvement and NHS research and development programmes are all making great demands upon clinicians. If these initiatives are to succeed within CAMHS, along with the complexity and the sheer volume of work, partnerships must be established with other agencies. One key partnership is the relationship between CAMHS and the local university or further educational establishment. Studies carried out by the health faculties of local universities can play a helpful role in providing training for all members of the CAMHS (www.skillsforhealth.org.uk/~/media/Resource-Library/PDF/CAMHS-core_functions.aspx). For example, team teaching and the development of the nurse/therapist/practitioner role can enhance the quality of taught courses and provide a potential source of income for further training. In addition, social policy departments can provide links in the dissemination of information regarding national policy and trends. Child and adolescent mental health services should actively foster good working relationships with these departments in order both to underpin their practice and to support them in the pursuit of lifelong learning.

References

Care Services Improvement Partnenrship & National Institute for Mental Health in England (2007) *Core Functions: Child and Adolescent Mental Health Services – Tiers 3, 4.* CSIP & NIMHE (http://www.skillsforhealth.org.uk/~/media/Resource-Library/PDF/CAMHS-core_functions.aspx).

Child and Adolescent Faculty Further Education and Curriculum Committee (2008) *A Competency Based Curriculum for Specialist Training in Psychiatry: Specialist Module in Child and Adolescent Psychiatry* (http://www.rcpsych.ac.uk/PDF/Curriculum-Specialist%20Module%20in%20Child%20and%20Adolescent%20Psychiatry.pdf). Royal College of Psychiatrists.

Commission for Health Improvement (2002) *The Experience of Service Questionnaire Handbook*. Department of Health (http://www.dh.gov.uk/en/Policyandguidance/Humanresourcesandtraining/Modernisingpay/Agendaforchange/index.htm).

Critten, P. (1993) *Investing in People: Towards Corporate Capability*. Butterworth.

Davies, G. & Thompson, P. (2008) *QNIC Annual Report: Review Cycle 6: 2006–2007*. Royal College of Psychiatrists Centre for Quality Improvement.

Department of Education and Skills (2005) *Common Core of Skills and Knowledge for the Children's Workforce*. TSO (The Stationery Office).

Department of Health (1993) *A Vision for the Future. Report of the Chief Nursing Officer*. HMSO.

Department of Health (1998) *A First Class Service: Quality in the New NHS*. TSO (The Stationery Office).

Department of Health (2004a) *National Service Framework for Children Young People and Maternity Services. The Mental Health and Well-being of Children and Young People*. Department of Health Publications.

Department of Health (2004b) *The NHS Knowledge and Skills Framework and the Development Review Process*. Department of Health Publications.

Department of Health (2005) *New Ways of Working for Psychiatrists: Enhancing Effective, Person-centred Services Through New Ways of Working in Multidisciplinary and Multi-agency Contexts. Final report 'but not the end of the story'*. TSO (The Stationery Office).

Department of Health (2008) *Agenda for Change*. Department of Health (http://www.dh.gov.uk/en/Policyandguidance/Humanresourcesandtraining/Modernisingpay/Agendaforchange/index.htm).

Department of Health, NHS University, Sainsbury Centre for Mental Health, *et al* (2004) *The Ten Essential Shared Capabilities: A Framework for the Whole of the Mental Health Workforce*. TSO (The Stationery Office).

Dugmore, O., Craig, M. & Thorpe, H. (2008) *QINMAC Quality Improvement Network for Multi-Agency CAMHS Service Standards* (2nd edn). College Centre for Quality Improvement, Royal College of Psychiatrists.

Edwards, E., Vostanis, P. & Williams, R. (2007) *Specialist CAMHS Training: Evidence-based Development of Guidelines for Providers, Commissioners and Children and Young people who Use Services*. University of Leicester, Care Services Improvement Partnership.

Falender, C. A. & Shafranske, P. (2004) *Clinical Supervision: A Competency Based Approach*. American Psychological Association.

Goodman, R. (1997) The Strengths and Difficulties Questionnaire: a research note. *Journal of Child Psychology and Psychiatry*, **38**, 581–586.

Hawkins, P. & Shohet, R. (2000) *Supervision in the Helping Professions*. Open University Press.

HM Government (2004) *Every Child Matters: Change for Children*. TSO (The Stationary Office).

Holloway, E. (1995) *Clinical Supervision: A Systems Approach*. Sage Publications.

Kadushin, A. (1992) *Supervision in Social Work* (3rd edn). Columbia University Press.

Lave, J. & Wenger, E. (1991) *Situated Learning: Legitimate Peripheral Participation*. Cambridge University Press.

Leung, W. (2002) Competency based medical training: review. *BMJ*, **325**, 693–696.

Miller, G. E. (1990) The assessment of clinical skills/competence/performance. *Academic Medicine*, **65**, S63–S67.

Morris, T. (2007) *New Ways of Working in Mental Health: Early Implementer Site Projects Up-date*. Care Services Improvement Partnership.

National Collaborating Centre for Mental Health (2005) *Depression in Children and Young People: Identification and Management in Primary, Community and Secondary Care. Clinical Guideline CG28*. British Psychological Society & Royal College of Psychiatrists.

NHS Institution for Innovation and Improvement (2006) *NHS Leadership Qualities Framework*. Department of Health (http://www.dh.gov.uk/en/Policyandguidance/Humanresourcesandtraining/Modernisingpay/Agendaforchange/index.htm).

Nixon, B. & Anderson, Y. (2006) *Child and Adolescent Mental Health Services: Workforce Design and Planning Tool*. National CAMHS Support Service & Health and Social Care Advisory Service.

Rethans, J. J., Norcini, J. J., Barón-Maldonado, M., *et al* (2002) The relationship between competence and performance: implications for assessing practice performance. *Medical Education*, **36**, 901–909.

Royal College of Psychiatrists (2008) *Postgraduate Training in Psychiatry: Essential Information for Trainees and Trainers. Occasional Paper OP65.* Royal College of Psychiatrists.

Schaffer, D., Gould, M. S., Brasic, J., *et al* (1983) A children's global assessment scale (CGAS). *Archives of General Psychiatry*, **40**, 1228–1231.

Stoltenberg, C. D. & Delworth, U. (1987) *Supervising Counsellors and Therapists*. Jossey-Bass.

Wheeler, S. & Richards, K. (2007) The impact of clinical supervision on counsellors and therapists, their practice and their clients. A systematic review of the literature. *Counselling and Psychotherapy Research*, **7**, 54–65.

CHAPTER 8

Multidisciplinary working

Ian Partridge, Greg Richardson, Geraldine Casswell
and Nick Jones

'All animals are equal ...'
George Orwell, *Animal Farm*

Introduction

Effective CAMHS are based on multidisciplinary working. Although such working is a fundamental strength of practice, it can cause division and discord if there is not a clear understanding of its nature and tensions. The egalitarian models of multidisciplinary teams in the 1970s have moved on. The roles of CAMHS members are defined not only by their professional training but also by their individual interest, development and expertise. A well-functioning team can be stronger than the sum of its parts, but requires commitment from individuals to a team ethos and to recognise the professional skill, experience and interest of other disciplines. As with families, boundaries and roles need clarity, communication needs to be open, and an ability of members to contain anxiety is essential. Child and adolescent mental health services differ from each other both in numbers and in disciplinary composition. Successful team working depends on a systemically informed approach to team dynamics, as well as personal and professional relationships. In moving away from a doctor-led, illness-based model, the central issue is that of the integration of all disciplines in a fashion that values, legitimises and supports both the parts and the whole (Box 8.1).

Integration as a principle has become core to government policy for the welfare of children, and the provision of the CAMHS modernisation grant to Local Authorities and health providers was dependent on integrated services and joint commissioning. This principle is based on the belief that the outcomes for the child will be better; however, the precise mechanisms by which this occurs has been less clearly articulated. Now that many CAMHS have embraced a multidisciplinary team, the ongoing task is to find a way to respect the richness of the disciplines while enabling forums and dialogue for differences to be aired. Fuggle (personal communication, 2008) suggests the need for a coherent framework that can address three levels – integration of explanatory models, integration of treatment delivery, and organisational integration to support the first two levels.

Box 8.1 Principles of multidisciplinary working

- Specific disciplinary functions are clearly delineated and understood within the CAMHS
- Each discipline has the skills to work at all tiers
- Interdisciplinary training
- Agreed operational policies for teams and services that are evolved and developed in a multidisciplinary forum
- Forums for multidisciplinary discussion of clinical matters, organisational structure and the strategic direction of the service
- Professional supervision within individual disciplines and access to multidisciplinary supervision
- Administrative support

If certain disciplines are limited to working at certain tiers, or less experienced team members of any discipline are denied the experience of working across the tiers, the whole system is likely to become defined by a hierarchy of regard that will undermine its operational efficiency.

One reason that Tier 3 working is important within CAMHS is that it requires joint working across disciplines to a specific objective (e.g. the treatment of eating disorders) and thereby entails a development of multidisciplinary familiarity and understanding.

The team will function badly if there are gulfs between members (Box 8.2), but equally if there is uncritical consensus. Many teams of professionals who employ a systemic and developmental approach to their clinical work

---

Box 8.2 Tensions in multidisciplinary working

- Clinical overlap in the skills of the differing professionals
- Differences in skill levels and diversity between disciplines
- Differentials in salary
- Differentials in both professional and social status
- The influence of agencies outside CAMHS that may have little understanding of, or respect for, the multidisciplinary model
- Interdisciplinary rivalries and resentments rooted in historical, personal and professional experiences
- Differing training perspectives in different disciplines (multidisciplinary training is in its infancy)
- Different disciplines having different roles, responsibilities and priorities, leading to varying notions of professional 'good practice' (e.g. confidentiality)
- Hierarchies of regard depending on personal attributes as much as professional ones
- High anxiety leading to regression to a medical model

---

seem to behave as if such mechanisms for understanding do not apply to them (Kraemer, 1994). Conceptual or explanatory frameworks do not just go away if they are not discussed; just as in the 'conflict avoiding' family, tensions find a way of surfacing, usually to the detriment of the children for whom services are being provided.

Each discipline is autonomous as it has its own hierarchy and is accountable for its own work with children, young people and their families. Traditionally, there has been a view that the buck of each discipline's work stops on the consultant psychiatrist's desk. It is important that this myth is erased from the thinking of all agencies and all employers, as well as individual disciplines and professionals within CAMHS. Teams will be undermined if individual members are too insecure or precious about their status, and ultimate power and responsibility is given to one profession. To function effectively, each professional within a CAMHS must have role adequacy, role legitimacy and role support (NHS Health Advisory Service, 1995). Child and adolescent mental health service work requires a great deal of overlap in the nature of the work done by all professionals and disciplines, but multidisciplinary work can only be effective if the functional differences and responsibilities are clear and accepted.

Role adequacy

The World Health Organization's (1992) categories of emotional and behavioural disorders in ICD–10 would appear to make the role of CAMHS quite simple by clearly defining psychiatric disorders, which CAMHS should be able to assess and manage. However, it is not only medically trained professionals who can assess and treat these conditions, and hence they are wisely called 'mental disorders'. In children, the term 'mental health problem', which has an even wider definition, has come to prominence. Please let us cease to use that contradiction in terms the 'mental health disorder'. Epidemiological work suggests that between 10 and 20% of young people have psychopathology (Fombonne, 2002). Where the criterion of need for treatment has been used, the estimates are nearer the lower end of this range (Vikan, 1985), but such numbers are still beyond the individual interventions of CAMHS. All CAMHS members therefore require skills in the management of young people, consultation and preventive work as well as in the many modes of therapeutic intervention. Maintenance and development of the core skills requires ongoing training and supervision if role adequacy is to be maintained.

Role legitimacy

This is the area where the vexed questions of traditional roles within a health service, medical responsibility, leadership and anxiety management arise. Psychiatrists may be considered fortunate in that they are well-paid, highly trained members of a profession which, despite recent publicity, remains highly valued by the public. They are in short supply and are members of one of the most powerful trades unions in the country, the BMA. This allows them to command public respect and a revered position in the health service. Like parents in a similar position, they have considerable rights, but with those go some heavy responsibilities. Other disciplines may not be so fortunate and may find the struggle for legitimacy to be a slightly more uphill one – they may appear, like the identity-seeking adolescent, to be in search of respect and a desire to be taken seriously. This demonstrates a serious lack of understanding of their maturity in their roles, which will be recognised only if those roles are clearly defined, respected and rewarded.

Traditional roles

Traditionally, consultant psychiatrists are viewed as the ultimate authority in CAMHS and hence the people to whom others turn when uncertain, and in view of their length of training, this may be legitimate. In CAMHS, problems are rarely purely medical, so the 'ultimate authority' of the consultant is far more questionable. This is recognised, in that some clinical psychologists and nurses are consultants. The traditional role also means that the psychiatrist will be expected to take on management roles in terms of strategic development and operational monitoring of CAMHS. Such a role, which may be formalised in the post of clinical director, provides a complex task in view of the different professions and personalities involved, and the need to maintain networks in the organisation's management structure. There is no reason why other professions cannot take on such directorial roles, but it will be difficult for them to operate without the cooperation of psychiatrists.

Medical responsibility

The concept of medical responsibility engenders more anxiety in psychiatrists and ill feeling in other disciplines than any other. Psychiatrists are not responsible for patients seen by other members of teams or services of which they are members. They are not responsible for young people who are discussed with them, although their advice must not be negligent. They do not have to vet every referral into their service, as this delays assessment and treatment, and is negligent in its own right. Most young people referred to CAMHS demonstrate their distress in their behaviour and a doctor cannot be medically responsible for behaviour unless it is clearly caused by a medical condition, which the doctor is managing. Referrals come to a team, so the most suitable member of CAMHS can deal with that referral. Child and adolescent mental health service members are trained professionals who can work with young people and their families without constant oversight from a psychiatrist.

Medical responsibility is essentially good medical practice (General Medical Council, 2006). Indeed, the term 'medical responsibility' no longer appears in GMC literature.

Leadership

The traditional expectations of psychiatrists may lead to an automatic assumption of their leadership. Such expectations may be unrealistic in that a particular psychiatrist may not have leadership qualities or may misunderstand the leadership role, leading to the rest of the CAMHS resenting the psychiatrist's assumption of this role. The effective multidisciplinary functioning of the CAMHS will then be disrupted. Leadership must be distinguished from management, coordination, supervision and professional hierarchy, all of which are easier to define and the place of each professional within them clearer. Leaders are primarily required at times of change or uncertainty. They may therefore be defined as the person to whom other members of CAMHS go when they are worried about something – the 'anxiety sump' or, as Napoleon put it, 'a dealer in hope'.

Five styles of leadership are described (Gatrell, 1996): those who tell, those who sell, those who consult, those who participate and those who delegate. In professional hierarchies, telling may be appropriate, but effective team functioning depends on participation and delegation. Chapter 33 outlines a dozen characteristics of good leadership from the perspective of a Chief Executive.

Anxiety management

The maxim for all those working in CAMHS should be the first lines of Britain's favourite poem:

> 'If you can keep your head while all about you,
> Are losing theirs and blaming it on you'. (Rudyard Kipling)

'Not keeping your head' perfectly describes the responses of adults to young people's very difficult behaviour when they are bereft of any idea of what to do to manage the situation. The idea of 'illness' provides a convenient repository for a lack of understanding. Finding calm, structural solutions among a seething, projecting, emotional maelstrom is the task of any CAMHS professional as the ultimate consultative task. The service member who can do this best, and to whom other members of the team turn in such situations, is the key member of the service and may even be the leader.

Role support

The support to provide a service comes from the organisation in which the professionals work. Such support arises from the disciplinary structure, the multidisciplinary team and the host organisation's management structure. Role support is very variable in different settings and the professional who is unable to obtain it must consider whether it is tenable to continue to work in such an organisation. Professionals often feel overloaded by conflicting clinical and managerial pressures. Methods of addressing this are described for adult psychiatrists (Kennedy & Griffiths, 2000) and have resulted in New Ways of Working for psychiatrists (Department of Health, 2005) and for other disciplines, which are steadily catching up with the innovative practices of child and adolescent mental health professionals. The acknowledgement of different roles can produce a high level of respect for professional differences. To deny them usually results in professional rivalries and a dysfunctional team.

The roles of individual disciplines

Clinical child psychologists

Following an undergraduate psychology degree, a 3-year doctoral qualification is obtained in clinical psychology. It is usual for 2 or more years of relevant practical experience to be sandwiched between the two. Specialisation follows generic training and the clinical psychologist will have:

> 'a wide range of skills in the assessment, treatment and management of psychological problems in children and young people with physical illness, disabilities, emotional, educational and other difficulties. Their training is primarily in the context of health care and related services and involves considerable attention to the process of child development. Clinical training will also involve supervised practice with a full range of adults with mental health and other problems, with older adults and people with learning difficulties. This generic training complements the specialist child related skills and enables a rounded and comprehensive approach to the assessment and treatment of children and their carers.' (British Psychological Society, 2008)

Trained also in the administration of psychometric testing, clinical psychologists develop expertise in neuropsychological assessments and are able to offer a range of assessment, management and treatment options which enable them to provide a service in all tiers of a CAMHS.

Community psychiatric nurses

The majority of community psychiatric nurses will be registered mental health nurses, although this training offers little specific in terms of the theory and practice of working with children and their families. Because of this, there is a need for post-qualification training in relevant areas. Specialist courses have evolved in child and adolescent mental health. Community psychiatric nurses operate as key members of a CAMHS and are able to offer a prompt response as well as key assessment and treatment options. They are highly skilled and all tiers benefit from their input; they should not be used solely as Tier 2 professionals to protect professionals who hold themselves in higher regard.

In-patient psychiatric nurses

Nurses working in the Tier 4 in-patient service will include registered mental health nurses, some of whom will have obtained post-qualification training in child and adolescent mental health, nurses who are general or children's nursing trained and qualified, and untrained healthcare assistants. The in-patient nursing staff are the key and backbone to any in-patient unit offering skilled nursing care and a range of therapeutic inputs to the young people under their care and their families. In-patient staff may have a role in Tier 3 teams that are closely associated with their Tier 4 function to benefit from their expertise and to develop their community skills.

Child, adolescent and family psychiatrists

Medically qualified, they will specialise in general psychiatry before completing Membership of the Royal College of Psychiatrists; a further 3 years of specialist training specifically in child and adolescent psychiatry will follow before they achieve consultant status. Psychiatrists should work within all tiers of a CAMHS, delivering social, psychological and medical treatments. Under the Mental Health Act 1983, consultant psychiatrists, having obtained Section 12 approval, may be required to detain and treat psychiatrically ill young people, although changes to the Act (in 2007) with the concept of the responsible clinician, mean other disciplines can take on this responsibility. For in-patients, consultant psychiatrists will be medically responsible.

The position of the psychiatrist in the team is often a source of difficulty and conflict. There has been considerable debate about what psychiatrists should spend their time doing (Goodman, 1998), as they are an expensive resource that should be directed to maximum effect. Psychiatrists spend longer in training than most other mental health professionals, and this allows them to become skilled at the assessment and management of mental disorders. The fact that such skills may overlap in part with other professionals' skills does not impair either the psychiatrist's or other disciplines' role adequacy. In the NHS generally, more money is allocated to the postgraduate and in-service training of doctors than that of any other profession, so the potential to maintain that role adequacy may be greater than for any other mental health profession.

Social workers

Social workers are usually employed by the local Social Services department and attached to the CAMHS. This means they will be independent of the trust administering the CAMHS and have distinct line management and accountability. Such an attachment should, where possible, be full time and exclusive, so that specialist skills can be developed and the CAMHS can operate in a fully integrated multidisciplinary fashion. Social workers are often, but not always, graduates who undertake postgraduate training that

75

results in the Diploma in Social Work or the Certificate of Qualification in Social Work; they often go on to obtain a Master's degree. Their training is generic; however, there is the scope for some specialisation during training. Social workers may follow-up their training with post-qualification training in specialist areas.

Social workers have statutory responsibilities in the field of safeguarding children. Their work is structured by the rule of law, specifically the Children Act 1989 and the Mental Health Act 1983 updated in 2007 (some will be 'approved mental health professionals' under the terms of the latter). Social workers should work within all tiers of the CAMHS.

Other disciplines

The professions highlighted represent the core of any CAMHS: with the lack of any of those disciplines, it is difficult for a CAMHS to function coherently. There are a range of other disciplines that can be successfully integrated into a CAMHS, and have valuable insights to offer to the mental health needs of children and families. Examples include occupational therapists, child psychotherapists, family therapists, and music, art and drama therapists, as well as educationalists (e.g. teachers, educational psychologists). As with the core disciplines, the task becomes initially a process of agreeing an interface between the different explanatory models. Integrated models tend to promote a number of change mechanisms (e.g. systemic change in family relationships, reduction of anxiety in a child) and in these circumstances the child and family can benefit from the skills and therapeutic models from different disciplines. The bringing together of new disciplines into CAMHS has promoted innovative models of service delivery but will only continue to flourish if journals, conferences and training courses allow for the cross-fertilisation of conceptual models.

Primary mental health workers

Primary mental health workers are drawn from a number of professions, but their seniority and training mean they have considerable knowledge of young people's mental functioning. In many CAMHS they are the public face of the service, working with those who have responsibility for children who have mental health problems and referring on when they consider specialist services are required (Hickey *et al*, 2007). For the integration of primary mental health workers into CAMHS and to prevent their professional isolation it is often helpful for them to work with specialist CAMHS professionals in a Tier 3 team.

Conclusion

Multidisciplinary working is at the heart of CAMHS, it ensures that there is a professional and a skill to reach every aspect of children's psychological function. Each discipline is occupied by a person with all the frailties that the human condition is subject to; they must each understand those frailties and understand and value the abilities of all the team members to ensure a comprehensive service for children and young people.

References

British Psychological Society (2008) *Directory of Chartered Psychologists*. British Psychological Society.

Department of Health (2005) *New Ways of Working for Psychiatrists: Enhancing Effective, Person-centred Services Through New Ways of Working in Multidisciplinary and Multiagency Contexts*. TSO (The Stationery Office).

Fombonne, E. (2002) Case identification in an epidemiological context. In *Child and Adolescent Psychiatry* (eds M. Rutter & E. Taylor), pp. 52–69. Blackwell.

Gatrell, J. (1996) Managing people. In *Textbook of Management for Doctors* (ed. T. White), pp. 127–134. Churchill Livingstone.

General Medical Council (2006) *Good Medical Practice*. GMC.

Goodman, R. (1998) *Child and Adolescent Mental Health Services: Reasoned Advice to Commissioners and Providers*. Institute of Psychiatry. King's College London.

Hickey, N., Kramer, T. & Garralda, E. (2007) *Primary Mental Health Workers (PMHWs) in Child and Adolescent Mental Health Services: A Survey of Organisation, Management and Role*. Department of Health.

Kennedy, P. & Griffiths, H. (2000) *An Analysis of the Concerns of Consultant General Psychiatrists About Their Jobs, and of the Changing Practices That May Point Towards Solutions*. Northern Centre for Mental Health.

Kraemer, S. (1994) *The Case for a Multidisciplinary Child and Adolescent Mental Health Community Service: The Liaison Model. A Guide for Managers, Purchasers and GPs*. Tavistock Clinic.

NHS Health Advisory Service (1995) *Together We Stand: Commissioning, Role and Management of Child and Adolescent Mental Health Services*. HMSO.

Vikan, A. (1985) Psychiatric epidemiology in a sample of 1510 ten-year-old children. I. Prevalence. *Journal of Child Psychology and Psychiatry*, **76**, 55–75.

World Health Organization (1992) *The ICD–10 Classification of Mental and Behavioural Disorders*. WHO.

CHAPTER 9

User and carer participation and advocacy

Jonathan Barrett

'Doctor – the patient will see you now.'
Caption to cartoon in *The Spectator*

Introduction

Service user participation has become more prominent in both NHS policy documents and CAMHS strategy over the past decade. Article 12 of the *Convention on the Rights of the Child* (United Nations, 1990) enshrines the right to 'express his or her own views freely in all matters affecting the child, the views of the child being given due weight in accordance with the age and maturity of the child'. In 1995, the NHS Priorities and Planning Guidance sought to deliver 'greater voice and influence to users of NHS services and their carers in their own care, the development and definition of standards set for NHS services locally, and the development of NHS policy both locally and nationally' (NHS Executive, 1995). As with many top-down initiatives, the influence of this rhetoric on grass roots practice has been variable, resulting in pockets of good practice, rather than a consistent national strategy.

The move away from the so-called 'medical model' of the expert on a distant and all-wise pedestal, with the child and family as seen but only selectively heard recipients of care, has been facilitated by a shift both in terms of professional attitudes and social and politically driven initiatives with the patient as the 'consumer' of care. Institutional and organisational shifts have enshrined user participation as part of the *Every Child Matters: Change for Children* agendas (Department for Children, Schools and Families, 2003).

Active, rather than passive involvement of service users has been advocated (e.g. YoungMinds), with service users facilitated in setting the agenda for change as well as providing feedback in the context of service evaluation. There has been a tendency to place organisations rather than user and carer needs at the centre of service development (Goss & Miller, 1995), with the focus shifted to emphasise user and carer views. *Putting Participation into Practice* (Street & Herts, 2005) provides a framework for integrating user involvement into CAMHS. The participation of children and young people is at the heart of the NSF for children initiative (Department of Health, 2004). The government has stated its intent to involve young people in the design, implementation and review of the services that affect them in *Learning to Listen* (Children and Young People's Unit, 2001), and it behoves CAMHS to respond appropriately.

This chapter introduces the concept and history of service user participation from a CAMHS perspective, and considers the more active involvement of young people and their families, and the benefits of such participation. Implementation of participation is considered, with reference to resources of utility to a practitioner embarking on local efforts to involve service users, and future developments and potential innovations are identified.

The ladder of participation: a model for understanding user involvement

The ladder of participation represents a continuum of options in terms of user involvement and participation; organisations are able to go both up and down the ladder in terms of their community involvement and the ongoing attempts at operationalising the proper 'authority' (Fig. 9.1). Involvement includes information-sharing and consultation on specific issues. Levels of involvement are determined by the amount of power and agency afforded to young people. The ladder of participation model (Street & Herts, 2005) outlines eight levels of involvement, ranging from non-participation to passive through to active involvement service planning and delivery.

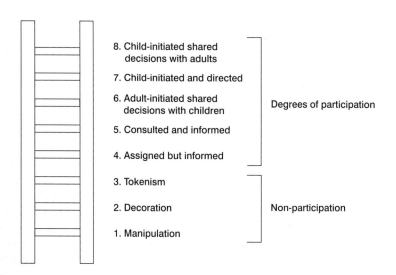

Fig. 9.1 The ladder of participation. Adapted from Street & Herts (2005).

At best, user and carer participation can reap dividends for all stakeholders; at worst, it can be patronising or tokenistic, paying lip service to the process of participation, risking diminished engagement and fostering resentment in service users. Not all young people and families will want to be involved, and there has to be a sense of realism about what can be achieved by CAMHS that are operating within finite resources. The level of participation requires mutual agreement between users, CAMHS workers and commissioners, depending on competing priorities, in order to stand a greater chance of success.

It must also be accepted that whatever form an intervention takes, however negotiated or informed, the question of clinical accountability does not disappear. However democratic our intentions as professional mental health workers, we cannot in good conscience succumb to the relativist mantra of the 'customer is always right' – although we may respect the desire for an inappropriate treatment option, we do not need to collude for it if the evidence suggests it to be either worthless or harmful. We should remember that on taking a faulty car to a mechanic we do not wish to provide and discuss repair options – we rightly expect the mechanic to diagnose and repair the problem. The point here is that negotiation and collaboration is a two-way process – a dialogue – the sins of the authoritarian past are not expunged by irresponsibly allowing the pendulum to swing into the arena of unfettered consumer choice.

Methods of involvement

The pros and cons of some currently employed participation strategies are presented in order of increasing engagement as suggested by the ladder of participation model.

Suggestion boxes are cheap, easy to implement and anonymous, but might not be accessible to those with literacy problems. Questionnaires are straightforward, allow anonymity and can be completed in the young person or carer's own time. They can reach a potentially large sample, but risk appearing faceless and can be prone to misinterpretation. Response rates might be low or skewed, and reading and writing skills are required. Computer programs can be more flexible than a written questionnaire; they can be tailored to local requirements with relative ease, and can ask questions in more or less detail contingent on previous responses. Information technology can facilitate rapid analysis of data to allow for a timely response to service user views. There are attendant concerns about confidentiality, and this approach may prove to be exclusive of those without information and communications technology (ICT) skills or access to a computer.

Telephone interviews can be advantageous, in that dedicated space for interviews is not required and they allow clarification of specific points. They are less prone to bias or leading questions if an independent person is employed, which can encourage people to share their views more readily.

However, it might be challenging to contact a young person at a mutually convenient time, and this might potentially result in difficulties maintaining confidentiality. Face-to-face interviews can improve response rates and overcome literacy problems. They allow the chance to facilitate discussion using non-verbal cues, but they are intensive of resources required to conduct interviews. The success or failure depends upon the establishment of rapport between the young person and interviewer.

Focus groups can facilitate synergistic development of ideas through discussion, but may be dominated by a particular prevailing view. They also require resources and planning to facilitate and to capture emerging ideas. More ambitious service user-involvement projects will facilitate service user involvement in planning groups. Involvement in planning develops empowerment and encourages ownership among service users. A prospective by-product is the opportunity for young people to develop their social skills and gain other transferable skills by virtue of team-working. Active and transparent involvement and appreciation of the decision-making process is an asset to higher levels of service user participation; however, care must be taken to support young people robustly to avoid this feeling symbolic. Involvement in service evaluation also allows for team-working and a shared commitment for both parties to act on the findings. Evaluation is not impartial though, as young people often have a vested interest in the outcome. Shifting the power base so that users are in charge of change has the merits of promoting enthusiasm and affords a youthful perspective, which can lend the service credibility. The process can also develop young people as role models. Maintaining boundaries can be challenging and it can be difficult to sustain momentum owing to other time commitments competing for young people's attention.

The mixed economy might be the most effective strategy; clearly the service will have to consider the appropriateness given the precise nature of their clinical work, as well as the openness to novelty among staff, young people and their families. The use of ICT can provide one route to increased user participation (e.g. short-messaging service (SMS) text messaging, email and internet-based discussion boards). Boundaries need to be maintained, and consideration given to concerns around stigma and confidentiality. Difficulties may arise with ensuring that service users are representative – perhaps the more educated or those with more social capital are more likely to come forward when views are canvassed. Advocacy might encourage those with learning or social communication difficulties, sensory impairments, looked-after children and those with language other than English. Special consideration needs to be given to how the opinions of hard-to-reach groups are gathered (e.g. those who attend sporadically or who drop out of CAMHS).

The timing of requests to engage young people and families must be considered to avoid them feeling obliged to participate when they might want to move on, while reconciling this with the practicalities of obtaining their responses efficiently.

Involving children and young people in the Children and Young People's Plan

In order to make the most constructive and positive use of user participation, it is important that an effective structure is formulated so that the process achieves its optimal potential. It is sensible not to act too quickly, putting on 'special events or consultations' – as there is a risk of duplicating existing work, a useful rule of thumb would be to capitalise on work that has already been done locally. This allows for integration with existing resources and attitudes, and avoids the impression of 'knowing what's best' for those you wish to engage with – it furthers the notions of continuity and evolution of ideas in service understanding and provision.

Many of the groups listed in Section 2.1 of the Children and Young People's Plan guidance (Department for Children, Schools and Families, 2009) will have already contributed to consultations, and often report that they feel overconsulted. Try to move on from consultation to their ongoing 'involvement'. This can be supported through their workers.

1   Don't allow tight timescales to prevent you from thinking creatively about work as part of an ongoing process. A plan of action that promotes a dialogue rather than a one-off consultation may better meet the needs of children and young people. Children and young people report that ongoing sessions enable them to see how their input has made a difference (Department for Children, Schools and Families, 2009).

2   Develop a clear, basic structure or strategy for involving children and young people with someone taking responsibility for ensuring that it is implemented (e.g. understanding of terminology varies: 0–13 years workers are often called participation workers, and 13+ years, voice and influence workers). This doesn't need to be complicated and can be principle-based. Try to agree a common understanding locally of 'participation', 'involvement' and 'voice and influence'. The structure allows the dialogue and it is the dialogue that is of paramount importance, i.e. the process is as important as the content – the means of engagement as important as that which is done. This reverts to the basic principle that all effective interventions are based upon well-established relationships. Workers report that working in the context of a local strategy places more importance on the work, and embeds it for the long term.

3   Get to know the workers who can help (including workers within the health and the voluntary sector as well as statutory services, Connexions (www.connexions-direct.com/) and Children's Fund (www.dcsf.gov.uk/everychildmatters/)), and contribute time and possibly resources. Utilise all of their skills to ensure that all children and young people are involved right across the age ranges.

4   The Children and Young People's Plan should be fit for purpose, and needs to be owned and agreed by children and young people, staff and

services. Your local participation and voice and influence workers can share their ideas on how this can be achieved. Joint area review will attempt to establish the extent to which children and young people are experiencing the right kinds of services. By having some ownership of the plan, children and young people will be likely to engage in the process of review.

Box 9.1 Participation resources available on the internet

- Young Advisors (www.youngadvisors.org.uk) provides details on an initiative to engage young people aged between 15 and 21 years in activities to inform community leaders and decision-makers.
- The CAMHS Outcome Research Consortium (www.corc.uk.net) uses outcomes data to encourage learning and improve practice in work with young people, families and carers.
- Expert Patients Programme (www.expertpatients.nhs.uk) provides some information on workshops for young people aged 12–18 years who are living with a long-term health condition. The website has some useful publications of relevance to setting up a participation project.
- Participation Works (www.participationworks.org.uk) provides a portal to resources on children and young people's participation. It provides an extensive hub of relevant resources, which is indispensable to busy CAMHS workers.
- YoungMinds (www.youngminds.org.uk) offers a wealth of resources on participation in CAMHS, including publications and details on training courses.
- The National Youth Agency (www.nya.org.uk) provides support to those involved in young people's personal and social development. They have produced standards for the active involvement of children and young people: 'Hear by Right', and 'Act by Right'.
- The *You're Welcome Quality Criteria* (Department of Health, 2007; www. dh.gov.uk) are principles defined by the Department of Health for creating services that are young-people-friendly. There is a section covering CAMHS and a companion toolkit is available as an aid to implementation.
- The Choice and Partnership Approach (www.camhsnetwork.co.uk) is an example of a framework for CAMHS, which integrates participation into everyday clinical practice.
- The Children's Society (www.childrenssociety.org.uk) is a national charity which has published various documents on advocacy and participation. Details of local participation projects are provided to serve as inspiration.
- The National Youth Advocacy Service (www.nyas.net) facilitates young people in having their views heard and effecting change. Their work includes encouraging children and young people's participation in the planning and development of services. The NYAS provides training for agencies.
- Although the responsibilities of the Care Services Improvement Partnership (www.csip.org.uk) have been subsumed by Regional Health Authorities in 2009, the document *High Impact Changes for Health and Social Care* (Care Services Improvement Partnership, 2008) emphasises the importance of including users and carers in planning and delivery of services.

Potential benefits of participation

Participation can improve relationships with young people and families in CAMHS, and can augment local initiatives, ensuring they have resonance with local service users. When implemented effectively, they can enhance job satisfaction for CAMHS workers and lead to a synergy between collaborators to boost creativity. There is the potential to generate self-esteem in young people, and a sense of ownership and empowerment. Child and adolescent mental health services retain responsibility for ensuring that adequate training is provided for participants. Exciting opportunities exist for services to incorporate service user participation in all aspects of CAMHS planning and delivery.

Future developments

Sharing experiences and evaluating the implementation of participation projects will allow other teams and populations to benefit from their efforts. Some resources, which will facilitate this process, are presented in Box 9.1.

Conclusion

Effective participation is valued and respected, and encourages diversity, empowerment and respect; it also leads to synergy and tolerance of different perspectives. It is an expected component of a comprehensive CAMHS, and can underpin all aspects of a well-functioning service.

References

Care Services Improvement Partnership (2008) *High Impact Changes for Health and Social Care*. Department of Health (http://www.csip.org.uk/silo/files/hics-doc-11th-march.pdf).

Children and Young People's Unit (2001) *Learning to Listen: Core Principles for the Involvement of Children and Young People*. Department for Education and Skills.

Department for Children, Schools and Families (2003) *Every Child Matters: Change for Children*. TSO (The Stationery Office) (http://www.everychildmatters.gov.uk/).

Department for Children, Schools and Families (2009) *Children and Young People's Plan Guidance 2009*. TSO (The Stationery Office).

Department of Health (2004) *National Service Framework for Children, Young People and Maternity Services*. TSO (The Stationery Office) (http://www.dh.gov.uk/en/Healthcare/NationalServiceFrameworks/Children/DH_4089111).

Department of Health (2007) *You're Welcome Quality Criteria: Making Health Services Young People Friendly*. TSO (The Stationery Office).

Goss, S. & Miller, C. (1995) *From Margin to Mainstream: Developing User and Carer Centred Community Care*. Joseph Rowntree Foundation.

NHS Executive (1995) *Priorities and Planning Guidance for the NHS: 1997/98*. NHS Executive.

Street, C. & Herts, B. (2005) *Putting Participation into Practice*. YoungMinds.

United Nations (1990) *Convention on the Rights of the Child*. UN (http://www2.ohchr.org/english/law/crc.htm).

CHAPTER 10

A comprehensive CAMHS[1]

Clare Lamb & Ann York

'Good order is the foundation of all good things.'
Edmund Burke (1729–1797)

Introduction

The jurisdictions of England, Ireland, Northern Ireland, Scotland and Wales have each produced CAMHS strategies that are at different stages of development and implementation. There are no significant differences in the prevalence and types of mental health problems experienced by children under the age of 15 years in England, Wales or Scotland. Hence, there is no justification for inequity of service provision. Ireland and Northern Ireland have a higher percentage of young people in their populations and require a higher number of whole time equivalent (WTE) clinicians in their teams. Child and adolescent mental health services must be equitable across the jurisdictions, and practitioners and policy-makers must share practice and learn from each other. The five jurisdictions all have services that are currently stretched. Recruitment and retention as well as the geography of an area are problematic in different places.

The Royal College of Psychiatrists has tried to guide the provision of specialist CAMHS at Tiers 2–4 by the NHS (Royal College of Psychiatrists, 2006). There is insufficient evidence to give detailed guidance on services for those with intellectual disability, substance misuse or forensic problems, or infant mental health services. However, services should be able to provide for these groups, and indeed the English NSF (Department of Health & Department for Education and Skills, 2004) and proxy targets for a comprehensive CAMHS had services for 16- and 17-year-olds and those with intellectual disability as core targets. The recommendations for staffing and remit for services are necessarily ballpark ones, based on rationalising the evidence. The guidance is meant to be living, evolving support for service development, open to local interpretation based on careful needs

---

1. The first part of this chapter is summarised from *Building and Sustaining Specialist CAMHS* (Royal College of Psychiatrists, 2006) and the second part from the *Working at the CAMHS/Adult Interface: Good Practice Guidance for the Provision of Psychiatric Services to Adolescents/Young Adults* (Lamb *et al*, 2008).

assessment and priorities. It should be used wisely, with care and authority, to shape local services to be the best possible for young people.

Specialist CAMHS

Tier 2 and 3 services are the core of specialist CAMHS and cannot be disaggregated if young people and families are to experience a seamless CAMHS, and they should have a single point of entry. Many current specialist CAMHS only see young people up to the age of 16 years. Psychiatric disorders increase in frequency above this age and specialist CAMHS that end at the 16th birthday will require significant extra resources to extend services to the age of 18. Capacity calculations based on providing an epidemiologically needs-based service for 0 to 16-year-olds suggest that team capacity for intervention is ideal at 40 new referrals per WTE per year.

Key working

Clinician keyworker case-load should average 40 cases per WTE across the service, varying according to the type of cases held and the other responsibilities of the clinician that impact on their job plan. However, some clinicians will be able to hold far larger case-loads, especially if those are co-worked, or are low intensity. Similarly, high-intensity, high-frequency interventions (e.g. individual psychodynamic psychotherapy) may mean lower case-loads can be held. A service model that calculates individual capacity according to job role is ideal (see Chapter 12).

Support to Tier 1

Specialist CAMHS work with Tier 1 professionals may be provided by dedicated primary mental health workers, ideally working as a team linked to and supervised within specialist CAMHS. However, all CAMHS professionals should have the skills to consult to and support Tier 1 (see Chapter 13).

Staffing of Tier 2/3

Specialist CAMHS require a minimum of 20 WTE clinicians for all those up to the 16th birthday in a total population of 100 000. Teams must ensure a range of clinical professionals who are able to deliver cognitive, behavioural, psychodynamic and systemic skills, complemented by psychiatric medical skills. Exact proportions of each skill will vary according to local need and commissioning arrangements. Each profession must have access to uniprofessional supervision and training and, ideally, never be the only professional from that discipline in the service. Additional staffing will be required for significant intellectual disability, substance misuse and dual diagnosis, forensic and infant mental health services.

Remit of specialist CAMHS

Services should be commissioned to provide mental health services for children and young people up to their 18th birthday, including liaison with and consultation to other agencies, and assessment and treatment of psychiatric and neurodevelopmental disorders including:

- psychosis
- depressive disorders
- ADHD
- autism-spectrum disorders
- Tourette syndrome and complex tic disorders
- self-harm and suicide attempts
- eating disorders
- obsessive–compulsive disorder (OCD)
- phobias and anxiety disorders
- mental health problems secondary to abusive experiences
- mental health problems associated with physical health problems and somatoform disorders.

The following services can also be provided by specialist CAMHS, but in some areas may be provided for by other agencies and specialists such as community paediatricians, health visitors and multi-agency teams, with input by specialist CAMHS workers.

- Services for under-5-year-olds with milder behaviour or sleep problems (e.g. provided for by health visitor sleep and behaviour clinics).
- Mental health problems associated with intellectual disability (e.g. provided by multi-agency teams).
- Disruptive behaviour and conduct disorders (e.g. youth offending teams and Local Authority services).
- Adjustment disorders (e.g. voluntary sector services dealing with parental separation).
- Elective mutism (e.g. speech and language therapy services).
- Elimination problems (e.g. paediatric and health visitor services).

In addition, specialist multidisciplinary teams may be commissioned to provide:

- second opinion service
- expert witness service
- parenting assessment in complex cases.

Tier 4

Tier 4 NHS mental health services are very specialised services in residential, day-patient or out-patient settings for children and adolescents with severe and/or complex problems requiring a combination or intensity of interventions that cannot be provided by community CAMHS. There is a need for coherent development and provision of comprehensive Tier 4 services across the five jurisdictions based on national plans, with particular focus on the provision of child and adolescent mental health in-patient services. Plans should be developed within a multi-agency, integrated commissioning agenda (see Chapter 29).

Tier 4 in-patient bed numbers

Overall, 20–40 in-patient CAMHS beds per 1 million total population are required to provide mental health services for young people up to the age of 18 years with severe mental health problems requiring emergency or very intensive treatments. The number of in-patient beds required for a given population must be based on a comprehensive needs assessment. The recognised optimal maximum number of beds for an adolescent in-patient unit is around 12. There is no minimum number of beds, but it is difficult for a stand-alone unit to be clinically and financially viable below six to seven beds. Bed occupancy should not be more than 85% if there is to be availability of emergency beds, and this percentage will be lower, the smaller the unit. Staffing of in-patient units is influenced by skill mix, task demands of a particular shift, case dependency/acuity and case mix.

Disorders commonly managed by Tier 4

The following disorders are those most commonly treated in CAMHS in-patient units:

- severe eating disorder
- severe affective disorder
- severe anxiety/emotional disorder
- severe OCD
- psychotic disorders
- other mental illnesses where physical, social and family variables operate to inhibit progress in the community.

In addition, commissioners must ensure that specialist out-patient and in-patient expertise is available for young people with:

- intellectual disability with comorbid mental illness and/or challenging behaviour
- severe eating disorders
- complex neuropsychiatric problems
- sensory handicaps
- rare paediatric disorders
- head injury/brain injury
- mother and baby in-patient provision
- severe/complex substance use problems and dual diagnosis.

Intensive treatment

Intensive community treatment should be developed in the context of, and closely linked with, well-resourced community CAMHS and accessible age-appropriate Tier 4 in-patient facilities. Such provision includes: day units; crisis teams/intensive community support teams/outreach teams/home treatment teams; enhanced paediatric ward/specialist adolescent ward; and liaison/transition community mental health teams for 16- to 18-year-olds (see Chapter 28).

CAMHS out-of-office hours

In England, there has been a target to provide out-of-hours mental health services for those with urgent mental health needs. Where out-of-hours cover exists, it tends to be provided by the consultant psychiatrist, although increasingly other senior members of the multidisciplinary team provide this service. Detailed discussions must take place between commissioners, CAMHS and adult mental health services in order to explore creative solutions in the light of the limited capacity of some CAMHS to provide comprehensive out-of-hours cover and joint protocols agreed. For example, initial emergency out-of-hours care may be provided by adult services who liaise with CAMHS.

CAMHS for 16- and 17-year-olds

The Royal College of Psychiatrists have agreed a number of points of consensus regarding good practice with respect to both the mental healthcare offered to young people and the transition of their care from child to adult services (Lamb *et al*, 2008). Finances and workforce capacity will have an influence on local developments and arrangements with respect to 16- and 17-year-olds, but whatever the resources available and whatever precise arrangements are in place, these vulnerable young people should receive good practice.

Models of service

In recent years there has been considerable impetus in the development of innovative services across the UK that promote greater working between child and adult mental health services (Maitra & Jolley, 2000). In order to combat the gaps in service and inequity of provision, an increasing number of mental health services have developed clinical liaison or link posts to facilitate joint working by CAMHS and adult mental health teams. Others have set up specific teams for older adolescents/young adults – some of these teams are generic, others are disorder specific (e.g. early intervention psychosis services). Many of these teams work across the traditional age range of transition. Research on service structure recommends any or a combination of the following types of transition service:
- designated transition service
- designated transition team within a service

- designated staff trained in adolescent work seconded to adult teams (Richards & Vostanis, 2004).

Most of the models cited below have improved the mental health service offered by forging strong working links or formal partnership agreements with other agencies involved with young people. Successful partnerships have been formed with non-statutory and voluntary organisations as well as those from the statutory sector.

Fully funded community-based multidisciplinary team

In some areas there are fully funded multidisciplinary teams designed to bridge and work jointly with CAMHS and adult mental health services to meet the generic mental health needs of older adolescents. In England, many of these teams link with, or are part of, the early intervention psychosis service and in addition have good working relationships with the local home treatment and crisis resolution teams as well as Social Services, education, the local youth offending team and substance misuse service. National surveys of community mental health services for older adolescents/young adults carried out in England between 1999 and 2005 (Lamb *et al*, 2008) explored the skills, capabilities and main characteristics of identified teams. There were variations in resources and different models of service delivery among the teams surveyed. However, there were key similarities. Common aspects included a multidisciplinary team with a mix of expertise from both CAMHS and adult mental health services, providing individual and family psychosocial and psychological interventions alongside medication. The teams promoted a youth-centred and flexible approach with an emphasis on effective engagement of young people through outreach and joint working with other agencies. They provided expertise to treat the range of mental disorders presenting in older adolescents. Many of the community services lacked age-appropriate day provision and psychiatric in-patient services.

Disorder-specific services

A number of disorder-specific services have been set up to span the traditional age range across CAMHS and adult services. In England, the adult mental health NSF (Department of Health, 1999) outlined the policy requirement for early intervention services for first-episode psychosis in 14- to 35-year-olds. This policy has been widely implemented across England and in some areas has acted as a catalyst to the further development of generic mental health services that bridge the transition age.

Designated liaison/link posts

A number of NHS trusts have funded 'transition' or 'liaison' posts that comprise one or two clinicians, often community psychiatric nurses with expertise in working with adolescents. These individuals carry out assessments and some face-to-face work, in addition to working jointly across both the adult mental health services and CAMHS to facilitate work with older adolescents.

Transition mental health teams for looked-after children

Other NHS trusts have joined with other agencies and implemented multi-agency commissioning to provide transition (16- to 18-year-olds) mental health teams for the sole use of looked-after children (i.e. those young people in care or in the process of leaving Social Services care).

'Virtual team'

Another example of a model linking both CAMHS and adult services is that of a 'virtual team' where designated members from the respective multidisciplinary services work together to provide a range of skills and expertise to help meet the developmental and mental health needs of older adolescents presenting to either service.

Workforce and capacity for 16- and 17-year-olds

Workforce and capacity requirements for specialist CAMHS working with children up to the age of 16 have been published (Kelvin, 2005; Royal College of Psychiatrists, 2006). The needs of the 16- and 17-year-old cohorts are widely held to be much greater than comparative year cohorts in the age periods up to the 16th birthday, and Kelvin (2005) has calculated the evidenced-based tariff of staffing required to deliver comprehensive CAMHS to this cohort. It is based on the model of specialist CAMHS (NHS Health Advisory Service, 1995) – a community-based multidisciplinary service offering specialised mental health services to young people with complex and severe mental health problems. Often, more than one professional is required in the management of these young people in view of their multiple needs. Comorbidities are common in young people referred to specialist services and often the input of more than one clinician is required. Work will necessarily involve re-integration into education, training or work. This model of a mental health team for older adolescents differs from the typical adult mental health team in that it includes interventions for neurodevelopmental disorders such as ADHD and Asperger syndrome, in addition to other disorders that might not usually meet the eligibility criteria for adult specialist care.

Kelvin's calculations produce a staff tariff for a service serving a total population of 100 000 (approximately 2222 16- and 17-year-olds) based on the known prevalence of psychiatric disorders, attendance fractions and the number of clinicians required to provide evidence-based interventions for a broad range of psychiatric presentations including: neurodevelopmental disorders, eating disorders, depressive disorders, adjustment disorders and emerging personality disorders, in addition to severe and enduring mental disorders such as bipolar disorder and psychoses.

The staffing required to provide comprehensive specialist CAMHS from 0 to the 17th birthday for a total population of 100 000 is 16 WTE for a non-teaching centre and 20 WTE for a teaching centre (Kelvin, 2005; Royal College of Psychiatrists, 2006), but does not include youth offending or substance misuse work. Kelvin compared his new data for 16- and 17-year-olds with the data for 0 to 16-year-olds (Kelvin, 2005) and calculated that comprehensive CAMHS for 16- and 17-year-olds for a total population of 100 000 not including youth offending and substance misuse work requires 6.6 WTE clinicians (1.45 WTE consultant psychiatrists) for a non-teaching centre and 8.4 WTE clinicians (1.8 WTE consultant psychiatrists) for a teaching centre. This equates to 3.3 WTE and 4.2 WTE clinicians per year (age cohort 16 or 17 years) per 100 000 total population for a non-teaching centre and a teaching centre respectively.

This information enabled Kelvin to estimate a ratio of the staff tariff for specialist CAMHS for year 16 or 17 compared with the staff tariff for any one single year group 0–15 years inclusive. For a non-teaching centre, the ratio is 3.9. For a teaching centre, the ratio is 3.8. He concludes that if we want to deliver equitable levels of service to 16- and/or 17-year-olds compared with the younger age cohorts, then 3.9 more staff for each year at 16 or 17 are required than for each year from 0 to the 16th birthday (0–15 years inclusive). This information can be used to calculate the extra staff required for a given CAMHS in order to extend their service up to the 18th birthday. Recommendations for the staffing tariff for a comprehensive CAMHS from 0 to the 18th birthday (not including youth offending and substance misuse work) based on Kelvin's calculations are $(16 + 3.3) = 19.3$ WTE for a non-teaching centre, and $(20 + 4.2) = 24.2$ WTE for a teaching centre.

Recommendations

In each primary care trust (England) or local health board (Scotland and Wales) area, commissioners for CAMHS and adult mental health services must work together to ensure provision of accessible and effective mental health services for 16- and 17-year-olds. They should ensure that in each NHS trust, agreement is reached between CAMHS and adult mental health services on the process of transition and the age at which it will occur. Further agreement will be required on which groups of young people will be referred on to adult mental health services and which will require alternative arrangements for ongoing treatment of a mental health problem. Alternative arrangements might include primary care counsellors, GP, clinical psychology, student counselling services, youth service counsellors or other non-statutory or voluntary sector provision. The key consideration is that the young people concerned can access mental health expertise for their particular difficulties and that their views are taken into account during the planning process.

The following diagnoses would generally fulfil the criteria for referral to adult mental health services:

- schizophrenia and related psychoses
- bipolar disorder
- severe OCD
- severe depressive disorder
- severe or chronic eating disorders.

The principles of integrated planning offer a useful model in ensuring that individuals at the transition between CAMHS and adult services obtain seamless care. For those presenting with severe mental disorder needing ongoing care with adult psychiatric services, discussion should take place between services at an early stage (at least 6 months prior to the age of transition). The young person must be consulted and involved in discussions. Where possible, prior to transfer of care, a period of joint working should be introduced, with the keyworker from each service linking to facilitate meaningful engagement of the young person. Formal handover of care should be marked by a specific multidisciplinary case conference. In England and Wales this should be by the care programme approach. Services should aim to have a degree of flexibility around time of transition in line with the developmental needs of the young person concerned. Specific agreement must be reached and protocols written regarding the transfer of care for young people who are in treatment with children's mental health services and are within the following diagnostic groups:

- ADHD
- autism-spectrum disorder (e.g. Asperger syndrome)
- emerging borderline personality disorder
- mild to moderate intellectual disability
- psychological sequelae of chronic physical illness (e.g. cystic fibrosis, diabetes)
- psychological sequelae of abusive experiences.

The process of transfer and provision of ongoing care to these groups can be complex as they may not fulfil the referral criteria for an adult mental health service that prioritises severe mental illness. Local arrangements should reflect good practice guidance regarding each of the diagnostic groups. Commissioners must be informed of gaps in service and of their responsibility to commission new services where resources are lacking. Within each NHS trust (in conjunction with local commissioners, senior practitioners and managers) CAMHS, adult mental health and other key agencies such as clinical psychology, Social Services, primary care and relevant non-statutory services should work together to draw up standard agreements with respect to care pathways and the programmes of transition for each of the disorders listed, involving young people and their families/carers in the process. Transition protocols should ensure that a planning meeting between agencies involved in the transfer of care takes place at an early stage. In areas where there is a long waiting list, for example in clinical psychology, this should be taken into account when planning the timing of referral. Formal transfer of care should be marked by a specific meeting or case conference.

Pathways of care and treatment protocols must also be agreed between the local CAMHS and adult mental health service with respect to self-harm and emergency presentations to accident and emergency departments. This should reflect good practice guidance (e.g. NICE guidelines) and the recommendations in the Royal College of Psychiatrists report (Kaplan, 2007) (see Chapter 15).

The Royal College Psychiatrists (2002), English and Welsh policy documents (National Assembly for Wales, 2001, 2005, 2006; Department of Health & Department for Education and Skills, 2004), as well as Scottish government documents (Scottish Executive, 2003, 2005, 2006) suggest that, ideally, no young person under 18 years should be admitted to an adult psychiatric unit, and that in-patient care should be in specialist, age-appropriate facilities. Until resources for adolescent services become available across the UK, specific agreement should exist between CAMHS and adult mental health services on protocols for the safe admission and management of 16- and 17-year-olds on adult psychiatric wards (Royal College of Psychiatrists, 2002; Office of the Children's Commissioner for England, 2007) and in *The National Service Framework for Mental Health in England* (Department of Health, 1999) and that for Wales. Admissions to adult wards should be for brief periods only. In most circumstances, an age-appropriate in-patient setting that provides access to education and expertise in child and adolescent mental health should be identified, and transfer of care arranged as soon as possible.

Where a 16- or 17-year-old is receiving treatment in an 'independent sector' adolescent psychiatric in-patient unit, the professionals involved must ensure that transition arrangements are addressed as outlined above for the NHS sector.

Conclusion

Significant work has been undertaken across the UK to establish guidelines for effective interventions, team skills and models of service delivery as well as the staff needed to provide those services. For those 0–15 and 16 and 17 years old, Kelvin provides some preliminary estimates of the workforce capacity that is required to provide a comprehensive community mental health service. Developments are underpinned by collaboration between child and adult services to facilitate successful transition planning and programmes that result in effective engagement of young people either with adult psychiatric services or alternative services such as clinical psychology or young people's counselling services that meet their needs. Further collaboration between providers and commissioning of new services will be necessary in order to meet the gaps in provision for young adults with enduring neurodevelopmental disorders such as ADHD and autism-spectrum disorders, and to fund transition arrangements. Significant investment is needed across all four jurisdictions of the UK in order to manage the deficits in age-appropriate crisis intervention and psychiatric in-patient services for young people with mental disorders, including those with intellectual disability.

References

Department of Health (1999) *The National Service Framework for Mental Health, Modern Standards and Service Models*. Department of Health.

Department of Health & Department for Education and Skills (2004) *National Service Framework for Children, Young People and Maternity Services*. Department of Health (http://www.dh.gov.uk/en/Healthcare/Children/DH_4089111).

Kaplan, T. (2007) *Child and Adolescent Mental Health Problems in the Emergency Department and the Services to Deal with These*. Royal College of Psychiatrists.

Kelvin, R. (2005) Capacity of Tier 2/3 CAMHS and service specification: a model to enable evidence based service development. *Child and Adolescent Mental Health*, **10**, 63–73.

Lamb, C., Hall, D., Kelvin, R., *et al* (2008) *Working at the CAMHS/Adult Interface: Good Practice Guidance for the Provision of Psychiatric Services to Adolescents/Young Adults*. Royal College of Psychiatrists.

Maitra, B. & Jolley, A. (2000) Liaison between child and adult psychiatric services. In *Family Matters: Interfaces Between Child and Adult Mental Health* (eds P. Reder, M. McClure & A. Jolley), pp. 285–382. Routledge.

National Assembly for Wales (2001) *Child and Adolescent Mental Health Services: Everybody's Business*. Primary and Community Healthcare Division.

National Assembly for Wales (2005) *National Service Framework for Children, Young People and Maternity Services in Wales*. Welsh Assembly Government (http://www.wales.nhs.uk/sites3/documents/441/33519%20Main%20Doc%20Complete%20LoRes.pdf).

National Assembly for Wales (2006) *Review of Youth Homelessness. Social Justice and Regeneration Committee papers SLJ(2)-17-06*. Welsh Assembly Government.

NHS Health Advisory Service (1995) *Together We Stand: Commissioning, Role and Management of Child and Adolescent Mental Health Services*. HMSO.

Office of the Children's Commissioner for England (2007) *Pushed into the Shadows – Young People's Experience of Adult Mental Health Facilities*. OCC.

Richards, M. & Vostanis, P. (2004) Interprofessional perspectives on transitional mental health services for young people aged 16–19 years. *Journal of Interprofessional Care*, **18**, 115–128.

Royal College of Psychiatrists (2002) *Acute In-patient Psychiatric Care for Young People with Severe Mental Illness: Recommendations for Commissioners, Child and Adolescent Psychiatrists and General Psychiatrists. Council Report CR106*. Royal College of Psychiatrists.

Royal College of Psychiatrists (2006) *Building and Sustaining Specialist CAMHS. Council Report CR137*. Royal College of Psychiatrists.

Scottish Executive (2003) *Mental Health (Care and Treatment) (Scotland) Act 2003*. Scottish Executive Health Department.

Scottish Executive (2005) *The Mental Health of Children and Young People: A Framework for Promotion, Prevention and Care*. Scottish Executive.

Scottish Executive (2006) *Delivering for Mental Health: The Mental Health Delivery Plan for Scotland*. NHS Scotland.

CHAPTER 11

Referral management

Sophie Roberts and Ian Partridge

'I'm playing all the right notes, but not necessarily in the right order.'
Eric Morecambe

Introduction

In CAMHS provision, managing referrals is perhaps the one area that illustrates most clearly the failure to understand and implement the principles of the tiered model of working. If there is one type of problem that generates concern and anxiety in families, commissioners and service providers, it is the management of the demand placed upon the service and how this demand is met.

Waiting lists in CAMHS are a common cause of distress to children's families, referrers and professionals within the service, and have been shown to increase rates of non-attendance (Subotski & Berelowitz, 1990). To avoid waiting lists and to provide an efficient service, a CAMHS must have an overt prioritisation and allocation process for its referrals. The process of allocation must be based upon managerially realistic and clinically relevant principles. As discussed previously, in the future, CAMHS should move away from a system based upon referrals, to one in which tiers are interacting and mutually supporting each other in such a fashion that the notion of referral becomes redundant and working together is integral. The effective functioning of the primary mental health worker will greatly facilitate this process. In the interim, the process of referral and allocation will be the first test of the efficiency of a CAMHS.

Where GPs have access to mental health professionals of different disciplines in adult psychiatric services, they tend to refer different patient groups to each professional (O'Neill-Byrne & Browning, 1996). It is uncertain whether these specific referrals are always geared to meeting the patients' needs. Studies have shown that there is a poor level of understanding among GPs (Markantonakis & Mathai, 1990; Thompson & Place, 1995; Jones et al, 2000; Foreman, 2001) and paediatricians (Oke & Mayer, 1991) of the different roles of disciplines within a CAMHS. General practitioners identify quick access to services as a top priority for them when they refer children and families with mental health issues (Weeramanthri & Keaney, 2000).

All systems of referral management, however labelled, should be based upon the principles of working together, working efficiently and working in a fashion that is informed by the best evidentially substantiated clinical practice. It is our argument that this is most realistically achieved by the informed implementation of the principles of the tiered system, and this involves a proper prioritisation of working into and with Tier 1. There are various ways of managing demand; one can look to process it more effectively, to minimise it by defining provision clearly via need and urgency, or to increase the supply side to meet the increase in demand, but in all cases it is the overriding philosophy of the service provision that will inform such a response. In terms of resources, organisational emphasis and service development, Tier 1 should at all times be prioritised. If CAMHS is centred upon and working around Tier 1, then demand is more easily managed and other tiers will be able to function more effectively.

In the present climate, great emphasis is based upon partnership, choice and speed of response. In terms of good practice, this is nothing new.

In the area of child and adolescent mental health, intervention is not a surgical procedure based upon notions of individual pathology and management; any systemically informed intervention is by definition collaborative with the family and other involved agencies and professionals. Equally, we are aware that it is families and professionals working at Tier 1 who have the greatest involvement and understanding of their patient's situation, and as such the involvement of CAMHS can be in a great number of cases indirect. Specialist CAMHS professionals can see their role as informing, educating and supporting those best placed to intervene in a family's life – and as such their 'workload' should include supporting the workload management of those operating in Tier 1.

The question of 'choice' is more problematic in that it is now taken as a given that choice is right and proper, and health service provision is more and more seen in a consumerist framework. This creates an unrealistic position in terms of the management of demands and needs to be seriously confronted on two fronts. First, the reification of choice as a universal evidentially validated 'good'. Although in other service industries the mantra that 'the customer is always right' may hold some water, in terms of mental health this is not the case. The child and the family are not always right – in some cases they are simply wrong. At this point we should note that there is an internal contradiction between the emphasis upon 'evidence-based practice' and 'choice' should the family choose to dismiss the evidence-based course of treatment indicated. The point is that although principles of accessibility and flexibility must inform our work, we must also remain responsible and accountable for both our clinical interventions and the organisational forms they take. Second, we must be aware of, and systemically understand, the reality of choice. In an ideal world, families would not choose to be involved with CAMHS – they are involved because something has gone wrong, is causing anxiety, distress or unhappiness. Most families would choose not to have a daughter with severe anorexia, a son suffering a psychotic breakdown, a child with autism or intellectual difficulties. Their choice would be for the condition to not exist. The role of CAMHS is not cure – their first choice – but management of the difficulties and containment of the anxieties. As such, choice is by definition limited and exists upon a spectrum.

Tier 1 functions most effectively when clinicians of different disciplines and levels of seniority support it. When working effectively, intervention at Tier 1 has two results. First, both Tier 1 professionals and families have greater confidence in the nature of the service provided for them and their children, and second, we reduce the level of unnecessary and possibly damaging referrals to the more specialist tiers of CAMHS, thus freeing them up to provide a speedier and more family-friendly service. Specialist services need to define what they do, but also clearly delineate what they do not do and how they prioritise the demands upon their services.

We detail below structural issues that arise from these principles but recognise that different organisational imperatives operate and reference will be made to these.

It has been recommended that services disseminate clear referral criteria to GPs, Social Services and other referrers to help them identify and appropriately refer children and young people (National Assembly for Wales, 2005). Some services use a medicalised model of severity of mental illness as a way of achieving this (Box 11.1). It can, however, also be argued that these in fact create a barrier to young people accessing specialist CAMHS. If the tiered system is functioning effectively then it is more appropriate to encourage referrers to contact primary mental health workers (operating at Tier 1/2) to clarify the nature and severity of the mental health issue and at which tier of the comprehensive CAMHS it should be managed to see if referral to Tier 2/3 is necessary; this, of course, also shares knowledge, decreases the sense of 'ivory tower' services, and builds good community networks and relationships. It might be appropriate

---

Box 11.1 Suggested criteria for prioritisation

- Psychotic disorder
- Severe depressive disorder
- Eating disorder
- OCD
- Emotional or neurotic disorder
- Psychosomatic disorder
- The mental health problems of those involved with Social Services
- The mental health problems of those involved with education support services

for the specialist CAMHS to issue some referral guidelines describing what the specialist team does work with and how (e.g. psychosis, depression) and what other difficulties (e.g. school-based behaviour problems) other services in the authority would have a primary role in as long as this has been with the local partner agencies at a strategic level.

Allocation meetings

The first structure in managing referrals is an allocation meeting. This should be organised on a weekly basis, at least, to ensure a prompt response to referrers. Allocation should be undertaken by a member of the service who has sufficient seniority and knowledge of the service to command the trust of those to whom the work will be passed. Alternatively, there may be a small allocation team of senior members of different disciplines working in the service. Allocation is not a task for a junior member of the administrative team. Whole team seances, where the referral is moved to a member of the service by some sort of mysterious motion, are not appropriate. Neither is a 'bran tub' of a filing cabinet drawer, from which service members take the referrals of their choice an efficient way of managing young people and their families. The idea that a psychiatrist must initially assess all referrals is anachronistic, devalues the skills of other service members and generates waiting lists.

All referrals, other than emergencies, should be allocated at this meeting. The remainder of this chapter discusses the criteria that will need to be considered.

The service's priorities

The fewer the staff in a CAMHS, the more important it is they have a priority list for referrals. An example is given in Box 11.1. A very small service, after realistic discussion with commissioners and partner agencies, may inform referrers that it only has the resources to assess and manage young people with possible psychotic illnesses and eating disorders, and work with young people in and leaving care. All other referrals then have to be returned, as the service does not have the resources to address them.

Urgency

The allocation team, or a member of it, should assess the validity of an urgent referral and allocate accordingly. Referrals of young people who have taken a drug overdose or otherwise seriously harmed themselves should be rapidly processed and seen within 24 hours of being physically fit. Referrals assessed as emergencies should be dealt with immediately by whichever member of the team has time, possibly through a multidisciplinary emergency duty rota. Certain disciplines (e.g. community psychiatric nurses or junior doctors) should have time for emergencies built into their weekly timetables. Such cases may not reach the allocation meeting but must be recorded as part of the CAMHS workload.

Sector

Sectorisation facilitates close liaison with Tier 1 workers and enables the establishment of networks and relationships with particular members of CAMHS. If referrals are taken only from the primary mental health worker, if one is allocated to that sector, there is an opportunity for effective management of referrals as well as more directly effective liaison with Tier 1 services.

Clarification

Contact between the referrer and the service preceding referral is of considerable help to the allocation team. Indeed, referral may be reframed as a request for consultation. Not infrequently, clarification is required and a nominated member of the allocation team should take responsibility for this liaison function and obtain the necessary further information to facilitate appropriate allocation. The involvement of other agencies involved with young people who are referred to the service is often unclear and may require further information from the referrer to avoid duplication of work or from agencies working at cross-purposes.

Inter-agency work

A number of other agencies may be involved with a referred young person and 'ownership' should be clarified. There is the danger that with a number of professionals involved with a young person and family, confusion can arise as to where responsibility and accountability lie. Consideration and discussion with other involved agencies can minimise such danger. Allocation team members may coordinate the CAMHS involvement, or allocate the task to another member of the service. It may be necessary to organise a professionals' meeting to discuss different agency involvement, current and intended. In such circumstances, it is important to ensure efficient use of time and resources, and to clarify and agree boundaries, communication networks and appropriate roles with the professionals from the other agencies. Close liaison with other agencies, both formal and informal, can also lead to more effective use of a CAMHS and increased awareness of its service provision.

Disciplinary function

The nature of the referral may dictate referral to a specific discipline acting as an initial filter. Inter- and intra-disciplinary specialties and areas of expertise and interest should be developed and understood by the allocation team to ensure the individual tailoring of assessment processes and management strategies to meet young people's needs.

Specialist teams

A number of specialist teams may be operating at Tier 3; areas covered by these teams may include eating disorders, bereavement, autism-spectrum disorders, attention-deficit disorders, paediatric liaison, risk assessment, and family therapy. Allocation may be direct to such a team or there may be a need for an initial assessment by a professional operating at Tier 2.

Individual workloads

An individual's current workload will be at the forefront of the minds of the allocation team; this promotes team cohesion and enables support for those under pressure of work. Occasionally, 'holding operations' or alternative allocations are necessary to protect individuals with too heavy a case-load.

Training requirements

Most CAMHS act as training centres for all disciplines, and training is required in Tier 2 and Tier 3 treatment programmes. Trainees are not service providers and therefore their case-loads should be carefully monitored, but they do require young people and families to be allocated to them to gain their experience and develop their expertise.

Co-working

Many referrals require an element of joint assessment or working that does not fit within the remit of a specialist team. Such *ad hoc* Tier 3 multidisciplinary working can enable a fuller assessment as well as provide training, staff support, protection and supervision.

Re-referrals

If a young person is re-referred, consideration should be given to the benefits or otherwise of seeing the same professional again. An alternative Tier 2 professional or Tier 3 team perspective may be indicated.

Awareness of the context of referrals

Contractual obligations to commissioners, GPs and primary care organisations, as well as pressure from referrers and families, are recognised as influences upon response rates, and, at times, evaluation and management of such external anxieties will be required.

Alternative models

The Choice and Partnership Approach (CAPA), developed by Kingsbury & York (2006), is covered in Chapter 12.

Another model is the consultation and advisory (2 + 1) model of working (Heywood *et al*, 2003), which was developed on the basis of work by Street & Downey (1996) as a way of managing demand and waiting lists in the absence of a primary mental health worker structure, and in recognition of the fact that the non-attendance at first appointments was high and that the average number of appointments within specialist CAMHS was three. The model is collaborative and client/parent centred. The approach:

- is brief and focused
- reflects on the process of the referral
- elicits parents' expectations and wishes
- identifies and works with ambivalence or blame
- assesses severity and need
- negotiates clear and realistic goals for the consultation and any further therapeutic intervention
- allows families to 'opt in' and give 'informed consent' to therapy.

In summary, the first session is offered within 4 weeks of referral after the family have opted in and completed a questionnaire. The first and second sessions are within 2 weeks of each other. In the initial sessions, the aim is to develop an interactive understanding of the referral process and the problem, to understand the family's ideology of the problem and their expectations of the consultation, and to develop a needs assessment. There is then a 1–3 month gap before the third/final session. The 'consultants' may offer 'expert' opinion or practical advice if requested, self-help literature or liaison with other agencies. After the initial meetings there may be a referral to specialist CAMHS. Often this model is run as a multidisciplinary clinic with time built in for case discussion and/or peer supervision.

Conclusion

A process of allocation based upon multidisciplinary consideration and flexibility allows for the clarification of priorities, and the maximal utilisation of resources, wherein the goals of effective and speedy response and supportive team functioning are facilitated.

References

Foreman, D. M. (2001) General practitioners and child and adolescent psychiatry: awareness and training of the new commissioners. *Psychiatric Bulletin*, **25**, 101–104.

Heywood, S., Kroll, L., Stancombe, J., *et al* (2003) A brief consultation and advisory approach for use in child and adolescent mental health services: a pilot study. *Clinical Child Psychology and Psychiatry*, **8**, 503–512.

Jones, E., Lucey, C. & Wadland, L. (2000) Triage: a waiting list initiative in a child mental health service. *Psychiatric Bulletin*, **24**, 57–59.

Kingsbury, S. & York, A. (2006) *The 7 HELPFUL Habits of Effective CAMHS and the Choice and Partnership Approach: A Workbook for CAMHS*, (2nd edn). CAMHS Network.

Markantonakis, A. & Mathai, J. (1990) An evaluation of general practitioners' knowledge and satisfaction of a local child and family psychiatric service. *Psychiatric Bulletin*, **14**, 328–329.

National Assembly for Wales (2005) *National Service Framework for Children, Young People and Maternity Services in Wales*. Children's Health & Social Care Directorate, Welsh Assembly Government (http://wales.gov.uk/docs/caecd/publications/090414nsfchildrenyoungp eoplematernityen.pdf).

O'Neill-Byrne, K. & Browning, S. M. (1996) Which patients do GPs refer to which professional. *Psychiatric Bulletin*, **20**, 584–587.

Oke, S. & Mayer, R. (1991) Referrals to child psychiatry – a survey of staff attitudes. *Archives of Disease in Childhood*, **66**, 862–865.

Street, E. & Downey, J. (1996) *Brief Therapeutic Consultations: An Approach to Systemic Counselling*. Wiley.

Subotski, F. & Berelowitz, M. (1990) Consumer views at a child guidance clinic. *Newsletter of the Association for Child Psychology and Psychiatry*, **12**, 8–12.

Thompson, A. & Place, M. (1995) What influences general practitioners' use of child psychiatry services? *Psychiatric Bulletin*, **19**, 10–12.

Weeramanthri, T. & Keaney, F. (2000) What do inner city general practitioners want from a child and adolescent mental health service? *Psychiatric Bulletin*, **24**, 258–260.

CHAPTER 12

Demand and capacity management

Ann York and Steve Kingsbury

'Do the right thing. It will gratify some people and astonish the rest.'
    Mark Twain

Introduction

The English NSF for children, young people and maternity services emphasises that CAMHS must be evidence-based, needs-led, accessible at the right time and working in partnership with children and their families to make decisions about their care (Department for Education and Skills & Department of Health, 2004). Services need to be prompt, personalised, give greater choice, be well coordinated, equally available to all, able to involve people in decisions about their care, and achieve good outcomes. Similar guidance in the other parts of the UK emphasise these service qualities.

Any service model must take into account the needs and wants of the individual and the reality of the capabilities and capacity of the service (Warner & Williams, 2005). Contact with families must involve the shared understanding of all these factors in deciding together what the plan for action should be. Isolated attempts to improve the quality of referrals, prioritise or select better, or change how services respond to demand do not usually make a long-lasting impact on the whole system (Williams *et al*, 2005). Box 12.1 summarises the frequent effects of some common service designs.

All clinical, administrative and managerial staff, and their commissioners and partner agencies, want to provide services that work for young people and their families. However, many CAMHS feel overwhelmed with what can seem a relentless workload. Child and adolescent mental health services commonly feel that if they had more time, money and staff, they could manage.

Although to some extent this may be so, there are many things that can be done to increase efficiency and effectiveness as well as to improve patient flow within existing resources. Applying demand and capacity analysis skills allows services to make the best use of what they have and to demonstrate what they may need more of. These techniques are not specific to CAMHS – the principles apply equally to car manufacturing, queuing in a supermarket and physical health services (e.g. Spear, 2004).

Box 12.1 Common strategies to cope with demand

Raising threshold of severity of disorder or complexity for acceptance into the service
- Referrers quickly realise how to 'throw over the bar' (e.g. by mentioning symptoms that indicate urgency).

Requesting more and more information to determine eligibility for service
- Families generally wait in limbo while the service tries to find out extra details such as the school's view of the child. Such processes create unacceptable delays in deciding whether a family will be accepted into the service.

Classic triage
- Assesses for eligibility and urgency and then places family at some priority level on a waiting list.
- Urgent cases are seen but all others usually face an unacceptable wait, in limbo, some receiving no intervention.

2 + 1
- The family is assessed and offered two sessions of brief intervention. This package is often offered to those who appear from the referral letter to be suitable for a brief intervention.
- The system works well for some families, with good user feedback as families are seen quickly. However, those that need more than three sessions or turn out to be not suitable for a brief intervention at assessment are usually placed on a waiting list for further help.

Demand and capacity management does not mean working harder, just better. Demand and capacity analysis does not undermine quality but allows a clearer focus on it. The major gains of quality and effectiveness are maximised by streamlining processes, and the capacity of the service can be calculated so that choices can be made to expand capacity to meet demand or to restrict demand to fit capacity.

Streamlining processes

Any CAMHS tier must be organised as efficiently as possible to maximise capacity. Imbalance between demand and capacity leads to waiting lists (or 'queues') and a common assumption is that increasing resources will reduce waiting lists. However, many queues are due to problems in patient 'flow' and increasing resources will not necessarily increase flow if a bottleneck is not dealt with. Variation in processes (i.e. how we do things) has been shown to have more impact on flow than natural variation such as patient or staff characteristics. Audits have shown that waiting list durations can be four times more to do with how a service deploys its resources (i.e. how many clinical sessions per referral) than how many referrals it receives (York & Kingsbury, 2009).

105

There are several processes that can help maximise capacity, with beneficial effects on waiting times without increased workload.

Process mapping

Process mapping involves analysing the steps a patient, with their help if at all possible, takes from referral to discharge, or for different parts of their journey such as only from referral to first appointment. The amount of time the steps take is described as the task time. Process mapping is traditionally done by taking a large piece of lining paper, lots of Post-it Notes and mapping out the steps, incorporating timescales and duplicating processes. Good ideas for improvement can be added to the 'diagram' using the Post-it Notes. It is especially helpful to process map at places in the journey that involve waits (bottlenecks). This can help identify whether the cause is a true lack of capacity (see below) or inefficient processes.

Process mapping can be very revealing of how many tasks happen because 'we always do it this way'. Usually these 'custom and practice' assumptions result in increased waiting times. Creating new processes requires discarding 'what ought to be' and prioritising 'what we and the patient would like'.

Demand

This is the amount of time it takes to process a referral from start to finish. To calculate existing demand: the requests for the service is equal to the number of referrals accepted multiplied by the amount of time a case 'consumes'. It is important to realise that the time a case 'consumes' is the same as the time offered by the clinician (i.e. demand is created in the interaction between the family and the therapist). Demand therefore varies according to what a patient 'receives'. For example a referral to a psychotherapy service may mean a demand for 50–100 hours of clinical time, whereas a referral to a brief therapy service may mean a demand for 3–4 hours of clinical time. A service that actively uses the child and family's own skills and resources may reduce their contact duration by even as little as one session, releasing capacity and effectively reducing their 'demand'.

Capacity

Capacity is the amount of clinical time available to meet demand. 'Skill' capacity is that which is available from clinicians for clinical work, whereas 'kit' capacity relates to equipment (e.g. psychometric testing tools) or space (e.g. the availability of rooms). The limiting factor is the smallest of these things. In some services, staff time is available but limitation on room bookings restricts what can be provided.

Bottlenecks

Bottlenecks impair the smooth flow of the patient on their 'journey'. It can be spotted by a 'queue' in front of it (i.e. a waiting list). Bottlenecks may be functional (e.g. due to inefficient processes) or skill based (e.g. due to lack of clinical time). In situations where there is low demand, a potential bottleneck may be masked. For example, there may be long waits for assessments, but if that was resolved then long waits for therapies may be uncovered.

In CAMHS, the most obvious bottleneck is the waiting list into the service, or for specific types of assessments or treatments. A waiting list of a constant size means that there was a demand and capacity imbalance in the recent past. In other words, the service is in balance now but wasn't then. A lengthening waiting list means there is a current imbalance. Uncovered maternity or sick leave is a common example: this may add roughly 50 patients per year to the waiting list. This bulge may remain constant until that staff member returns.

A common cause of a clinical skill bottleneck is an internal referral to a specialist skill. In these instances it's likely that there are no extended core clinical skills ahead of the bottleneck. For example, all referrals to CBT may go on a waiting list for a clinical psychologist with diploma-level CBT skills with no one else in the team viewed as capable in core-level CBT. So one solution to the bottleneck is to develop within the team some extended core skills in CBT (not confined to one profession) and reserve the diploma-level CBT for those that need it. Bottleneck fixed.

National targets for first appointments have resulted in many CAMHS moving to an early assessment or triage model. However, unless this incorporates a whole-system approach to demand and capacity-based service redesign, many services find they develop a different bottleneck – a treatment waiting list.

Carve out and segmentation

Carve out occurs when a certain amount of capacity is reserved for a specific purpose. It ensures good provision for those who can access the carved-out capacity but is inefficient for the service as a whole. For example, bus lanes are great for buses in rush hour when demand is high for the road capacity. However, car drivers have to wait longer as they have less road capacity available. When the road is fairly empty, the bus lane makes no difference to flow of either cars or buses. A rough rule of thumb is that if a specific portion of capacity is under-utilised then this may be a carve-out, resulting in an inefficient use of capacity. A CAMHS example could be new patient slots only reserved for priorities/emergencies, unless the capacity exactly matches the demand so that all slots are used.

In contrast, segmentation is effective in providing streamlined provision for many patients. Segmentation occurs when those with similar needs and so with similar, predictable pathways, are grouped together. An example is swimming pool lanes reserved for slow, medium and fast swimmers. In CAMHS, a medication review clinic may group patients with similar process and skill needs (psychiatry or nursing, growth monitoring, side-effect monitoring). Other needs (e.g. for parent skills training) may be best met at a different time in the service, with a patient group who may not be on medication. Segmenting according to processes, rather than diagnoses is useful. Attention-deficit hyperactivity disorder is often managed in a clinic where multiple needs and skills are needed. Segmentation may be more efficient, holding a medication review clinic and attending to other needs alongside families who need similar processes (e.g. parenting skills groups).

A whole-system approach

The 7 HELPFUL Habits of Effective CAMHS (Box 12.2; York & Kingsbury, 2009) incorporate demand and capacity theory with practical ideas for service redesign, providing a broad framework for service improvement and delivery that incorporates most of the ten high-impact changes for service improvement and delivery (NHS Modernisation Agency, 2004; Care Services Improvement Partnership, 2006). Within the seven HELPFUL habits sits a clinical system, the Choice and Partnership Approach (CAPA). The CAPA helps services to do the right things with the right people at the right time. The stance is collaborative, ensuring informed consent and choice, and incorporates care planning and evidence-based practice. It is flexible for families and clinicians. It allows services to be clear about what they do and how much they do as a team and as individuals.

Together, CAPA and *The 7 HELPFUL Habits* provide a practical framework for services to develop to meet the agendas for *Our Choices in Mental Health* (Care Services Improvement Partnership, 2005), healthcare standards (Department of Health, 2004), New Ways of Working (Royal College of Psychiatrists & National Institute of Mental Health England, 2005), and *You're Welcome* standards (Department of Health, 2007).

Box 12.2 The seven HELPFUL habits

- Handle demand
- Extend capacity
- Let go of families
- Process map and redesign
- Flow management
- Use care bundles
- Look after staff

Reproduced from York & Kinsbury, 2009

Each habit has sub-items of changes that will help with that area. In total, there are 35 items covering areas such as having a service-level agreement, extending clinical skills, and roles and appraisal. They are not meant to be prescriptive, but a menu of ingredients to work from. There is an emphasis on services developing a culture of curiosity about their practice, self-enquiry and confidence about change.

The strength of the habits seems to be their clarity, practicality, and applicability to CAMHS and validation in clinical services (York & Kingsbury, 2009). They have been written up as a practical workbook, alongside a description of how to implement CAPA (York & Kingsbury, 2009). *The 7 HELPFUL Habits* is supported by a service development questionnaire, which CAMHS can use to self-review. A website, www. camhsnetwork.co.uk, provides additional information, including about team job planning and capacity calculation.

The CAPA puts into practice many of the seven HELPFUL habits. It is user-focused, satisfying for clinicians to work in, and sits well with the evidence of factors that improve outcomes for children with mental health problems. It has three key stages.

1   Choice appointments as initial contacts: the family books a choice appointment at a time and venue to suit them. The appointment focuses on what they want to change, choice about how to think about the problem and whether they need and want any help, and what type of intervention would be best. It combines assessment, facilitation of informed choice and motivational enhancement in a strengths-based approach. The professional stance is to facilitate client choice informed by clinical expertise. It involves the clear discussion and agreement of a joint understanding leading to an intervention plan, using a care-planning approach.

2   Core partnership work: the aim is to link from the choice goals and to build on the work the family have done between choice and partnership ('pre-partnership work'). This intervention may include further assessment. It relies on families being active agents in their own change. This is an especially important experience for those families and young people who have previously felt unengaged by service contact. Clinicians will be using extended core clinical skills such as working in a systemic framework or with threshold CBT techniques.

3   Specialist or specific partnership work (if necessary): this is clinical work that is specifically reserved in individual clinicians' job plans. It is often using higher level skills in a specific methodology (e.g. diploma-level CBT for depression or systemic therapy using a screen and a reflecting team). This work is supported by extended core clinical skills of the same therapy type to avoid internal waiting lists (bottlenecks).

The CAPA is enhanced by careful team job planning that ensures clarification of the nature of core work by clinicians with extended clinical skills and specialist work and this being incorporated into individual job plans. This enables best use (and protection) of specialist and core skills, and easy calculation of capacity for new and intervention work in a service. There are ten key components (Box 12.3) and CAPA is most effective when all are in place.

Box 12.3 Ten key components of CAPA

Choice
1 Language change, moving away from the passivity of 'assessment' and 'treatment'
2 Full booking to choice (i.e. does not go on a waiting list)
3 Choice framework to all contacts (CHOICE: being Curious, using our Honest Opinion, seeking their Informed Consent and encouraging their Engagement)
4 Care planning and goals

Partnership
5 Selecting a clinician with the right clinical skills that match the family goals for partnership
6 Full booking to partnership (i.e. does not go on a waiting list)
7 Extended core and specialist skills in team

Service factors
8 Individual and team job planning completed
9 Regular multidisciplinary peer-group discussion
10 Team away days – at least quarterly

Conclusion

Demand and capacity analysis can help services redesign themselves to work better for both users and staff. Whole-system approaches based on the care pathway, the patient experience and the systemic functioning of the service (such as CAPA) avoid only improving part of the service for some children and families. More information can be found in Box 12.4.

References

Care Services Improvement Partnership (2005) *Our Choices in Mental Health*. CSIP (http://www.csip.org.uk).

Care Services Improvement Partnership (2006) *10 High Impact Changes for Mental Health Services* (http://www.csip.org.uk).

Department for Education and Skills & Department of Health (2004) *National Service Framework for Children, Young People and Maternity Services*. Department of Health (http://www.dh.gov.uk/en/Healthcare/Children/DH_108).

Department of Health (2004) *Standards for Better Health*. Department of Health Publications.

Box 12.4 Demand and capacity resources available on the internet

- Institute of Healthcare Improvement (www.ihi.org): not-for-profit organisation in Boston. Dynamic website with lots of ideas and case studies.
- *10 High Impact Changes* (Care Services Improvement Partnership, 2006) and leadership improvement guides (e.g. Pursuing Perfection; www.ihi.org/IHI/Programs/StrategicInitiatives/PursuingPerfection.htm).
- Knowledge Community for the National Institute for Mental Health (http://kc.nimhe.org.uk): lots of information on service development, including CAMHS. Primarily of relevance in England but this site is worth a look at wherever you are based.
- Participation Works (www.participationworks.org.uk) provides a portal to resources on children and young people's participation. It provides an extensive hub of relevant resources, which is indispensable to busy CAMHS workers.
- CAMHS Network (www.camhsnetwork.co.uk): information about the seven HELPFUL habits, CAPA, service improvement in CAMHS and online community forums.
- National CAMHS Support Service (NCSS) for England (www.camhs.org.uk).
- Improving patient flow (http://www.steyn.org.uk): computer models to illustrate demand and capacity principles. Allows you to change factors and see what the effect is.

Department of Health (2007) *You're Welcome Quality Criteria: Making Health Services Young People Friendly*. Department of Health Publications.

NHS Modernisation Agency (2004) Improvement leader guides. NHS Institute for Innovation and Improvement (http://www.institute.nhs.uk/building_capability/building_improvement_capability/improvement_leaders%27_guides%3a_introduction.html).

Royal College of Psychiatrists & National Institute of Mental Health England (2005) *New Ways of Working for Psychiatrists: Enhancing Effective, Person-Centred Services Through New Ways of Working in Multidisciplinary and Multi-agency Contexts*. Department of Health (http://www.dh.gov.uk/prod_consum_dh/groups/dh_digitalassets/@dh/@en/documents/digitalasset/dh_4122343.pdf).

Spear, J. S. (2004) Learning to lead at Toyota. *Harvard Business Review*, **82**, 78–86 (http://www.ihi.org/IHI/Topics/Improvement/ImprovementMethods/Literature/LearningtoleadatToyota.htm).

Warner, M. & Williams, R. (2005) The nature of strategy and its application in statutory and non-statutory services. In *Child and Adolescent Mental Health Services: Strategy, Planning, Delivery, and Evaluation* (eds R. Williams & M. Kerfoot), pp. 39–62. Oxford University Press.

Williams, R., Rawlinson, S., Davies, O. & Barber, W. (2005) Demand for and use of public sector child and adolescent mental health services. In *Child and Adolescent Mental Health Services: Strategy, Planning, Delivery and Evaluation* (eds R. Williams & M. Kerfoot), pp. 445–469. Oxford University Press.

York, A. & Kingsbury, S. (2009) *The Choice and Partnership Approach: A Guide to CAPA*. CAMHS Network.

CHAPTER 13

Strategies for working with Tier 1

Greg Richardson, Ashley Wyatt and Ian Partridge

'In the beginning was the word and that word may well have been anxiety.'
Jules Masserman

Introduction

Mental health problems in children are best understood as being affected by and presenting in the children's constitutional functioning and in all areas of their interaction with their environment. Parents, families and teachers have a major role to play in the maintenance of mental health. Professionals such as childminders, teachers, school nurses, educational psychologists, social workers, GPs and health visitors make a substantial contribution to the promotion and maintenance of the mental health of children if they come in contact with them. They also play a role in the early identification of mental health problems, children's vulnerability thereto and in the management of those mental health problems once identified. However, Tier 1 professionals often feel at a loss as to how to manage children's mental health problems and all the emotional baggage that goes with them.

Mental health professionals, who provide a small part of the mental healthcare of children, classify the more serious mental health problems as mental disorders (World Health Organization, 1992). These disorders represent a small proportion of mental health problems produced by constitutional, family, educational, social and environmental factors, illness or developmental delay, all of which may impair future psychological functioning.

The epidemiological evidence is that mental disorders affect about 10% of children (Ford *et al*, 2003), although estimates range from 10 to 20% (Fombonne, 2002). If all those children were referred to CAMHS, the service would be overwhelmed. Child and adolescent mental health services see only about 20% of these children. The alternative of providing support to Tier 1 professionals from primary mental health workers, or other CAMHS professionals ensures:

- children with mental health problems, and their families, are dealt with by those with whom they already have a relationship;
- more children than could be seen by individual mental health professionals have the benefit of mental health expertise;

- increased confidence and expertise among Tier 1 professionals dealing directly with young people and their families (Richardson & Partridge, 2000).

The Audit Commission (1999) review of CAMHS in England and Wales demonstrated that child and adolescent mental health professionals at that time spent 1% of their time supporting Tier 1, which was a worrying finding as 80–90% of children and young people with a recognisable health problem were never seen by child and adolescent mental health professionals (Offord, 1987; Cox, 1993), and those that were seen were not necessarily the most needy (Offord, 1982). The Audit Commission review also showed that where primary mental health workers are in place, referrals to Tiers 2, 3 and 4 are reduced. Although this 1% figure will have increased since 1999, the proportion of time devoted to supporting Tier 1 is still small for most CAMHS. If parents are asked how they would feel if their child was referred to a CAMHS, the feelings of being blamed, stigmatised, incompetent, bewildered and frightened often outweigh those of relief or feeling the problem is being taken seriously. The referral process has therefore seriously assaulted their mental health and self-esteem, even if it was poor prior to referral, although, generally, mental health professionals are aware of the vulnerability of referred families. The input of Tier 1 professionals may therefore be considerably more helpful to the mental health of a young person and family than referral into Tier 2 or 3.

Tier 1 professionals are those who, by virtue of their job, have regular daily contact with children with whom they work directly, and therefore impinge to a greater or lesser extent on their mental health in the normal course of the children's lives, and may have a profound effect on children's psychological development. These professionals in turn decide when it is necessary to involve professionals from Tier 2 or 3.

Working with Tier 1 professionals is therefore the major priority for CAMHS if they are to lay any claim to meeting the needs of the majority of young people with mental health problems and to do effective preventive work. Such work requires considerable thought and planning. The expectations, understandings, beliefs and sophistication of those working at Tier 1 are varied. Basic lessons about 'incurability', allied to the need for management of certain disorders to be the responsibility of all involved in the care of young people, need to be owned and understood by all those working at Tier 1 to avoid unrealistic demands and expectations.

The increased emphasis given to the consultation and training role of CAMHS is a key theme of both *Every Child Matters* (Department for Children, Schools and Families, 2003) and Standard 9 of the children's NSF (Department of Health, 2004). Both stress that mental health is 'everybody's business' – with the explicit assumption that all children's services staff across all agencies should have access to both training and consultation from other staff who have more expertise in such matters. This is clearly a longer-term aim, but does provide a challenge to every local CAMHS along with all the competing demands such as delivering on waiting time targets.

Challenges to effective working with Tier 1

Referral system and other perverse incentives

There is a tendency for Tier 1 workers to seek referral of children to specialist agencies when they develop a concern regarding mental health problems. The tendency arises because they undervalue both their own relationships with the families and their abilities in the management of the difficulties being presented. The problem of Tier 1 professionals feeling deskilled or disempowered is one for which CAMHS professionals must take a degree of responsibility. A common understanding of terms such as 'mental health problem', 'a child in need' or 'emotional and behavioural difficulties' is necessary across all agencies, so that each takes their part in trying to restore the well-being of the child.

Mental health has always been an issue for all agencies who deal with children, and this has recently been given a higher priority through *Every Child Matters* (Department for Children, Schools and Families, 2003). Without accessible support and a shared language, the needs of the individual child can get lost in the process of institutional dialogue and discord. This will produce a fragmented and compartmentalised approach to mental health, and the application of a simplistic model of linear causality and problem-solving, in which children's mental health problems can be seen and 'treated' in a vacuum by specialists offering a 'cure'. Child mental health should not be regarded as a curative science but rather as offering more or less helpful advice and management in liaison with those involved with the developing child, be they parents or other professionals. The common factor behind all referrals to CAMHS is the anxiety of the referrer. If this is understood and addressed, it is more likely that confidence will be given to the referrer and hence to the person who is engendering anxiety. Referrals to other agencies or personnel relieve anxiety but also absolve responsibility, and can mean a loss of skills delivered to the child, the loss of a relationship, and the stigmatising of the child. Referral may, none the less, be an appropriate response to the anxiety, but discussion is required beforehand to determine whether this is so.

Ignorance of the involvement of other agencies

The referral system encourages children to be moved within agencies as well as across them, but lack of liaison often leads to an ignorance of such involvement. General practitioners may not be aware that education support services or Social Services are involved with the child, whom they have referred on to a health-based CAMHS. The agencies may then be working in ignorance of each other's input, and so confusing the family, possibly contradicting each other and multiplying resource use.

The future development of ContactPoint (Department for Children, Schools and Families, 2009), through which it is intended that agencies will access information about other agencies involvement, as well as the Common Assessment Framework (Department for Children, Schools and Families, 2008) will in theory address these difficulties. The Common Assessment Framework in particular may assist the decision being made as to whether local CAMHS either provide consultation to professionals already involved, or agree to a referral.

Resources

The development of the consultation model raises an extra dimension in terms of allocating the resource of a CAMHS. First, the proportions to be allocated to direct service provision and to the training of and consultation to others has to be agreed (between commissioners and providers). Second, a realistic spread of consultation has to be agreed within the overall resources allocated to this task: should most resources be directed towards providing consultation to targeted services (e.g. looked-after services, substance misuse services, youth offending services) or should resources be directed towards the support of universal services (e.g. in schools and early years settings)? Each locality will have to make decisions in the light of local circumstances.

If consultation is to be delivered successfully, there must be explicit agreement with the managements of the services to which consultation is provided. All of this takes up often scarce management resources within the CAMHS.

Effectiveness of interventions

Management strategies are to a limited extent guided by national bodies such as NICE, but many interventions have a limited evidence base. It is therefore the responsibility of each service to audit and develop in response to evidence of efficacy rather than due to ideology or personal preference on behalf of members of CAMHS or other professionals. It is an important principle of inter-agency work that expectations are both clarified and evaluated. Consultative and liaison interventions with Tier 1 professionals need to be subjected to the same critical scrutiny that is given to clinical interventions. Ways of achieving this are being developed by the CORC (Ford et al, 2006) building on small-scale local initiatives.

Stigma of mental health

The general public view is still that the local CAMHS is the place where 'nutters' go, and where families are told it is their fault that their children have difficulties. Mental health remains tainted with 'madness' to pupils, families and teachers. Overcoming such stigma will have to precede effective mental health work and little progress is being made (Yamey, 1999).

These are complex and emotionally difficult issues, which must be confronted if children's mental health problems are to be addressed in the situations in which they arise. It is erroneous to assume that referral to CAMHS will solve all problems. Traditional 'medical' referral pathways provide security for those bewildered and made anxious by the children, young people and families with whom they have to deal. Ultimately, the only reason that referrals are made to a CAMHS is the existence of anxiety on somebody's part – be it the child, family or professional – and the belief that 'something must be done'. Those trying to break down institutionalised referral pathways often find themselves at the receiving end of Tier 1 professionals' frustrations, and are perceived as instituting blocking strategies and failing to meet the legitimate needs of their clients, whereas they are in fact ensuring that children are not stigmatised unnecessarily and that resources are effectively allocated to those in most need.

Mental health or emotional well-being

Closer working with Tier 1 services raises issues of differing 'languages'. With the development of the Healthy Schools initiative (Department for Education and Skills, 1999; Department for Children, Schools and Families & Department of Health, 2009), terms such as 'emotional well-being', the development of self-esteem, and the importance of the concept of 'resilience' mean that there is much scope for mutual misunderstanding concerning the relative roles of professionals in those different services. A specific example concerns the use of the terms 'conduct disorder' and 'challenging behaviour'. Do these terms mean the same thing? Are they being applied to the same group of children? Does education deal with the latter and CAMHS with the former?

Initiatives in Tier 1 working

Methods of practice outside clinics are described by Nicol (2002). Considerable liaison work needs to be done at Tier 1 to prevent these initiatives merely becoming elaborate referral routes into CAMHS, but if successfully achieved it may move Tier 1 support to the forefront of CAMHS. When working with other agencies, information sharing will raise issues about confidentiality, which will need to be addressed in order that all agencies are aware of each other's involvement with young people. Inter-agency information-sharing protocols are already being developed in local settings, and these will need to take into account the specific information-sharing issues raised by inter-agency working.

Primary mental health workers

The role of the primary mental health worker was suggested in *Together We Stand* (NHS Health Advisory Service, 1995). This worker is a professional from CAMHS who develops relationships in a particular locality and empowers Tier 1 professionals in their work with the mental health of children with the aims listed in Box 13.1.

Over the past 8 years there has been a steady expansion of primary mental health worker posts described in work commissioned by the Department of Health (Hickey *et al*, 2007). This is a carefully undertaken observational study of the progress that has been made in this area over the past few years, by identifying how many primary mental health workers are operating in England and surveying them regarding their roles, with particular reference to the markers of job satisfaction in the role. Primary mental health workers generally have one of three bases:

- primary care-based services including those based in educational or social care settings as well as GP services;

Box 13.1 Aims for a primary mental health worker

- Ensure that all who work directly with children and families have access to information about mental health services, advice, support and training for the mental health aspects of that role and understand the working of their local CAMHS
- Ensure that professionals who support children and families, from statutory and non-statutory agencies, work closely together in a coordinated way
- Ensure greater benefit for those receiving services (this can be achieved through multi-agency assessment of need, case management, multi-agency information systems, cross-agency supervision and joint study days or exchanges)
- Ensure young people and families within the locality are fully aware of the support and services available to them (e.g. by collecting information on local services and ensuring it is readily available in schools)
- Ensure that services promote the development of positive emotional and mental health, both as a product of the way they are organised (their process) and through the specific direct initiatives targeted at this goal (their content), using methods such as joint initiatives with voluntary organisations, working with schools, working with health promotion services, developing parent advice services, working with health visitors, working with school nurses and reviewing referral processes
- Ensure that young people, their families and carers are routinely and systematically involved by agencies and can express their views on current services and their development, through discussion with users and Tier 1 staff, and inform families about the processes that are happening to them
- Ensure referrals to CAMHS are necessary to meet the child's and family's mental health needs
- Discuss potential referrals with Tier 1 workers
- Effectively prioritise cases requiring intervention through community knowledge
- Ensure referrers are kept in contact with the progress made by families involved with CAMHS

- independent services separate from CAMHS and other CAMHS and child care agencies;
- CAMHS-based primary mental health workers.

This provides a useful way of understanding how these posts have developed and may well reflect the different funding streams that have come into CAMHS over recent years and the cooperation between health commissioners, providers and Local Authorities in different localities. It is reassuring that 'many had reached a senior level within their original discipline' (Hickey *et al*, 2007), as the job of a primary mental health worker requires sophisticated understanding of mental health development and interpersonal interaction.

Primary mental health workers are seen by some authorities as cheap 'quick fixes' for the ailments of CAMHS. They are not. To function effectively they must have limited catchment areas (maximum 50 000 total population) if they are to develop useful and trusting relationships and networks. The catchment area may be demarcated as the area served by a secondary school with its feeders, or a mental health or Social Service sector, or the combined catchment area of a group of general practices. School catchment areas seem the most natural localities for children and young people.

Primary mental health workers must be experienced and skilful mental health professionals who command the respect of all Tier 1 professionals in their patch, from GPs to head teachers to service managers in Social Services. They must have good administrative support, so that they can communicate quickly with those with whom they work. They must be closely connected with the local CAMHS, possibly by involvement in one of the CAMHS Tier 3 teams, or by grouping primary mental health workers into teams to avoid isolation and to ensure continuing skill development. The local CAMHS must give priority to referrals from primary mental health workers, as they provide the referral conduit into CAMHS from their locality and they are employed for their judgement on such matters. Equally, they must not be bypassed by the community CAMHS taking direct referrals from 'preferred' professionals. Those with whom they work will then see primary mental health workers as effective.

Tier 1 specialisation

Tier 1 specialisation recognises that certain staff such as health visitors and school nurses already perform a considerable amount of mental health work and with appropriate supplementary training and supervision could take on work that might otherwise be referred to CAMHS. School nurses and health visitors find they are dealing with children's psychological problems but often consider themselves ill-trained to do so. Training and consultation allow them to fulfil that function more effectively and confidently; these workers may then feel able to provide a within-school or surgery service (Richardson & Partridge, 2000). Recent initiatives have resulted in wide-ranging reviews of the role of school nurses and health visitors (Adams, 2007) in relation to emotional health. These are likely to lead to increased calls for support to these groups from CAMHS. In some parts of the country, either or both groups play a key role in screening referrals to CAMHS, and the need to support them in this role is therefore paramount.

With the new GP contract (Department of Health, 2009), some GPs are developing a special interest in child and adolescent mental health. Similarly, there has also been an initiative by the Royal College of Paediatrics and Child Health (2006) to develop a training specialism in mental health. However, there still remain stigmatisation issues for children who choose to go to see these professionals, especially if they are known to have taken on this mental health role.

Consultation

The varieties of mental health consultation are described by Nicol (2002). However, they often seem unappreciated by those devoted to the referral system. Consultation is a primary tool in the mental health professional's armoury and requires certain principles to be effective.

- Clarify the aims of the consultation.
- Clarify the constraints on the consultation.
- Clarify the areas in which consulters feel their strengths and the strengths of their service lie.
- Clarify the areas in which the consulters feel deficient or bad about their service.
- Clarify who has the problem.
- Clarify what are the intended benefits for the young person and family from the consultation.
- Identify who else is involved with the child and family.
- Explain that problems are managed, not cured.
- Clarify where the responsibility for change lies.
- Encourage change in functioning rather than diagnosing dysfunction.

It is difficult to measure change in target children or families who are consulted about, but it is possible to assess change in Tier 1 professionals' confidence in dealing with situations involving a young person's mental health. The value of the consultation process, for example through the use of questionnaires and analogue scales developed with the consultees has been assessed (Richardson & Partridge, 2000; Wyatt & Richardson, 2006 (details available on request from the author)). This has now been developed by CORC (see www.corc.uk.net). Effective consultation cannot be undertaken without the development of relationships, or the whole exercise becomes a responsibility shifting sham. Consultation cannot be done by computer. In order to coordinate community services and prevent stigmatising referral to mental health services, it may be possible to reach a stage whereby there is no referral into CAMHS without prior consultation. This will ensure that interventions at the Tier 1 level can be suggested and the concerns of the referrer discussed and addressed.

A range of other services are now also making requests to CAMHS to provide them with consultation: these include early years services, with the development of national rollout of children's centres, integrated youth support services, youth offending teams, substance misuse services, and young carers services. A local CAMHS has to make decisions as to the extent of consultation it will provide, how consultation relates to referral pathways, and whether CAMHS clinicians have the required skills to provide consultation in these more specialised settings. Local CAMHS will need to take decisions as to whether one CAMHS professional will provide consultation to a range of different services in one geographical area, or whether this will be undertaken on the basis of the type of service receiving the consultation (i.e. whether to 'split' on a geographical or functional basis). The more important the role of consultation becomes, the more the question will need to be asked as to whether all CAMHS clinicians now have to be able to provide consultation and/or training as part of their overall skill set. Again, local partnerships need to decide whether this consultation role is primarily to be delivered by primary mental health workers or should be developed by most of its CAMHS workforce. This will be partly determined by the views of other services that contribute to the CAMHS partnership group. The provision of consultation to another service is linked to the provision of training to that service. Many CAMHS now have distinct training projects that provide a range of multidisciplinary training on emotional and mental health. It is the messages coming from the provision of consultation that can often determine the priorities for training.

There will need to be congruent supervision and management across agencies, so that locality workers are not given conflicting instructions on how to manage their workload in terms of the differing priorities of differing agencies. Agreements for the provision of consultation need to be explicit as to the relative roles of the CAMHS professional providing the consultation, and the line manager of the staff member in that particular children's service. This should include protocols around communication between the consultant and the line manager. These arrangements will need to be congruent with other arrangements in place concerning case management and assessment (e.g. the Common Assessment Framework and the role of the lead professional).

Information distribution

The Royal College of Psychiatrists and patient support groups publish management guidelines for a range of conditions. Information is also available on the internet, but this is often conflicting and variable in quality. Local CAMHS may therefore consider it worthwhile to publish guidelines on the management of common mental health problems for Tier 1 professionals, as well as letting them know the sorts of problems for which there are effective interventions.

Liaison to schools

Until relatively recently, the emphasis given to literacy and numeracy, and to league tables, had resulted in the neglect of the emotional and social aspects of education. The fact that schooling affects all areas of children's functioning, including their mental health, seems now to be generally accepted and the important positive factors required to make a school effective recognised (Mortimore, 1995). Teachers are second only to parents and families in affecting children's mental health for good or ill. However, most teachers are unconscious of their role as mental health workers. For the past 30 years 'in marking work, assessing personality, streaming, setting and selection [teachers]... are determining the whole future of the child, not only his success in school' (Shipman, 1968). As a result, 'the teacher may be subject to impossible demands, being required to ensure success regardless of ability, and having his ability as a teacher criticised on non-educational grounds' (Shipman, 1968). Supporting teachers as mental health workers is a core task for CAMHS enabling them to 'bridge the divide between cognitive and social development' (Dunn, 1996) in the interests of the mental health of pupils.

A major step forward in determining which factors improve a school's effect on young people's mental health was the publication of *Fifteen Thousand Hours* (Rutter *et al*, 1979), which clarified what made a good school. The fact that schooling affects all areas of children's functioning, including their mental health, seems now to be generally accepted and is helpfully explained in books for the lay public (e.g. Skynner & Cleese, 1994), as well as in publications directed at teachers (e.g. YoungMinds, 1996). The important positive factors required to make a school effective have been described (Mortimore, 1995). However, the place of mental health work in school is apparently unrecognised.

With the current emphasis on integration, the pressure on teachers to deal with children with special educational needs in large classes is increasing. Techniques for dealing with children with emotional and behavioural difficulties in the classroom have been described (Howlin, 2002), but there are considerable barriers to implementing them. In an educational system in which academic prowess and the results of standard assessment tasks are the gold standard, teachers, understandably, are not well motivated or able to put extra effort into dealing with difficult and often unrewarding children, especially if the outcomes of such interventions show up in years rather than hours. The result is often the 'Pontius Pilate' quotation: 'We have procedures in school for dealing with misbehaviour, yet X desperately needs the sort of help that we cannot provide.' The more honest (and legitimate) response is: 'X is beyond our understanding and control, and we are desperate to be supported in helping him with his difficulties or we shall exclude him.' Non-stigmatising interventions based on current teacher–pupil and teacher–parent relationships arise from their confidence that they have appropriate and accessible support. School nurses are often drawn into these issues in school and appear to gain confidence in their mental health role if they are provided with regular consultation (Richardson & Partridge, 2000). Schools play a major part in developing the mental well-being on which their pupil's adult psychological functioning will be based. Child and adolescent mental health professionals have an obligation to support, not displace, teachers in that work, but considerable work needs to be done before teachers view CAMHS professionals as supportive colleagues rather than psychic wizards or work-shy cranks.

The publication of *Promoting Emotional Health and Well-being Through the National Healthy School Standard* (Department of Health & Department for Education and Skills, 2004) marked the beginning of a somewhat frenetic period of developments concerning emotional health in relation to schools. A key strand of Healthy Schools is 'emotional health' and this led to a range of emotional health initiatives that have recently been developed.

The SEAL initiative (Department for Education and Skills, 2005) has resulted in significant levels of training being delivered to primary-school staff and, from 2007, to high-school staff as well. Other initiatives such as Second Step (Larsen & Samdal, 2007) have also addressed specific aspects of emotional health in schools (e.g. conflict resolution). In addition, it is in school settings that the blurring of a distinction between consultation and referral has begun to occur. The development of behavioural and educational support teams (Halsey *et al*, 2005) has led to CAMHS staff being employed within multidisciplinary school-based teams. They have undertaken a mixture of consultation to other members of the team, consultation and training to the wider school staff team, as well as some direct service provision to children and their families. The position has been further developed by the creation of a range of new types of staff who take on emotional health-promoting tasks in schools (e.g. learning mentors, parenting support advisors)

The concept of schools as the base for 'extended services' is likely to further blur the distinction between consultation from CAMHS to Tier 1 professionals, and schools as settings where health-based staff and school-based staff both provide a range of emotional health/mental health services. In 2007, the 'Mental Health in Schools' pilot was announced by the then newly created Department for Children, Schools and Families (Department for Children, Schools and Families & Department of Health, 2008). This is pump priming finance to clusters of schools to develop 'Wave 2' (group-based early intervention) approaches, and 'Wave 3' (individual work with children and their families) approaches, all delivered by a mixture of school-appointed, CAMHS-seconded, and voluntary sector staff. This marked a shift away from mental health finance being allocated through health or social care agencies, and places clear expectations on CAMHS to increase the proportion of their resources allocated to supporting Tier 1 services.

Liaison to Social Service's children's departments

Many, if not most, children in contact with social care will have emotional health aspects to their difficulties. When the demands made by Social Services on CAMHS for individual work with these young people are questioned, the CAMHS professionals are perceived as unsupportively avoiding 'problem' children. Social workers, in their search for support, can also be undermined by CAMHS. Their understanding and assessment of a situation are often in danger of being placed in a subordinate relationship to that of the consulting 'expert'. There is a consequent devaluing of professional status and the disempowering and deskilling of that agency on an institutional level. Such a process is also apparent in legal and court work. The generation of such a hierarchy of regard does not facilitate the management of children in their environment and is not an effective and efficient use of resources, although it may bolster the ego and social status of individual CAMHS professionals. Children and adolescent mental health services cannot accept this hierarchy of regard and then complain about referral rates, lack of resources and the inadequacies of other agencies.

Again, the development of *Every Child Matters* (Department for Children, Schools and Families, 2003) and *Care Matters: Time for Change* (Department for Education and Skills, 2007) leads to a much higher priority for the mental health needs of looked-after children in particular. Many residential units now have regular consultation from CAMHS professionals. Some areas of the country have developed prioritised access to CAMHS by looked-after children. The development of the Multi-Agency Looked After Partnerships (MALAP; Department of Health, 2002) aims to promote a range of developments concerning the provision of consultation to these settings.

The SDQ (Goodman, 2001) is now being used to measure the mental disturbance of looked-after children, which could lead to either an increase in referrals of looked-after children or an increase in those caring for looked-after children.

Liaison to primary healthcare services

Primary care services are often disengaged from, if not ignorant of, the many agencies and systems that work with children, but there are many techniques for working with them (Garralda, 2002). Their understanding of educational support systems is often poor, so they may be manipulated by schools into avoiding using those systems in the hope of getting a more rapid and effective response from a CAMHS. It is helpful to enquire from all primary care referrers where a child is at school and what educational support they are receiving, as well as about the involvement of other agencies. Children and adolescent mental health services' contact with those other agencies then enables the support of children, and a discussion of the benefits and purpose of a referral to CAMHS.

It is difficult for GPs to attend regular consultation sessions; however, primary mental health workers can visit practices regularly to discuss mental health issues and can always ring to discuss a referral they have received. Similarly, telephone discussions with health visitors and GPs help develop relationships with CAMHS professionals and increase understanding of mental health issues. Children and adolescent mental health service professionals must always be aware of the difficulties in a surgery of a very emotional, distressed or angry parent or child, and be prepared to talk through the management of that situation. General practitioners take continuing medical education very seriously and multidisciplinary presentations to them reinforce the message that children's mental health problems are rarely managed exclusively by medical methods. An example of a protocol for GPs to follow when considering a referral to CAMHS is given in Box 13.2.

Conclusion

Every Child Matters (Department for Children, Schools and Families, 2003) has clarified that the needs of children should be met by all agencies

---

Box 13.2 Handy hints for GPs

- Try to determine who has the problem (it is rarely the child) and what they are really worried about. You can then direct your interventions accordingly
- What do the family hope to gain from this appointment.
- A telephone call for advice or discussion is often preferable to referral to another service. A primary mental health worker can be very helpful.
- Always ask who else is involved with the child (e.g. social worker, school special needs department). They may know far more about the child and be in a better position to help than any medical agency. Referring the family back to them may be the most useful intervention.
- Encouragement of what parents are doing right in their child rearing is more effective than diagnosing what is going wrong. Encourage the parents and they will encourage the child; criticise the parents and they will criticise the child.
- Be sure the family want a referral to CAMHS and are not going to be desperately undermined by it because they already lack confidence in their child rearing.
- Schools have support services to deal with educational problems and problems in school. Families should be directed to use them if they are worried about problems in school.
- There are information fact sheets available from the Royal College of Psychiatrists and other sources.

---

working together, as close to the child and family as possible, so many agencies can justifiably call on CAMHS for their perspective or input. It is the role of the CAMHS Partnership Group at local level to agree how their resources are to be deployed overall, and how to respond to new initiatives as they emerge.

Children's health depends on their physical and mental well-being. Schools, primary health groups, Social Services and other children's services have a large part to play in developing their mental well-being, on which children's adult psychological functioning will be based. Current government policy is further promoting the role child and adolescent mental health professionals have in assisting other professionals in that work, by developing relationships with them. Consultation and liaison provide a regular structure in which these relationships can flourish, and is already playing a more significant role within a local CAMHS.

References

Adams, C. (2007) Health visitor's role in family mental health. *Journal of Family Health Care*, **17**, 37–38.

Audit Commission (1999) *Children in Mind*. Audit Commission Publications.

Cox, A. (1993) Preventive aspects of child psychiatry. *Archives of Disease in Childhood*, **68**, 691–701.

Department for Children, Schools and Families (2003) *Every Child Matters: Change for Children*. TSO (The Stationery Office).

Department for Children, Schools and Families (2008) Common assessment framework. Department for Children, Schools and Families (http://www.dcsf.gov.uk/everychildmatters/strategy/deliveringservices1/caf/cafframework/).

Department for Children, Schools and Families (2009) Contact Point. Department for Children, Schools and Families (http://www.dcsf.gov.uk/everychildmatters/strategy/deliveringservices1/contactpoint/contactpoint/).

Department for Children, Schools and Families & Department of Health (2008) *Targeted Mental Health in Schools Project. Using the evidence to inform your approach: A practical guide for headteachers and commissioners*. Department for Children, Schools and Families Publications.

Department for Children, Schools and Families & Department of Health (2009) Healthy schools. Department for Children, Schools and Families & Department of Health (http://www.healthyschools.gov.uk/).

Department for Education and Skills (1999) *Healthy Schools: How the National Healthy School Standard Contributes to School Improvement*. DfES Publications.

Department for Education and Skills (2005) *Excellence and Enjoyment: Social and Emotional Aspects of Learning Guidance*. DfES Publications.

Department for Education and Skills (2007) *Care Matters: Time for Change*. TSO (The Stationery Office).

Department of Health (2002) *Promoting the Health of Looked After Children*. Department of Health.

Department of Health (2004) *National Service Framework for Children, Young People and Maternity Services. The Mental Health and Well-being of Children and Young People*. Department of Health Publications.

Department of Health (2009) General Medical Services (GMS) contract. Department of Health (http://www.dh.gov.uk/en/managingyourorganisation/Humanresourcesandtraining/modernisingpay/GPcontracts/index.htm).

Department of Health & Department for Education and Skills (2004) *Promoting Emotional Health and Well-being Through the National Healthy School Standard*. NHS Health Development Agency.

Dunn, J. (1996) Children's relationships: bridging the divide between cognitive and social development. *Journal of Child Psychology and Psychiatry*, **37**, 507–518.

Fombonne, E. (2002) Case identification in an epidemiological context. In *Child and Adolescent Psychiatry* (eds M. Rutter & E. Taylor), pp. 52–69. Blackwell.

Ford, T., Goodman, R. & Meltzer, H. (2003) The British Child and Adolescent Mental Health Survey 1999: the prevalence of DSM-IV disorders. *Journal of the American Academy of Child and Adolescent Psychiatry*, **42**, 1203–1211.

Ford, T., Tingay, K., Wolpert, M., *et al* (2006) CORC's survey of routine outcome monitoring and national CAMHS dataset developments: a response to Johnston and Gower. *Child and Adolescent Mental Health*, **11**, 50–52.

Garralda, M. E. (2002) Primary health care psychiatry. In *Child and Adolescent Psychiatry* (4th edn) (eds M. Rutter & E. Taylor), pp. 1090–1100. Blackwell.

Goodman, R. (2001) The psychiatric properties of the strengths and difficulties questionnaire. *Journal of the American Academy of Child and Adolescent Psychiatry*, **40**, 1337–1345.

Halsey, K., Gulliver, C., Johnson, A., *et al* (2005) *Evaluation of Behaviour and Education Support Teams. National Foundation for Educational Research Report RR706*. Department for Education and Skills.

Hickey, N., Kramer, T. & Garralda, E. (2007) *Primary Mental Health Workers (PMHWs) in Child and Adolescent Mental Health Services: A Survey of Organisation, Management and Role*. Department of Health.

Howlin, P. (2002) Special educational treatment. In *Child and Adolescent Psychiatry* (eds M. Rutter & E. Taylor), pp. 1128–1147. Blackwell.

Larsen, T., & Samdal, O. (2007) Implementing Second Step: balancing fidelity and program adaptation. *Journal of Educational and Psychological Consultation*, **17**, 1–29.

Mortimore, P. (1995) The positive effects of schooling. In *Psychosocial Disturbances in Young People* (ed. M. Rutter), pp. 333–364. Cambridge University Press.

NHS Health Advisory Service (1995) *Together We Stand: Commissioning, Role and Management of Child and Adolescent Mental Health Services*. HMSO.

Nicol, A. R. (2002) Practice in non-medical settings. In *Child and Adolescent Psychiatry* (4th edn) (eds M. Rutter & E. Taylor), pp. 1077–1089. Blackwell.

Offord, D (1982) Primary prevention: aspects of program design and evaluation. *Journal of the American Academy of Psychiatry*, **211**, 225–230.

Offord, D. (1987) Prevention of emotional and behavioural problems in children. *Journal of Child Psychology and Psychiatry*, **28**, 9–19.

Richardson, G. & Partridge, I. (2000) Child and adolescent mental health services: liaison with tier 1 services. A consultation exercise with school nurses. *Psychiatric Bulletin*, **24**, 462–463.

Royal College of Paediatrics and Child Health (2006) Child in Mind. (http://www.rcpch.ac.uk/Education/Education-Courses-and-Programmes/Child-In-Mind). RCPCH.

Rutter, M., Maughan, B., Mortimore, P., *et al* (1979) *Fifteen Thousand Hours*. Open Books.

Shipman, M. D. (1968) *Sociology of the School*, pp. 13–14. Longman.

Skynner, R. & Cleese, J. (1994) *Life and How to Survive It*. Mandarin.

World Health Organization (1992) *The ICD–10 Classification of Mental and Behavioural Disorders*. WHO.

Yamey, G. (1999) Young less tolerant of mentally ill than the old. *BMJ*, **319**, 1092.

YoungMinds (1996) *Mental Health in Your School: A Guide for Teachers and Schools*. Jessica Kingsley Publishers.

CHAPTER 14

Structuring and managing treatment options

Barry Wright, Sarah Bryan, Ian Partridge, Nick Jones and Greg Richardson

'Life is short, the craft long to learn, opportunity fleeting, experiment deceptive and judgement difficult. Not only must the physician be ready to do his duty but the patient, the attendants, and external circumstances must all conduce to a cure.'

Hippocrates

Introduction

The routine problems presenting to a CAMHS are likely to be addressed by those working at Tier 2 by an individual specialist mental health professional working with the problem. The demands of this everyday CAMHS work require all the specialist skills available in the service. No professional, unless at a very inexperienced stage, should not be available for Tier 2 work. To some extent the expenditure of energy on the development of the more high-profile 'specialist' Tier 3 teams is secondary and needs to be carefully managed to maintain availability of Tier 2 specialist provision. Treatments such as CBT are often offered by Tier 3 teams, although service members with relevant skills will do this as part of their Tier 2 work. The system needs to be coordinated and managed so that there is equity of access for required services at the most effective tier.

Requisites of Tier 2

'Critical mass' of staff

Meeting the needs of the community and providing a comprehensive range of services requires a critical mass of CAMHS staff with a multidisciplinary skill mix and a clear recognition of professional function.

Assessment

Assessment represents the first stage of any therapeutic relationship and professionals working at Tier 2 need a clear model of assessment.

Continuum of care

The Tier 2 professional, who may link up with Tier 1 workers, will also be in a position to access and make use of Tier 3 and Tier 4 provision where required. This highlights the importance of communication both within CAMHS and with other agencies, as well as underpinning the principle that all disciplines should be involved in this area of service provision.

Training and supervision

Staff of all disciplines require access to affordable and relevant training. Training budgets are limited and unequal in their distribution. It may be that units develop alternative funding strategies to support less well-resourced disciplines. In-house training initiatives and multi-agency and multidisciplinary training programmes are effective and keep costs down. Professional supervision is a prerequisite for effective professional functioning. Supervision requires consideration of the areas of clinical management and practice, the management of workload and case-load, and personal and professional development. Supervision will usually take place within the hierarchical structures of disciplines in which there are clear lines of responsibility and accountability. Within a CAMHS, cross-disciplinary supervision and support are part of multidisciplinary working, but cannot replace professional supervision (see Chapter 7).

Treatment options within a CAMHS

Parent support and management

Most families at some stage of their lives need support and advice from others, although this is usually from the extended family and neighbourhood. For those requiring more support than this, a progression through telephone help-lines, the internet, voluntary organisations and primary care may result in contact with CAMHS. The initial approach is to ask the question 'Whose problem is this – the child's, parents', family's or referrer's?' If it becomes evident that the parents do require support, it will be necessary to address three fundamental issues:

- the level of the parents' understanding of the child's developmental pathway;
- the parents' level of awareness of how to manage the child's behaviour;
- the effectiveness of the parents' management, and matters that interfere with that effectiveness.

From this starting point, a template of intervention strategies can be developed, aimed at education, advice on management tactics or reassurance. If the parents' understanding and awareness of their child's and their own difficulties are being undermined by lack of consistency in their approach to the problem, further questions may need consideration.

- What is the nature of the attachment between parent and child?
- Is there a need for parent training?
- Do the parents encourage and facilitate resilience in their child?
- Do the parents fail to manage one or more than one (or all) of their children?
- What models of parenting have the parents experienced?
- Do the parents have a history of loss, trauma or abuse?
- Are there current indications of parental depression, substance misuse or mental health problems?
- Are the parents being adequately mutually supportive?
- Are the parents being adequately supported?

This process enables pragmatism in utilisation of resources and allows the negotiation of a package of focused intervention. Consideration needs to be given to the motivation and ability of the parents to undertake a focused piece of work. Before embarking on Tier 2 work, it may be helpful to clarify the following with the parent(s), as an integral part of user and carer involvement.

- Can the parent(s) manage to attend a clinic or out-patient setting?
- Are there travel considerations that make home visiting a preferred option?
- Are there problems taking time off work or school?
- Is there insurmountable stigma attached to CAMHS attendance?
- Are there gender issues or professional skills required in allocation?
- Is there a healthy working partnership between family and professionals?
- Do the young person and family members consent to the process that is being undertaken?

A careful exploration of the practical issues will often avoid unattended later appointments and will allow the Tier 2 professional to be in a position to match the requirements of the parent(s), child and family to the most useful treatment approach, which could involve any of the following, singly or in combination:

- a behavioural programme
- individual work with or more general support for the parent(s)
- structural work with the parent(s) (e.g. parent advisor model)
- referral to adult mental health service
- referral to a voluntary agency (e.g. Home-Start, www.home-start.org. uk; New Pin, www.newpin.org.uk – now part of the Family Welfare Association, www.fwa.org.uk)
- referral to a Local Authority support programme (e.g. family centre, family aide)
- referral to a Tier 3 team in relation to parent skills training (based on, for example, Webster-Stratton (1994), Mellow Parenting (www.

mellowparenting.org) or work on parent–child dynamics through a relationship play group

- parent training and attachment work through such techniques as Theraplay (Jernberg & Booth, 1999).

Guidance is available on which interventions have an evidence base (Fonagy *et al*, 2002; Wolpert *et al*, 2006). The National Institute for Health and Clinical Excellence regularly produces and updates guidance to CAMHS practitioners on topics as varied as the treatment of depression and ADHD (National Collaborating Centre for Mental Health, 2005, 2008), as well as borderline and antisocial personality disorders (National Institute for Health and Clinical Excellence, 2009*a*,*b*), but certain conditions and predicaments still present to CAMHS for which there is little evidence of effective interventions. In this situation the principles in Box 14.1 become even more important.

Casework and inter-agency liaison

Frequently, a referral to CAMHS may come from more than one source. These situations commonly arise when a young person's difficulties have created concern and anxiety in different settings. As a result, agencies respond by referring or otherwise requesting help from CAMHS. In such complex but not uncommon situations, mental health specialists often finds themselves key players in managing the case or facilitating inter-agency liaison. Although this is not a skill uniquely owned by mental health professionals, they often have considerable experience in providing containment for families and professionals alike in situations involving chronic or persisting difficulties or those that incite high levels of anxiety.

Tier 2 professionals can offer containing casework strategies such as:

- the pulling together of all relevant information
- effecting communication between agencies and disciplines
- facilitating professional planning meetings
- providing psychological containment in crises.

Box 14.1 Principles of clinical practice

- Seeing all problems within a developmental context
- Seeing all problems within a relational context
- Avoiding an approach based upon notions of individual pathology
- Taking an approach that is focused upon problem-solving, and that facilitates and 'fits' with the needs of the young person and family

---

Psychopharmacological treatments

Although there is an overlap of specialist mental health skills within a CAMHS, multidisciplinary working requires an acknowledgement of specific therapeutic functions. Certain conditions (e.g. attentional disorders, affective and psychotic disorders) may require treatment with medication. Although the psychopharmacological brief will be undertaken by the medical specialist who will retain medical responsibility for the treatment, it is also possible that other Tier 2 workers may be involved in the monitoring of the condition. For example, the use of methylphenidate for ADHD may be administered by the GP, with the Tier 2 professional occasionally monitoring the functioning of the child at home and school, and offering support and management advice. Similarly, a young person on psychotropic medication may receive relapse prevention work from a Tier 2 professional of any discipline, although often the involved professionals constitute an *ad hoc*, inter-agency, patient-orientated Tier 3 team.

Behavioural therapy

Most Tier 2 workers can be expected to have a working knowledge of behavioural techniques. The role of the therapist is to facilitate a relearning process which examines existing learning patterns, sets new goals and alters behavioural contingencies in order to encourage the building up of desired behaviours. In the absence of more pernicious factors (e.g. abuse, neglect, severe family dysfunction) such techniques are effective and have the advantage of teaching parents the process of managing their child's behaviour rather than just offering a short-term solution to a specific behaviour. In considering a behavioural approach, the professional should assess:

- the scale of the difficulties – for example whether the behaviours are being maintained by the parental responses and how much motivation to change there is within the family system;
- whether the problems are being correctly defined;
- whether goals are specific, measureable, achievable and realistic;
- whether effective parent–professional partnerships have been established;
- whether behavioural treatments are being correctly and consistently applied.

Cognitive therapy

Young people presenting with symptoms caused or maintained by maladaptive cognitive habits or schemata are ideally suited to work that will explore the meaning of events and test alternative thinking habits. This approach is of particular benefit for late childhood and adolescence, wherein collaborative work may be used to explore the 'faulty' cognitive assumptions all too common during this developmental phase. It has the value of being focused and short term, as well as a problem-solving technique that needs minimal involvement with and pathologising of the young person (Graham, 2000). Motivational enhancement may be useful in young persons wishing to address their substance misuse or in those with eating disorders (Schmidt & Treasure, 1993).

Cognitive–behavioural therapy

Cognitive and behavioural therapies are combined in CBT, whereby the feelings engendered by certain thoughts are examined and certain behaviours tried out to alter those thoughts and feelings. The biopsychosocial model of illness lends itself to this therapeutic approach. The aim is for the young person to actively combat the thoughts often called 'cognitive distortions' or 'automatic thoughts' and behaviours that are problematic to them, and so improve how they feel. The effectiveness of CBT in anxiety and some depressive disorders is recognised (Brent *et al*, 2002; Fonagy *et al*, 2002; Wolpert *et al*, 2006), although its benefits over selective serotonin reuptake inhibitors in major depression have been questioned (Goodyer *et al*, 2007). Cognitive–behavioural therapy is often helpful in other conditions when one of the individuals in the family wishes to work on the difficult feelings they have about themselves or the way they behave in relationships. Social problem-solving work and coping strategy work fall within this therapeutic model, and can be empowering for children with paediatric illness (e.g. chronic fatigue syndrome), low self-esteem, anger/stress management problems or other child mental health difficulties.

Individual psychotherapy

Child psychotherapists are few in number and their work can be time intensive. However, although different psychotherapists may set different referral criteria and work from differing psychotherapeutic paradigms, it is clear that certain groups of young people may benefit from individual psychotherapy if they have problems such as:

- internalising disorders (e.g. anxiety)
- a history of loss and bereavement
- an abusive background
- struggles with their own development
- marked separation difficulties
- difficulties arising from adoption or fostering.

Allied to such work, the ability to offer psychotherapeutic consultation and perspectives to carers and parents of young people facing difficulties, as well as to fellow professionals operating within and without the service, is valuable.

Other individual therapies

A range of other therapies and variants of therapies have been developed that have a growing evidence base and may be included in available therapeutic options such as cognitive analytic therapy or interpersonal therapy. The important point here is not to list all the myriad of available named options, but more that clinicians and their managers need to be monitoring the evidence base and seeking to fund training for proven treatments, and seek the correct environment for evidence-based innovation to thrive and be adequately commissioned.

Counselling

Counselling depends on an equal relationship between counsellor and client; this can never be the case when working with children. The word is also used in many different ways such as to 'tell off' or advise, as well as the 'therapeutic' definition. Not surprisingly, there is little evidence that individual counselling is effective with children and young people, despite the high demand by parents and adults in the child's world who wish to distance themselves from and pathologise the child. Supportive or reflective techniques may help a child develop autonomy and adaptive coping, but needs careful monitoring and supervision. Because of the unequal power relationships between adults and children, such counselling may in some circumstances be abusive.

Creative therapies

Other therapeutic models making additional use of non-verbal mediums such as play, music, art and drama can be helpful options within CAMHS. These may be particularly helpful for non-verbal children. Alternative methods of working with a child acknowledge the internal and external realities through different media and provide a safe space for a young person to find a way of making sense of and managing traumatic events or inadequate levels of care, which also must be addressed by the CAMHS.

Family therapy

Family therapy is a labour-intensive central service of CAMHS, in that systemic and developmental insights inform all interventions with children and their families. It offers a potent training arena for trainees and new members of staff, and facilitates the development of closer working practices among staff. The opportunity for live supervision also enhances the development of critical and supportive working patterns. With limited resources and with increasing demands upon CAMHS, such a provision must be effectively managed and clinically relevant (Partridge *et al*, 1999).

Family therapy should attempt to offer some flexibility as to when it operates and should recognise families' work commitments and schooling.

Teams should be of a multidisciplinary composition, with at least two experienced core members and two regular practitioners, as well as professionals in training, and coordinated by a senior clinician. Referrals will be either direct, from GPs, social workers or education personnel through the allocation process, or indirect via a member of the CAMHS who has already been involved with the family. Families should be asked to confirm their attendance by a given date; similarly, if families fail to attend subsequent appointments, a letter requesting their commitment to future sessions may be required. Such a system does increase administrative time, but it enables the service to be more cost-effective. The points to consider when allocating family therapy are listed in Box 14.2.

With the development of effective primary mental health workers, family therapy teams may be decentralised and developed on an inter-agency basis in localities. Child and adolescent mental health service staff will have a role in this process, supporting the primary mental health worker in the development of the team, by their active involvement in the team and in the training of professionals from other agencies.

At times, when it is considered economical in terms of time or useful in engaging a family, a pre-assessment interview or contact by a member of the CAMHS may be used. Families' expectations and experiences of family therapy must be considered in the overall organisation of the service to ensure confident engagement by the family. Efforts should be made to keep the families fully informed at all stages of the process, from the information leaflet they receive with their first appointment to decision-making

---

Box 14.2 Considerations in allocation to family therapy

- The nature of the presenting problem and its relation to family functioning.
- Family therapy intervention has to be geared to the developmental level of the children, or the children can be excluded if adult issues need addressing.
- The nature and quality of the referral must be considered, especially if reference is made to interactional family factors. Further clarification from the referrer may be necessary to decide the relevance of family therapy.
- The urgency of response required may mean that the family cannot wait for a family therapy appointment, although, in a crisis, family therapy may be effective in helping a family to gain confidence in their own resources rather than their relying on 'help' from outside agencies.
- Alternative responses may be more effective or economical, such as a visit by a community psychiatric nurse.
- Practical issues for the family such as access to the service base in terms of transport or financial considerations need to be examined.
- Any previous contact with the family by the CAMHS may inform the decision as to whether family therapy would be a helpful intervention.
- The recognised indicators and counter-indicators for family therapy should be reviewed (Skynner, 1976; Lask, 1987).

regarding discharge. Monthly appointments for out-patient family therapy are routine in busy services and give time for families to work on issues raised in the session.

Family therapy has many and varying clinical modalities (Jacobs & Pearse, 2002); a brief, focused and structural model (Minuchin & Fishman, 1981; de Shazer, 1988) has many advantages within a busy CAMHS, service delivery being as important as clinical purity. Key points regarding the management of a family therapy team are listed in Box 14.3.

Group psychotherapy

Similar principles to those discussed in relation to family therapy also apply to the management of a group work team. The time needed for coordination, invitation and planning of groups cannot be underestimated, making them a lot more resource intensive than the idea that a lot of people are being seen together might imply. Groups may consist of young people or parents/carers with a shared difficulty or a shared goal, or it may combine group work with adults and group work with children. Their efficacy is addressed by Fonagy *et al* (2002).

Self-regulation

Sensory integration (or processing function) is the neurological process that organises sensation from the body and from the environment and makes it possible to use the body effectively within the environment (Ayres, 1989). Sensory integration provides a crucial foundation for later, more complex learning and behaviour. For most children, sensory integration develops in the course of ordinary childhood activities. When the process is disordered

---

Box 14.3 Managing a family therapy service

- Set clear and explicit criteria for allocation.
- All families who appear from the referral to be suitable for family therapy could first be seen by a member of the team for initial assessment and engagement. The 'personal touch' may be more effective in engaging the family than the impersonality of written information to a family in 'need' or 'crisis'.
- Distinguish overtly between seeing a family for family therapy and offering a family assessment.
- Involve the families in the process of treatment as equal partners (they are the experts on their family and the team are experts on family functioning), and emphasise clear explanations and engagement throughout treatment.
- Use an opt-in system for appointments as this reduces waiting times and minimises non-attendance rates.
- Be flexible about activating alternative treatment resources.
- Establish clear supervision and training arrangements.
- Establish ongoing evaluation of the service.

a number of problems in attention control, emotional development, self-regulation, learning, language, motor skills and behaviour may be evident. Increasingly, occupational therapists in CAMHS are applying the growing body of knowledge and research on sensory processing disorder to children referred to their services, most particularly with pervasive developmental disorder (including autism and Asperger syndrome), ADHD, learning disorders (i.e. specific learning difficulties such as dyslexia), developmental disabilities, fragile-X syndrome, and developmental coordination disorder (including dyspraxia).

Assessment will usually involve standardised testing, structured observations, a detailed developmental history and interviews with carers and teachers. The findings give an additional insight into sometimes difficult-to-explain behaviours and provide alternative and at times more helpful strategies for parents and teachers. Treatment within CAMHS is most likely to centre upon:

- developing an individualised treatment plan recommending sensory–motor strategies to support the young person at home, school, work or social settings (Greenspan & Wieder, 2005);
- group treatment programmes such as the Alert Programme for Self-Regulation (Williams & Shellenberger, 1996).

These approaches depend upon carefully adapting the environment to support the young person with sensory processing difficulties. For example, the sensory-avoidant child with low thresholds for sensory stimuli is easily overwhelmed and is likely to function optimally in a less stimulating environment.

Conclusion

The evidence base for many interventions in CAMHS is lacking, but new research is helpful in allocating resources to effective interventions. However, the basic interactional tools of genuineness, warmth and empathy remain therapeutic in their own right, and without them no intervention is going to have a sound foundation for effectiveness. No therapy will be effective if the person or persons in need of the work does not consent to or engage with the work, although detention under the Mental Health Act or via a secure order may lead to a successful outcome by forcing therapy on the person detained, but even then the relationship between the patient and therapist is of paramount importance.

References

Ayres, A. J. (1989) *Sensory Integration and Praxis Tests Manual*. Western Psychological Services.

Brent, D. A., Gaynor, S. T. & Weersing, V. R. (2002) Cognitive-behavioural approaches to the treatment of depression and anxiety. In *Child and Adolescent Psychiatry* (eds M. Rutter & E. Taylor), pp. 921–937. Blackwell.

De Shazer, S. (1988) *Clues: Investigating Solutions in Brief Therapy*. Norton.

Fonagy, P., Target, M., Cottrell, D., *et al* (2002) *What Works for Whom*. Guilford Press.

Goodyer, I., Dubicka, B., Wilkinson, P., *et al* (2007) Selective serotonin reuptake inhibitors (SSRIs) and routine specialist care with and without cognitive behaviour therapy in adolescents with major depression: randomised control trial. *BMJ*, **335**, 142.

Graham, P. (2000) *Cognitive–Behaviour Therapy for Children and Families*. Cambridge University Press.

Greenspan, S. I. & Wieder, S. (2005) *Interdisciplinary Council on Developmental and Learning Disorders – Diagnostic Manual for Infancy and Early Childhood (ICDL–DMIC)*. Interdisciplinary Council on Developmental and Learning Disorders.

Jacobs, B. & Pearse, J. (2002) Family therapy. In *Child and Adolescent Psychiatry* (eds M. Rutter & E. Taylor), pp. 968–982. Blackwell.

Jernberg, A. M. & Booth, P. D. (1999) *Theraplay*. Jossey-Bass.

Lask, B. (1987) Family therapy. *BMJ*, **294**, 203–204.

Minuchin, S. & Fishman, H. C. (1981) *Family Therapy Techniques*. Harvard University Press.

National Collaborating Centre for Mental Health (2005) *Depression in Children and Young People: Identification and Management in Primary, Community and Secondary Care. Clinical Guideline CG28*. National Institute for Health and Clinical Excellence.

National Collaborating Centre for Mental Health (2008) *Attention Deficit Hyperactivity Disorder: Diagnosis and Management of ADHD in Children, Young People and Adults. Clinical Guideline CG72*. British Psychological Society & Royal College of Psychiatrists.

National Institute for Health and Clinical Excellence (2009a) *Borderline Personality Disorder: Treatment and Management. Clinical Guideline CG78*. NICE.

National Institute for Health and Clinical Excellence (2009b) *Antisocial Personality Disorder: Treatment, Management and Prevention. Clinical Guideline CG77*. NICE.

Partridge, I., Redmond, C., Williams, C., *et al* (1999) Evaluating family therapy in a child and adolescent mental health service. *Psychiatric Bulletin*, **23**, 531–533.

Schmidt, U. & Treasure, J. (1993) *Getting Better Bit(e) by Bit(e)*. Lawrence Erlbaum.

Skynner, A. C. R. (1976) *One Flesh, Separate Persons*. Constable.

Webster-Stratton, C. (1994) *Troubled Families, Problem Children*. John Wiley & Sons.

Williams, M. S. & Shellenberger, S. (1996) *'How Does Your Engine Run?' A Leader's Guide to the Alert Program for Self-Regulation*. Therapy Works.

Wolpert, M., Fuggle, P., Cottrell, D., *et al* (2006) *Drawing on the Evidence*. CAMHS Publications.

CHAPTER 15

CAMHS in the emergency department[1]

Tony Kaplan

'The chapter of accidents is the longest chapter in the book.'
John Wilkes

Introduction

A UK study showed that of 107 young people with mental health problems presenting to the emergency department, a third presented following self-harm (Healy *et al*, 2002). Most of these cases were young girls. After specialist assessment (and brief intervention), most were not admitted for further treatment but were seen for urgent follow-up (75% within 2 weeks) in out-patients. Of the attenders who had not self-harmed, the most common problem was psychosis, including hypomania (a third of this group), followed by adjustment and other anxiety-related disorders, and problems related to intellectual difficulties. Also seen were problems related to conduct, drug and alcohol misuse, and depression (without self-harm).

Historically, perhaps because of lack of training, the American experience has been that:

> 'the atmosphere towards psychiatric patients is often negative and hostile. The problems of the children and family are perceived as self inflicted, deserved outcomes that are evidence of weak, disorganised families, making poor life choice.' (Thomas, 2003)

The NICE (National Collaborating Centre for Mental Health, 2004) guidelines on self-harm would suggest that this attitude, at least with regard to self-harm, is prevalent in UK hospitals also. There is little research on how decisions are made in the emergency department about young people with mental health problems, the different levels of tolerance in different parents and assessing professionals, the application of specific threshold criteria within care pathways, or to the negative effects of hospitalisation.

---

1. Based on *Child and Adolescent Mental Health Problems in the Emergency Department and the Services to Deal with These* (Royal College of Psychiatrists Child and Adolescent Faculty, 2006) and *Emergency Department Handbook: Children and Adolescents with Mental Health Problems* (Kaplan, 2009).

Requirements

There is a requirement in England, within the children's NSF (Department of Health, 2004) and in Scotland through the recommendations (Scottish Government, 2005) for commissioners and Local Authorities to ensure that policies and protocols for the treatment of children and young people with emergency mental health needs are developed in partnership. The level of service provided and the criteria for referral also require clarification. There is an expectation that arrangements are in place to: ensure 24-hour cover to meet children's urgent needs; that, where indicated, specialist mental health assessment is undertaken within 24 hours or the next working day; and that all staff likely to be called upon to carry out the initial social and mental health assessment receive specific training. On-call and 24-hour specialist CAMHS are not yet provided in many areas.

Emergency departments are one of the range of provisions that address the needs of children, adolescents and families with acute biopsychosocial problems. Other provisions to meet this need include: specialised paediatric emergency departments; primary care out-of-hours assessment centres; specialised mental health emergency and assessment centres; crisis intervention outreach/home visiting services, sometimes available to young people over the age of 16; and 'drop-in' community-based crisis services provided independently or in partnership with voluntary sector organisations. Although this chapter will deal only with hospital-based services, other models of emergency and crisis intervention in CAMHS will need addressing in the longer term.

Presentations to the emergency department

Context

Children and young people present to the emergency department when what they are doing becomes intolerable to the people who feel responsible for caring for them. Their behaviour may become intolerable when it is too upsetting, too frightening or too confusing to be coped with by the physical and emotional resources of the supporting system; we should, however, recognise that children's emotional and behavioural problems may exceed the parents' capacity to cope as a consequence of impairments in the adults' functioning rather than an escalation in the child's behaviour. These things often go together, interacting in a mutually reinforcing circular causality (Gutterman *et al*, 1993; Pumariega & Winters, 2003). Furthermore, 'while the child's ecological context influences the time, nature and severity of the crisis, the organisation of emergency mental health services in the ecology of a health care system may influence the outcome of the crisis' (Thomas, 2003). The author points out that 'psychiatric emergency services are brief windows of time in which the child or adolescent and the family are coming

139

for the first time, ready to receive help and engage in change'. However, commonly the organising assumption with mental health presentations to the emergency department is that separation from their care-giving environment (usually their families) is the desirable solution, in the short term at least. To some extent this is because the emergency department staff who see children, young people and their families in crisis are relatively untrained in being able to include in their assessment an understanding of cognitive and emotional development, family/systemic dynamic influences on the child, and even the significance of certain symptoms in the child; hence, the tendency to admit children and young people for further assessment by a qualified CAMHS professional within the next working day. The initial emergency department assessment 'screens' patients, with an emphasis on examining for pathognomonic indicators and overt presenting symptoms and risk. It is easier in that context to admit than to discharge. Little attention is given to crisis intervention to produce change that would limit risk, de-escalate crisis, enhance support and may even produce dramatic and fundamental change in the young person's support structures.

Presenting problems

- Self-harm: this is by far the most common presenting problem requiring CAMHS intervention (Fox & Hawton, 2004).
- Acute psychiatric disorders, which cannot be coped with by the carer and cannot be managed by normal out-patient services, such as:
  - depression (e.g. because of suicidality, self-neglect, agitation, starvation);
  - psychosis (e.g. because of overwhelmingly high arousal, fear, distress, aggression or unpredictability, or because of inexplicable, socially embarrassing or risk-taking behaviour);
  - anxiety syndromes (e.g. because of panic symptoms, often manifesting as physical complaints, insomnia, exhausting demands for reassurance and emotional support, or overwhelming, intrusive mental symptoms possibly as part of OCD or post-traumatic stress disorder (PTSD));
  - hypomania (e.g. with disinhibition, over-activity).
- Acute exacerbations of behavioural symptoms associated with chronic developmental disorder, such as:
  - autism-spectrum disorder (e.g. insomnia, aggression/frustration reactions);
  - ADHD (e.g. risk or injuries related to dangerous impulsivity, overwhelming over-activity related to social/environmental context).
- Eating disorders (especially because of medical complications, for example fainting, weakness and coldness).
- Delirium, confusional and toxic states.

- Complications of drug/substance/alcohol misuse/withdrawal including unconsciousness, psychosis, anxiety, behavioural dyscontrol.
- Side-effects of psychotropic medications.
- Medically unexplained symptoms (e.g. psychosomatic/conversion symptoms).
- Signs or reports of abuse or neglect, including factitious or induced disorders.
- Children may also present when their parent is the referred or identified patient, for example a parent presenting serious mental illness or where the parent is the victim of domestic violence.
- Behaviour problems, especially violence – when there is no other obvious place for the carers to get help from, or because there is a previous involvement with the hospital (e.g. previous admissions to paediatric departments) and/or a CAMHS history.

Referral pathways

Children and young people will often be brought to the emergency department by parents, although in some cases they will be brought by non-parental carers and/or friends. Older teenagers may refer themselves. They may be referred by a professional referrer, most commonly the GP or primary care practitioner. They may also be referred by their school or college (including school nurse), Social Services, community or residential team, and other Tier 1 professionals. They may be brought to the emergency department by the police, as the gateway for what may be seen as benign social control through mental health services.

Function, competencies, roles and responsibilities

CAMHS first-line staff

Function

Child and adolescent mental health services are required to consult to the paediatric or psychiatric front-line staff, to provide advice on the emergency treatment of young people in the emergency department, and provide advice on their emergency treatment.

Where consultation is insufficient to resolve the problems presented and where resources permit, CAMHS contribute to the assessment and emergency intervention and management directly. Child and adolescent mental health services also contribute to the referral on to a specialist Tier 4 in-patient unit if required (if no other disposal is available that would ensure the patient's safety and protect against serious deterioration in their condition until they could be seen by a suitable qualified CAMHS professional). Most commonly, however, CAMHS offer assessment, not in the emergency department but on the next working day, to children and young people admitted to a paediatric ward.

Competencies

- Take a referral on a child or teenager in a calm, thoughtful and organised way.
- To consult to other professionals, especially understanding what problems that professional needs to resolve, and through a process of systematic questioning helping to reach a set of conclusions about the best way(s) forward.
- Engage and interview children and young people on their own and with their family/carers.
- Interview parents to get collateral history in a respectful, patient and thoughtful way.
- Take a full history of the presenting problem and its antecedents (highlighting the salient aggravating and ameliorating factors and events) to understand the young person's family and social circumstances and how these may influence outcome, and to understand how the young person copes with adversity, specifically the kind of adversity that has led to the current crisis.
- Take a full developmental history, understanding the implications and predictive value of early events, attainments, difficulties and relationships in the child's life.
- To have specialist knowledge about child and adolescent mental health and behavioural problems and their presentations, including the alerting signs and symptoms of child abuse.
- To conduct a mental state examination.
- To assess the risk to which the child, their carers and the community are exposed by being aware of the known risk and protective factors for suicidality and self-harm in young people.
- To intervene effectively in the current crisis.
- To develop a risk management plan in consultation with other professionals if necessary, including other (senior) CAMHS colleagues – this may include referring on for urgent admission to a Tier 4 adolescent in-patient unit or to a CAMHS community team for out-patient follow-up.
- To use the law as it relates to children and young people:
  - to understand 'parental responsibility', the powers parents/guardians have to make decisions for the child and who by right needs to be involved in accessing further services;
  - to make a formal determination of the young person's 'capacity' and competence to give and withhold consent to treatment;
  - to make decisions about the right to confidentiality and information sharing;
  - to know and understand the local safeguarding children policy and be able to implement this;
  - to understand the applicability of the Children Act 1989 or the relevant Mental Health Act to detain a young person in hospital

against their wishes if so indicated by the risk management plan.

- To be aware of local resources relevant to the needs of children and young people with mental health crises and if necessary where to refer on to and how, and what funding arrangements are in place for specialist services.
- To establish that the young person's needs for protection and care may be met on an adult mental health ward if the patient is admitted there because no more suitable placement is available.
- To know when limits of knowledge or skills are reached and then who to call for advice.

Roles and responsibilities of the consultant in child psychiatry

- Advising governments, policy makers and public sector authorities that are responsible for commissioning services and any public, independent, voluntary or private sector providers of healthcare who deliver services (including after- and longer-term care) for children and young people who present with mental health crises to the emergency department.
- Providing consultation and advice to providers of acute care, emergency, paediatric and mental health services, within the context of comprehensive CAMHS.
- Working with staff of child health, emergency departments, and within other units that deliver services to develop, implement and monitor protocols for the psychosocial assessment and treatment of children and young people presenting to the emergency department in crisis. This should involve close liaison and cooperation between the medical, nursing and other relevant professional staff of specialist CAMH, adult mental health, paediatric, emergency, general medical, substance misuse, and Social Services.
- Identifying the staffing levels and training required to provide comprehensive services for children and young people who are seen in the emergency department.
- Advising on and being involved in delivering training for CAMHS staff and the staff of the paediatric, child health, emergency, social and education service departments in order to ensure that young people, their families and carers receive immediate responses and aftercare relevant to their mental health crisis. In particular, this should include involvement in developing and implementing modular programmes for training staff of primary healthcare, ambulance, emergency, paediatric and child health, and CAMHS in comprehensive psychosocial and risk assessment.
- Being available to teach and supervise junior medical staff, and to consult with non-medical staff who are involved in assessing and treating children and young people who need emergency assessment

and intervention as a consequence of a mental health crisis, including those who harm themselves.

- In certain cases and circumstances, being involved directly in the clinical care of children and young people.
- Working with local commissioners and service providers to review implementation of this advice.

Role and function of the paediatric liaison CAMHS team

- To coordinate and advertise the on-call CAMHS.
- To draw up protocols with the emergency department and paediatric teams, for example for the management of alcohol intoxication and of self-harm in young people.
- To contribute to training of medical, nursing and other staff in the emergency department (and paediatrics).
- To contribute to audits concerning child and adolescent mental health, paediatrics and the emergency department (e.g. audit of management of self-harm).
- To be part of identification and analysis of risk and serious incidents concerning children, young people and their families who present with mental health problems in the emergency department and to developing plans for the future to avoid or deal effectively with such incidents.
- To ensure a clear line of communication between CAMHS, paediatrics and the emergency department.

Interface with other agencies

Police

Place of safety

Whether the emergency department is suitable as a designated place of safety for adolescents who may be violent is something that needs to be agreed locally. Child and adolescent mental health service or paediatric staff may be well placed to provide de-escalation because they are usually more used to talking to upset teenagers than their adult colleagues, but issues of security/safety of staff and other children need to be considered. Where a young person is brought to the emergency department as a place of safety, the police should agree to wait to provide assistance in the event of violence, to wait until the matter is resolved and, if necessary, to remove the young person (and their family) from the emergency department if they do not require urgent medical treatment.

Powers of arrest and willingness to act

Until they are admitted, the emergency department is to be regarded as a public area. As such, any law that applies to behaviour in a public place applies to the emergency department. This includes the use of Section 136 of the Mental Health Act.

Domestic violence

All staff who are aware of violence between the adults caring for a child are expected to be proactive in supporting victims of this violence and in protecting children who are exposed to witnessing or experiencing violence. Safeguarding children procedures should be initiated. The domestic violence unit of the police (usually, in England at least, this is a subunit of the community police unit) are trained to deal sensitively with those involved in domestic violence, whether as victims or perpetrators.

Social Services

Mental Health Act assessments

In the Mental Health Act 2007, the role of the approved social worker is expanded to include approved mental health professionals from other disciplines who have had approved training in applying the Mental Health Act. In practice it is likely that social workers will still do the bulk of the work. Approved mental health professionals are required to assess people of all ages and to know the law and how it applies to young people and children. However, most work primarily with adults and will have little experience of working with and interviewing young people. It would be good practice for assessments to be conducted by an approved person with expertise in dealing with children, or jointly by an approved mental health professional and a children and families social worker, although out of hours an approved mental health professional working alone may have to suffice. In this latter case, it is especially important for the approved mental health professional to have access to advice and consultation from a senior CAMHS professional. The local CAMHS should have a part in the training of approved mental health professionals locally, and should at the very least check that there is a CAMHS module in the training.

Emergency placements

The social worker will have knowledge of and access to emergency placement of children and young people, whose presentation to the emergency department is predicated on threats, dangers, inadequacies and/ or stresses in their home placement or the absence of a reliable place to stay. Emergency placement through Social Services may obviate the need for a hospital admission in some cases. There is a statutory duty on Social Services to provide for children under the age of 16 who have no (safe) home to live in – the predicament for 16- and 17-year-olds is well known, and it may be particularly important for there to be clear and explicit local agreements on the scope and threshold for Social Services' responsibility for this age group. The Children Act applies to anyone under the age of 18, and 16- and 17-year-olds may be defined as 'in need' under this Act.

Safeguarding children

The duty social worker must be involved in all cases of confirmed or suspected child abuse and neglect, if only to be consulted about the first steps to ensure the safety of the child, and to advise on the application of the local child protection policies and procedures. The emergency department will usually house or have access to the Child Protection Register, and this should be referenced in all cases of children presenting to the emergency department. The social worker will also have access to the Social Services database, which may have useful information on children and families known to be at risk or requiring support services. The social worker's holistic assessment will also identify resilience and strengths in the family and in their support networks, which might be enhanced to reduce the risk of abuse or neglect.

Family support

The duty social worker will be able to provide information on resources to support families in need. Knowing which resources may become available may reduce the sense of desperation of some families with ill or disturbing children, and allow them to cope a little longer and tolerate a little more in the short term. Resources may include day centres, home-visiting support (social) workers, the potential for respite placements, women's refuge placements for families experiencing domestic violence and/or financial support, and support with getting appropriate social security benefits for families stressed by poverty, where the stress of impoverishment is having an adverse effect on the mental health and socioemotional development of the child.

Management and liaison

A number of Royal College of Psychiatrists' College reports (1998, 2004*a*,*b*) and the NICE guidelines on self-harm (National Collaborating Centre for Mental Health, 2004) all recommend the establishment of an emergency department liaison committee. Where this has been implemented, it will be a local decision as to whether CAMHS and paediatric/child health services join this forum to discuss all cases presenting to the emergency department with special mental health needs whatever their age, or whether it would be more effective for there to be a separate children and young people's liaison committee. The latter may be indicated where there is a separate paediatric emergency department, as long as the needs of 16- and 17-year-olds are addressed. A CAMHS consultant should be nominated as having lead responsibility for liaising with the emergency department. The Royal College of Psychiatrists (1998) recommends that a CAMHS consultant and a paediatric consultant take joint responsibility for setting up and chairing a liaison committee: this committee will supersede any liaison committee overseeing policies and procedures regarding self-harm only.

The agencies, disciplines and departments potentially involved – primary care, police and the ambulance service, the emergency department, adult and child and adolescent mental health services, paediatrics and health visiting, Social Services, and, where relevant, voluntary sector representatives – should have a formally constituted group in which to:

- discuss and authorise robust working arrangements, written agreements and protocols for accepting and making (cross-) referrals;
- improve communication and develop a shared understanding of certain difficult presentations and their institutional responses;
- confirm management and administrative arrangements;
- agree responsibility for and plan training and induction of junior staff, new staff, agency and locum staff;
- agree standards and set up joint inter-departmental and inter-agency audit and evaluation cycles.

Resources

Every emergency department should have interview facilities which are safe, child and adolescent friendly, quiet, private, clean, reasonably comfortable, and large enough to allow a meeting of professionals with the child/young person and their family.

Information management, medical records and databases

Rapid access to the child or young person's medical records is essential for the provision of good and safe services. Protocols need to be in place for access to notes between trusts, respecting the patient's right to confidentiality. Electronic databases will in the future make it technically feasible for notes to be shared, but this ease of access will make it even more crucial for the portals of entry to be restricted in accordance with the Data Protection Act and the GMC (2004) rules on confidentiality and disclosure of patient information. Data should be collected in a way that allows audit studies to be facilitated.

Consideration should be given to a system for filing community care plans, in accordance with locally agreed community programme approaches, on young patients with mental health problems who are likely to attend the emergency department in crisis, especially for those classed as 'frequent attenders'.

The operation of a 'flag' or 'green card' system, whereby identified highly vulnerable patients who are not likely to abuse the system are admitted more or less directly to the designated ward (usually this applies to paediatrics), should be considered.

Access to the Child Protection (Safeguarding Children) Register is a problem in some areas. All emergency departments should have direct access to their local register, but this is not always the case. In some areas the Child Protection Register is held by the Local Authority, and access is via the duty social worker, which can introduce an unacceptable delay in establishing whether the child is on the register or not. The hospital may serve more than one Local Authority area; the Child Protection Register may only be available for the area in which the hospital is situated (even when most of the patient population is drawn from the neighbouring area). There is currently no national child protection database and no system for electronically ascertaining whether the child is subject to child protection surveillance. This needs to be remedied.

Commissioning

The commissioning primary care trusts in England, the local health boards in Wales, and the health boards under the leadership of child health commissioners in Scotland should establish the following.

24-hours a day, 7-days a week CAMHS cover to the emergency department

Commissioners should ensure that standards and levels of care and treatment for children and young people attending the emergency department with mental health problems are in line with national recommendations.

There should be a sustainable working day and out-of-hours rota of senior CAMHS professionals, available for direct intervention (usually provided by junior doctors or CAMHS liaison nurses) where resources allow and where this would be cost-effective relative to demand, or alternatively and at the least, available to offer specialist consultation by telephone. Supervision arrangements should be in place.

Services for 16- and 17-year-olds

Commissioners should ensure that agreements are in place between paediatric, adult mental health and CAMHS for the assessment and treatment of 16- and 17-year-olds, including agreeing thresholds for admission and the provision of suitable designated beds if they need admission.

If they are to be admitted to an adult psychiatric bed, written arrangements for this to happen in a way that best protects the young person from abuse and humiliation and meets their developmental needs should be in place. This should include advice on dealing with the young person's and the family's understandable fears and misgivings. The recommended arrangement would be for the young person to be nursed in a single room with 1:1 nursing by nurses who are CRB checked and preferably with experience of dealing with young people, jointly managed by, or at least with access to advice from, a CAMHS consultant or senior CAMHS nurse. The young person should be transferred to a designated adolescent unit bed at the earliest opportunity (Royal College of Psychiatrists Child and Adolescent Faculty, 2006; Kaplan, 2009).

Emergency psychiatric in-patient provision

Commissioners should ensure that local and regional arrangements for the emergency admission of a child or young person are in place and known to the emergency department. Children under 16 needing admission should always be admitted to a paediatric ward. Protocols, including inclusion and exclusion criteria, for this should be written and available to on-call paediatric junior staff seeing the child in the emergency department.

Commissioners should block-purchase specialist acute adolescent unit beds or make available sufficient funds for acquiring beds in the independent sector in an emergency. The number of beds should be established by a needs assessment, taking into account the fluctuations in bed utilisation over at least 3 years and published advice (Lamb & York, 2006). Each strategic health sector should move to commission through a consortium of primary care trusts its own NHS acute adolescent in-patient facility. In Scotland, health boards, and now regional planning groups, would commission these services.

Waiting times

The 4-hour waiting time in the emergency department for resolution of a mental health crisis for children and young people is, in many cases, impractical, and may lead to ineffective, minimising or unduly restrictive outcomes. Exclusion criteria will need to be agreed with the commissioners and if necessary with the strategic health authorities who are charged with performance monitoring. It may be advisable to have locally agreed response times for triage, for first assessment by paediatric first-line staff (for under-16s and where applicable all under-18s), for mental health first-line staff (where there is agreement to see over-16s) and for CAMHS consultation.

Interpreting services

For those whose first language is not English and also for those with sensory difficulties, interpreting services should be available.

Conclusion

Young people presenting in the emergency department are often not well understood by staff. The rapid support of skilled CAMHS professionals is essential for the well-being of the child and family, and to reassure the emergency department staff. The provision of such support must be built in to the operational policy of any CAMHS.

References

Department of Health (2004) *National Service Framework for Children Young People and Maternity Services. The Mental Health and Well-being of Children and Young People.* TSO (The Stationery Office).

Fox, C. & Hawton, K. (2004) *Deliberate Self-Harm in Adolescence*. Jessica Kingsley.

General Medical Council (2004) Confidentiality: protecting and providing information. GMC (http://www.gmc-uk.org/guidance/current/library/confidentiality.asp).

Gutterman, E. M., Markowitz, J. S., LeConte, J. S., *et al* (1993) Determinants for hospitalization from an emergency mental health service. *Journal of the American Academy of Child and Adolescent Psychiatry*, **32**, 114–122.

Healy, E., Saha, S., Subotsky, F., *et al* (2002) Emergency presentations to an inner-city adolescent psychiatric service. *Journal of Adolescence*, **25**, 397–404.

Kaplan, T. (ed.) (2009) *Emergency Department Handbook: Children and Adolescents with Mental Health Problems*. RCPsych Publications.

Lamb, C. & York, A. (2006) *Building and Sustaining Specialist CAMHS. Council Report CR137*. Royal College of Psychiatrists.

National Collaborating Centre for Mental Health (2004) *The Short-Term Physical and Psychological Management and Secondary Prevention of Self-Harm in Primary and Secondary Care. Clinical Guideline CG16*. National Institute for Health and Clinical Excellence.

Pumariega, A. J. & Winters, N. C. (2003) Trends and shifting ecologies: Part 3. *Child and Adolescent Psychiatric Clinics of North America*, **12**, 779–793.

Royal College of Psychiatrists (1998) *Managing Deliberate Self-Harm in Young People. Council Report CR64*. Royal College of Psychiatrists.

Royal College of Psychiatrists (2004a) *Psychiatric Services to Accident and Emergency Departments. Council Report CR118*. Royal College of Psychiatrists.

Royal College of Psychiatrists (2004b) *Assessment Following Self-Harm in Adults. Council Report CR122*. Royal College of Psychiatrists.

Royal College of Psychiatrists Child and Adolescent Faculty (2006) *Child and Adolescent Mental Health Problems in the Emergency Department and the Services to Deal with These.* Royal College of Psychiatrists (http://www.rcpsych.ac.uk/college/faculties/childandadolescent/newsandinformation.aspx).

Scottish Government (2005) *Children and Young People's Mental Health: A Framework for Promotion, Prevention and Care*. Scottish Executive.

Thomas, L. E. (2003) Trends and shifting ecologies: Part 1. *Child and Adolescent Psychiatric Clinics of North America*, **12**, 599–611.

CHAPTER 16

Paediatric liaison

Barry Wright, Sebastian Kraemer, Kate Wurr
and Christine Williams

'What is the matter with Mary Jane?
She's perfectly well and she hasn't a pain,
And it's lovely rice pudding for dinner again!
What is the matter with Mary Jane?'

A. A. Milne

Introduction

The first of the five outcomes in *Every Child Matters* (Department for Children, Schools and Families, 2003), a government aspirational document, is 'Be healthy' and clearly refers to 'enjoying good physical and mental health'. These go hand in hand and services should be integrated to achieve these aspirations.

Children with mental health problems and psychiatric disorders or psychological morbidity frequently present in paediatric clinics and wards. Those with medical disorders have a higher incidence of mental disorders (Green *et al*, 2004; Hysing *et al*, 2007). These are sometimes not identified in paediatric services (Slowik & Noronha, 2004) and where they are, paediatricians rarely have the time or training to deal adequately with them (Garralda & Bailey, 1989). Without mental health provision and training, these children's needs will not be addressed. There are initiatives to address training by provision of mental health training specifically for paediatricians (www.rcpch.ac.uk/Education/Education-Courses-and-Programmes/Child-In-Mind) and this should also improve collaboration with paediatric colleagues. The opportunity for early intervention is crucial to prevent longer-term problems or unnecessary paediatric intervention and hospitalisations.

Despite evidence of need and effectiveness, most paediatric departments are still without any meaningful CAMHS input (Woodgate & Garralda, 2006), yet the most pressing need for CAMHS in general (Potter *et al*, 2005) is for precisely the cases that are found in hospital paediatric and child development departments: children with medical ill health, intellectual disabilities, developmental disorders, autism-spectrum disorders, self-harm, child abuse and comorbid cases. Between a quarter and a half of children in paediatric out-patient clinics have conditions in which psychological factors play a major role (Lask, 1994). Only a quarter of such children are likely to have received any CAMHS help (Glazebrook *et al*,

2003). The children's NSF recommended paediatric liaison (Department of Health, 2004), and the report on the implementation of Standard 9 of that NSF (Department of Health, 2006) outlines the need for CAMHS paediatric liaison as 'an essential service for the ill child, siblings, parents and carers in cases where the presenting illness has a psychological component, or where psychological distress is caused as a result of the illness'. The case for paediatric liaison is increasingly supported by evidence (Academy of Medical Royal Colleges & Royal College of Psychiatrists, 2009) and NHS policy, yet it is far from universally provided or widely understood (Kraemer, 2009). The benefits of paediatric liaison are summarised in Box 16.1.

Establishing a liaison team

For a paediatric liaison team to be successful, it must have commitment from paediatric services, CAMHS and, where possible, from hospital Social Services. The support of senior people in these various organisations ('top of the office ownership') is essential for the endeavour to be successful. Social work collaboration is vital, since there will be social or safeguarding concerns about a significant proportion of paediatric patients with complex needs (Ford *et al*, 2007). A starting discussion between interested representatives from services and disciplines should clarify the potential benefits of regular liaison, anticipating the complexity of service involvement whenever psychosocial issues are taken seriously. From the start it has to be clear who is to own such involvement and who will

---

Box 16.1 Advantages of liaison between paediatric services and CAMHS

- Better outcomes for children and young people
- A greater understanding of the respective services (Brown & Cooper, 1987; Cottrell & Worrall, 1995)
- Benefits for children and families referred to both services (Schwamm & Maloney, 1997)
- Development of a common understanding and common language relating to the psychosocial aspects of physical illness (Vandvik, 1994), for both career professionals and trainees
- Greater ability to put family and psychological issues on the agenda (Bingley *et al*, 1980)
- Mental health professionals are kept up to date with paediatric issues (Leslie, 1992)
- The sharing of ideas (Mattson, 1976)
- Opportunities for consultation (Jellenik *et al*, 1981), liaison and the regulation of workload between services (Black *et al*, 1990)
- Excellent training opportunities for new staff
- Greater sophistication and better morale in paediatric and associated staff

---

lead the discussion of its mutual benefits with their staff to ensure their commitment and interest.

Although paediatricians want to have better mental health services, there may be some mutual misunderstanding. Child and adolescent mental disorders are disturbing, both because emotional and behavioural symptoms may seem willful and also because they often include concerns about parenting or safeguarding children. Children and families may be reluctant to discuss emotional or mental health concerns with paediatricians (Briggs-Gowan *et al*, 2000).

Multidisciplinary liaison meetings are often the most useful forum for liaison staff to work with paediatric services. Exploratory discussions should address the following.

- Who will meet? Should there be one large meeting for medical and nursing staff, and other specialists such as speech and language therapists, physiotherapists, ward teachers, occupational therapists and liaison health visitors? Alternatively, it may be useful for specific disciplines or teams to have separate meeting times that could include, for example, specific liaison meetings for services in paediatric oncology, haematology (Woodgate & Garralda, 2006), paediatric surgical wards (Geist, 1977), nephrology services (North & Eminson, 1998) or paediatric intensive care units (Kasper & Nyamathi, 1988).

- When will it be best to meet to ensure that as many relevant professionals are able to attend as possible? During busy working days it may be hard to find a mutually agreed time, hence building on fora that already exist could be most economical. A useful model may be for the liaison team to join the paediatric team towards the end of their weekly ward round, when the team are already together and issues are fresh in their minds (Black *et al*, 1999).

- What is the purpose of the paediatric liaison meeting and are the staff of both services committed to that purpose? Clarifying the purposes of the team in an operational policy will be helpful. One primary task of multidisciplinary review meetings is to share impressions and information about clinical cases. This improves collective understanding and reduces the risk of splits between staff.

- How will the meeting be structured to allow maximum benefit for those attending, but ensuring that sufficient time is allocated to discuss complex problems? Any work discussion group should have a clear starting and finishing time and be chaired by an individual whose authority is accepted by staff. All colleagues, especially the most junior and inexperienced, should feel supported in expressing concerns, even when these are not yet clearly understood or articulated. In order to encourage free discussion, it is necessary to emphasise confidentiality and to keep a record only when decisions are made.

- What evaluation or audit processes will be used to assess the functioning of the paediatric liaison service? Whatever criteria are used, some measures of staff development and cohesion should be included.

- What records of discussions and agreed actions will be kept? Decisions about individual children may be recorded in the children's notes, but the paediatric liaison team may wish to keep a record of the themes of consultations without attributing observations to specific individuals so as to preserve confidentiality. Policy matters will require separate documentation, possibly by continual updating of the operational policy. It will need to be clear who has responsibility for such recording.

Structure of the paediatric liaison team

If there is agreement and commitment to the development of a paediatric liaison team, as with all Tier 3 teams described in this handbook, it should be multidisciplinary. In practice, the size and make-up of the team will depend on:

- the local catchment population;
- the nature of the local paediatric service (e.g. does it have specialist regional responsibility or facilities);
- the expertise, experience, interests and availability of staff within the local CAMHS. Acute NHS trusts are at liberty to recruit suitably experienced CAMHS staff to their hospitals and clinics;
- the will of service commissioners to have a paediatric liaison mental health service. The principal pressure to establish or develop liaison teams must come from paediatricians themselves (in collaboration with CAMHS). Neither national guidance nor published evidence will alone impress commissioners.

Similarly, the model of management varies from service to service. Some teams exist as Tier 3 teams within generic CAMHS, some are stand-alone services. Many services separate self-harm assessments (see Chapter 17) from other types of paediatric liaison. Some paediatric services fund individual professionals (e.g. psychologists) to work within certain clinics or on the wards. New paediatric liaison services should be judged against criteria such as multidisciplinary working, integration with existing services, the avoidance of professional isolation, continuing professional development needs, systems that leave no gaps in services, and good supervision and management structures.

The core liaison professions may include primary mental health, psychiatry, psychology, child mental health nursing, child psychotherapy, family therapy, occupational therapy and social work, but others may be co-opted. Not all multidisciplinary services will include all disciplines, but no liaison team should be newly commissioned as a unidisciplinary provision. It is recommended that the team includes a psychiatrist, essential when psychosis or threat of suicide or homicide presents itself. Understanding medical jargon can be useful, but all team members develop this. All team members' expertise and contribution should be valued, with efforts made to prevent any discipline associating too powerfully with their counterpart in the other team (perhaps most likely to occur between doctors). Each profession has special skills, many of them gained in the hospital over time, but also have much in common, so teamwork is flexible. Many staff will be part time, with posts in other areas of child and adolescent/family services. Research and training are part of the liaison task. Where services have been historically commissioned piece-meal, the integration of CAMHS input to paediatric services is desirable to create a healthy system and to avoid rivalry.

Services are often based on different geographical sites, and strategies such as those described in Box 16.2 are required to foster relationships between services.

Effects of a paediatric liaison team

Box 16.3 gives clinical scenarios where children may benefit from good cooperation between paediatric services and CAMHS.

More referrals and fewer referrals

Patterns of referral and usage of CAMHS by paediatric professionals change after the establishment of a paediatric liaison team (Black *et al*, 1999). Inter-service discussion provides new ideas and support for those already involved with families and may avert the need for formal CAMHS involvement. There should be no barrier, such as a referral protocol, to informal enquiries to the liaison team. Paediatric and associated staff should be encouraged to converse with the liaison team about any case they are concerned or curious about, even when these concerns are not clear or when mental health problems do not seem particularly prominent (Kraemer, 2008). Liaison staff also have a role in discussing ethical questions, for example in the treatment

---

Box 16.2 Strategies of liaison

- Establishment of a formal paediatric liaison team within the CAMHS
- A date, time and place when the paediatric liaison team meets with the paediatric multidisciplinary team to consult, liaise, discuss cases and refer between the two services
- Transfer of staff (nursing or medical) from one environment to the other on secondment or by mutual arrangement
- Attendance of CAMHS members at the paediatric grand ward round or educational meetings to discuss patients and topics of mutual interest.
- Telephone or email between teams, either at specified times or on an open-access basis

Box 16.3 Presentations in paediatrics where liaison is necessary or likely to be helpful

- Self-harm
- Stress causing or exacerbating physical symptoms (e.g. headaches, abdominal pain)
- Acute psychiatric disturbance
- Chronic illness such as diabetes, epilepsy, neurological disorder, asthma, rheumatic disorder, chronic anaemias
- Life-limiting illnesses such as cancers, cystic fibrosis, neurodegenerative and metabolic disorders
- Children who have mixed presentations of physical and emotional symptoms (e.g. Huntington's disease, eating disorders)
- Child protection including situations where the mental health or functioning of parents is a factor (the extreme case being induced or factitious illness)
- Intellectual disabilities with complex presentations
- Drug or alcohol misuse
- Disorders with a need for complex rehabilitative interventions (e.g. chronic fatigue syndrome)
- Somatisation, conversion disorder and other physical presentations with psychosocial aetiology
- Psychological or psychiatric presentations associated with physical illness (e.g. encephalitis, Paediatric Autoimmune Neuropsychiatric Disorders Associated with Streptococcal infection (PANDAS))
- Post-traumatic stress after trauma or injury
- Attachment and its impact upon physical presentation and care
- Psychological aspects of perinatal care
- Developmental problems including psychosocial or communicative delay (e.g. autism-spectrum disorders)
- Sensory impairments
- Family dynamics and health decision-making

of dying children. Discussion with the liaison team should be helpful in itself and may lead to increased paediatric confidence in managing the case, with or without a subsequent referral to the liaison team. It may also indicate that another agency may be more helpful to the child and family, and so ensure that referrals are directed to the most relevant services. Social Services, educational services, health visitors and speech and language therapists may be able to meet the child's needs better than the CAMHS, although a full multidisciplinary liaison discussion may be necessary to clarify this. A clearer understanding of CAMHS functioning by paediatric professionals, as a result of working with a liaison service, means greater use of specialist resources such as the CAMHS Tier 3 teams. Similarly, there may be more referrals for psychosomatic problems (Black *et al*, 1999), reflecting an increased awareness of the biological and psychosocial factors involved with many children in paediatric services.

Urgent cases

Good relationships help to facilitate the process of urgent referrals in both directions through understanding and discussion of each other's priorities. It means that at least one member of the liaison team staff must be readily available from CAMHS whether or not they are on site.

Unlike the case in adult psychiatry where acutely ill patients are seen directly by mental health staff, many acutely disturbed young people will first present to health services at hospital emergency departments, from where they may be admitted to a paediatric ward for examination and investigation. This pathway is not widely understood, yet is necessary to exclude organic or metabolic causes for their illness, to allow for social work exploration in many cases, and because there are hardly any child and adolescent psychiatric beds directly accessible from hospital emergency departments (Cotgrove *et al*, 2007). When it is required, arranging the admission of children and young people to specialist psychiatric units itself requires the specialist knowledge and skills of the liaison team, including familiarity with the Mental Health Act. Audit of the numbers of urgent referrals can lead to time being allocated prospectively to deal with the work generated.

Joint working

Regular liaison between CAMHS and paediatric professionals permits the integration of psychosocial, psychological and physical interventions. This is particularly helpful with children who have a chronic condition such as diabetes, epilepsy, asthma or cystic fibrosis, for which joint clinics run by the paediatric staff with a member of the paediatric liaison team may be considered. In general, co-location of CAMHS in the paediatric department is an advantage: 'The team is situated within the paediatric unit to allow easy and prompt referral and access' (Department of Health, 2006). Informal contacts ('corridor consultations') can occur frequently, encouraging familiarity and mutual learning between colleagues. The NSF encourages joint work and in-house CAMHS liaison, although ensuring the commissioning and providing the space for such services is not straightforward (Department of Health, 2006). By its very nature, paediatric liaison tends always to be marginalised in health policies. Although the principles are clear, there is no detailed advice for commissioners nor any guidance as to who should fund these services. Paediatrics may assume that CAMHS will pay, and vice versa. It has been suggested that 'Commissioners of paediatric services and CAMHS collaborate to ensure that a Paediatric Liaison service is provided with agreed apportioning of costs to the relevant budgets' (Department of Health, 2006).

Ownership of the liaison service includes responsibility for funding and managing it, and providing physical and administrative resources for the work of the team.

Cooperation and mutual respect

Established paediatric liaison provides opportunities for two-way learning, both for professionals in training and for qualified staff (Leslie, 1992). Respect for various working models enriches the quality of service to young people and their families. Where needs are jointly highlighted, ventures such as training workshops, presentations and other multi-agency forums are more easily organised (Williams *et al*, 1999). 'Child and adolescent mental health is part of the core training for all nurses, paediatricians, social workers and teachers' (Department of Health, 2006).

Multi-agency assessment

Joint assessments will be required in complex cases whether to clarify a child's psychosocial needs or as part of a more formal statutory assessment (Sturge, 1989). Joint assessment of specific conditions such as ADHD (Voeller, 1991), autism (Keen & Ward, 2004), chronic fatigue syndrome (Wright & Beverley, 1998; Garralda & Rangel, 2006) and psychosomatic illness (Dungar *et al*, 1986) should ensure integrated care packages that diminish the risk of parallel and even contradictory interventions from different agencies. Although now routinely recommended in all government policies, 'working together' is much more complicated than it appears. Even the most skilled professionals can get caught up in interagency struggles that may on occasion have some resonance with those of the family being treated. This phenomenon is most marked in cases of serious child abuse (Reder *et al*, 1994), but also occurs when the diagnosis is not clear or where there are ethical, moral or religious disagreements about treatment.

Paediatric liaison and staff support

Many families may resist referral of their child to a mental health professional. An alternative and helpful model is to see the paediatrician as the one requiring help with an insoluble problem (Kraemer, 2008). Aside from the obvious provision of advice to clinicians and services for children and families, another process that CAMHS professionals may facilitate for paediatric colleagues is that of staff support. Serious illness and death in children are very stressful to deal with on a day-to-day basis. Affording containment and support and enhancing coping in those who work in this context is no easy job in itself. Like the rest of paediatric liaison, the task is best undertaken in the context of an ongoing relationship with the paediatric team, and can be delivered individually or in work discussion groups, and on a regular or *ad hoc* basis.

The CAMHS ideal way of doing things (planned, holistic, systemic, timely, reflective) is often at odds with the necessarily event-driven nature of paediatrics, but can be complementary to this style by allowing the opportunity to think about things differently in a contained way. Some paediatric colleagues may well derive support from liaison with CAMHS in other, more indirect, ways. It is likely that if a culture is encouraged where to accept support is seen as a strength (rather than a weakness), more people are likely to avail themselves of it. Some useful strategies for staff support are listed in Box 16.4.

Paediatric liaison in other settings

The opportunities for CAMHS professionals to work with paediatric professionals outside formal paediatric liaison settings include the following.

- Multidisciplinary, multi-agency forums for discussing children with autism-spectrum disorders.
- Multidisciplinary work in child protection.
- Meetings set up to discuss children with complex needs where child health problems (mental or physical) are affecting educational or social functioning, at which representatives from agencies such as school, health and education may be required, in addition to paediatric and CAMHS staff, to discuss, with parental or carer permission, how best to help young people (Williams *et al*, 1999).
- The assessment of children whose needs cross boundaries between child mental health and Social Services (Wheeler *et al*, 1998).
- Jointly run bereavement and palliative care services (see Chapter 22).
- On-the-spot teaching from CAMHS members in joint clinics (Williams, 1983).

Box 16.4 Useful approaches and skills in staff support

- Flexibility in approach
- Non-judgemental stance – accepting that paediatric nurses and doctors are not mental health staff and that their different approach to assessment or treatment may be entirely appropriate to the context
- Active listening – rather than leaping to direct advice too quickly
- Getting a detailed story; 'what precisely happened?' not just 'how did you feel about it?' (the latter naturally follows from the narrative in most cases)
- Facilitating reflection as well as problem-solving
- Understanding rather than confronting or criticising. This can be achieved by positive connotation, often demonstrated by highlighting the staff's motivation (e.g. a professional's desire to protect a child from harm or humiliation) rather than focusing on actions of which the liaison clinician feels critical
- Encouraging team-based problem-solving (but not do it for them too readily)
- Ability to accept different professional styles – the model of multidisciplinary/ professional team working may not be the same as CAMHS

Child and adolescent mental health staff in hospitals also have a role beyond the care of paediatric patients:

- in the assessment and care of child patients in the hospital who have been seriously injured or burned or who have had major surgical interventions
- the children of parents disabled by chronic or terminal illnesses who are patients elsewhere in the hospital
- the newborn infants of mothers with perinatal anxiety or depression
- children of adults with serious mental illness if their treatment is taking place on the same campus.

Conclusion

Paediatric services and CAMHS overlap in their client groups and must work together to ensure that the children they serve have an integrated service in which their mental health needs are understood by their paediatric carers and their physical needs are understood by the CAMHS. Both everyday clinical work and statutory work involve paediatric as well as CAMHS staff. They will work more efficiently to the benefit of their patients if there are formal working arrangements, for which a paediatric liaison service provides a firm foundation.

References

Academy of Medical Royal Colleges & Royal College of Psychiatrists (2009) *No Health without Mental Health. The ALERT Summary Report*. Academy of Medical Royal Colleges.

Bingley, L., Leonard, J., Hensman, S., *et al* (1980) The comprehensive management of children on a paediatric ward – a family approach. *Archives of Disease in Childhood*, **55**, 555–561.

Black, D., McFadyen, A. & Broster, G. (1990) Development of a psychiatric liaison service. *Archives of Disease in Childhood*, **65**, 1373–1375.

Black, D., Wright, B., Williams, C., *et al* (1999) Paediatric liaison service. *Psychiatric Bulletin*, **23**, 528–530.

Briggs-Gowan, M. J., Horwitz, S. M., Schwab-Stone, M. E., *et al* (2000) Mental health in pediatric settings: distribution of disorders and factors related to service use. *Journal of the American Academy of Child and Adolescent Psychiatry*, **39**, 841–849.

Brown, A. & Cooper, A. F. (1987) The impact of a liaison psychiatry service on patterns of referral in a general hospital. *British Journal of Psychiatry*, **150**, 83–87.

Cotgrove, A., McLoughlin, R., O'Herlihy, A., *et al* (2007) The ability of adolescent psychiatric units to accept emergency admissions: changes in England and Wales between 2000 and 2005. *Psychiatric Bulletin*, **31**, 457–459.

Cottrell, D. & Worrall, A. (1995) Liaison child and adolescent psychiatry. *Advances in Psychiatric Treatment*, **1**, 78–85.

Department for Children, Schools and Families (2003) *Every Child Matters*. TSO (The Stationery Office)

Department of Health (2004) *Getting the Right Start: National Service Framework for Children. Standard for Hospital Services*. TSO (The Stationery Office).

Department of Health (2006) *Promoting the Mental Health and Psychological Well-Being of Children and Young People. Report on the Implementation of Standard 9 of the National Service Framework for Children, Young People and Maternity Services*. TSO (The Stationery Office).

Dungar, D., Pritchard, J., Hensman, S., *et al* (1986) The investigation of atypical psychosomatic illness: a team approach to diagnosis. *Clinical Pediatrics*, **25**, 341–344.

Ford, T., Vostanis, P., Meltzer, H., *et al* (2007) Psychiatric disorder among British children looked after by local authorities: comparison with children living in private households. *British Journal of Psychiatry*, **190**, 319–325.

Garralda, E. & Rangel, L. (2006) Paediatric Liaison work by child and adolescent mental health services. *Child and Adolescent Mental Health*, **11**, 19–24.

Garralda, M. & Bailey, D. (1989) Psychiatric disorders in general paediatric referrals. *Archives of Disease in Childhood*, **64**, 1727–1733.

Geist, R. (1977) Consultation on a pediatric surgical ward. *American Journal of Orthopsychiatry*, **47**, 432–444.

Glazebrook, C., Hollis, C., Heussler, C., *et al* (2003) Detecting emotional and behavioural problems in paediatric clinics. *Child: Care, Health and Development*, **29**, 141–149.

Green, H., McGinnity, A., Meltzer, H., *et al* (2004) *Mental Health of Children and Young People in Great Britain, 2004*. Palgrave MacMillan.

Hysing, M., Elgen, I., Gillberg, G., *et al* (2007) Chronic physical illness and mental health in children. Results from a large-scale population study. *Journal of Child Psychology and Psychiatry*, **48**, 785–792.

Jellenik, M., Herzog, D. & Selter, F. (1981) A psychiatric consultation service for hospitalised children. *Psychosomatics*, **22**, 27–33.

Kasper, J. & Nyamathi, A. (1988) Parents of children in the pediatric intensive care unit: what are their needs? *Heart and Lung*, **17**, 574–581.

Keen, D. & Ward, S. (2004) Autistic spectrum disorder. *Autism*, **8**, 39–48.

Kraemer, S. (2008) Paediatric liaison. *Psychiatry*, **7**, 371–374.

Kraemer, S. (2009) 'The menace of psychiatry': does it still ring a bell? *Archives of Disease in Childhood*, **94**, 570–572.

Lask, B. (1994) Paediatric liaison work. In *Child and Adolescent Psychiatry: Modern Approaches* (eds M. Rutter, E. Taylor & L. Hersov), pp. 996–1005. Blackwell Scientific.

Leslie, S. A. (1992) Paediatric liaison. *Archives of Disease in Children*, **67**, 1046–1049.

Mattson, A. (1976) Child psychiatric ward rounds on pediatrics. *Journal of the American Academy of Child Psychiatry*, **15**, 357–365.

North, C. & Eminson, M. (1998) A review of a psychiatry–nephrology liaison service. *European Child and Adolescent Psychiatry*, **7**, 235–245.

Potter, R., Langley, K. & Sakhuja, D. (2005) All things to all people: what referrers want from their child and adolescent mental health service. *Psychiatric Bulletin*, **29**, 262–265.

Reder, P., Duncan, S., Gray, M., *et al* (1994) *Beyond Blame*. Routledge.

Schwamm, J. S. & Maloney, M. J. (1997) Developing a psychiatry study group for community paediatricians. *Journal of the American Academy of Child and Adolescent Psychiatry*, **36**, 706–708.

Slowik, M. & Noronha, S. (2004) Need for child mental health consultation and paediatricians perception of these services. *Child and Adolescent Mental Health*, **9**, 121–124.

Sturge, J. (1989) Joint work in paediatrics: a child psychiatry perspective. *Archives of Disease in Childhood*, **64**, 155–158.

Vandvik, I. H. (1994) Collaboration between child psychiatry and paediatrics: the state of the relationship in Norway. *Acta Paediatrica*, **83**, 884–887.

Voeller, K. K. (1991) Clinical management of attention deficit hyperactivity disorder. *Journal of Child Neurology*, **6**(suppl.), S51–S67.

Wheeler, J., Bone, D. & Smith, J. (1998) Whole day assessments: a team approach to complex multi-problem families. *Clinical Child Psychology and Psychiatry*, **3**, 169–181.

Williams, J. (1983) Teaching how to counsel in a pediatric clinic. *Journal of the American Academy of Child Psychiatry*, **22**, 399–403.

Williams, C., Wright, B. & Smith, R. (1999) CHEAF (Child Health and Education Assessment Forum): a multidisciplinary powwow for children. *Psychiatric Bulletin*, **23**, 104–106.

Woodgate, M. & Garralda, M. (2006) Paediatric liaison work by child and adolescent mental health services. *Child and Adolescent Mental Health*, **11**, 19–24.

Wright, J. B. & Beverley, D. W. (1998) Chronic fatigue syndrome. *Archives of Disease in Childhood*, **79**, 368–374.

CHAPTER 17

Self-harm

Sophie Roberts, Phil Lucas, Barry Wright
and Greg Richardson

'It isn't as if there was anything wonderful about my little corner. Of course for people who like cold, wet, ugly bits it is something rather special, but otherwise it's just a corner.'

A. A. Milne, *The House at Pooh Corner*

Introduction

Suicide has long been recognised as a societal phenomenon as well as an individual one (Durkheim, 1970) and national strategies have been developed to address this (Department of Health, 2002).

Approximately 7–14% of adolescents harm themselves at some point; 20% will think seriously about it (Madge *et al*, 2008; O'Connor *et al* 2009), representing a considerable workload for CAMHS, both numerically and in terms of the risk posed and anxiety generated, and it is recognised that many such young people do not even reach the attention of health services (Hawton & Rodham, 2006). The most common forms of self-harm are cutting, scoring, scratching, overdosing and less commonly burning or punching. Most young people describe that they self-harm to forget about stress, relieve anxiety and, less commonly, to kill themselves (Young *et al*, 2007).

Most are not suffering from mental illness, although it is the responsibility of CAMHS to assess and treat these young people, as well as the anxiety engendered in others. Around 0.5–1% of young people who present following an episode of self-harm complete suicide, and 40% of those who survive a first attempt will repeat it; CAMHS should aim to reduce these figures.

Such young people may be referred to a CAMHS at a number of points in the cycle of self-harm (Box 17.1). Clinical and epidemiological information is readily available to inform practice in the management of self-harm (Rutter, 1990; Kerfoot *et al*, 1996; Meltzer *et al*, 2001; Wood *et al*, 2001; Gould *et al*, 2003; Fox & Hawton, 2004).

Providing a service

The assessment of the young person who has primarily self-harmed should be regarded as part of the everyday work of CAMHS. A speedy response can help alleviate anxieties. Competence, calmness and clarity

---

Box 17.1 Referral routes

- From a GP or other professional who is concerned about the possibility of self-harm because of stated intent or a history of self-harm, although less than a tenth of self-harm referrals to CAMHS come in this way (Nadkarni *et al*, 2000)
- From the emergency department soon after an episode of self-harm
- From a hospital ward after admission for self-harm
- After discharge from hospital following an episode of self-harm
- For in-patient care because of recurrent self-harm, serious suicidal intent or a life-threatening suicidal attempt

---

of thinking is more important than the professional background of the assessor. National Institute for Health and Clinical Excellence guidance (National Collaborating Centre for Mental Health, 2004) states that assessments should be undertaken by a healthcare practitioner working in CAMHS. Most services now have a multidisciplinary team that undertake assessments under the supervision of senior clinicians. Some services still rely on psychiatrists, junior and senior, to undertake the assessment, although this is not always logical since junior doctors on placement in CAMHS are likely to have least experience of working with young people and families. National Institute for Health and Clinical Excellence guidance (National Collaborating Centre for Mental Health, 2004) is clear that the professionals who undertake these assessments must be skilled in risk assessment and it is recommended that they receive regular supervision of this work as well as having access to consultation with a senior colleague.

Although there has been a drive for CAMHS to work on a preventative strategy for self-harm, the evidence for efficacy is limited. Prevention becomes problematic when suicidal ideation is relatively common among adolescents, with around 15% having these thoughts (Hawton & Rodham, 2006), and precipitating events are often non-specific, acts are often impulsive, and secrecy and denial are common.

Assessment and management

Child and adolescent mental health services, emergency departments and paediatric services should have a clear, mutually agreed protocol for treating these young people (Box 17.2) that ensures a clear and rapid care pathway. All young people who self-harm should be properly assessed and treated, including triage by children's health professionals who have received training in mental health issues.

National guidance (Royal College of Psychiatrists, 1998; National Collaborating Centre for Mental Health, 2004) recommends that all

---

Box 17.2 Treating those who self-harm

- Full psychosocial assessment
- Formulation of recent events (acute, chronic, behavioural disturbance)
- Mental state examination
- Comprehensive risk assessment
- Strategies for prevention of recurrence
- Intervention and follow-up
- Liaison with families and relevant agencies
- Preparation and provision of reports

---

children and young people (under 16) who self-harm should be admitted to hospital after they have self-harmed for:

- assessment of mental state, both by ward staff observing over a period of time and by a visiting member of CAMHS;
- time to obtain further information, from family, school, GP and Social Services. About a third of young people who self-harm and present in the emergency department are not accompanied by close family, and a fifth present on their own (Nadkarni *et al*, 2000);
- a cooling-off period for the young person and family, particularly where family breakdown has occurred (this may produce the opportunity for discussion of the reasons for the episode; conversely, it may allow time for the reasons to be repressed and not disclosed, potentially leading to a further episode of self-harm);
- observation of medical condition, particularly with respect to those who may have lied about the severity or nature of self-harm;
- time for professionals to engage with the young person and family or carers to smooth the path for any further care;
- time to set up an intervention package (e.g. medical treatment, family meeting, psychosocial follow-up, Social Services involvement, school involvement).

As CAMHS nationally provide for young people up to their 18th birthday, protocols with medical services may need to be re-negotiated as most paediatric departments only work up to 16, and medical teams may be reluctant to admit young people seen to be medically fit for discharge. It remains best practice for these young people to be admitted if they agree, for the reasons listed above.

The aims of assessment are the following.

- Assessment of continuing risk which is based on the circumstances of the self-harm such as planning and steps taken to avoid discovery, as well as the presence of ongoing suicidal ideation or plans. The objective circumstances of the act are a much less accurate indicator of suicidal intent than in adults due to cognitive immaturity and impulsivity. The subjective account of the episode should be given relatively more weight. In particular, questions about whether the young person believes they took enough tablets or engaged in a harmful act that might kill them and whether if they intended to die they believe that this is a permanent state, are often useful.

- Assessment of presence or absence of current mental illness through a full mental state examination is necessary, although only a minority of those who self-harm are suffering from mental illness. An episode of self-harm without an apparent trigger should increase the assessor's suspicion of a mental illness.

- Assessment of reasons for the event – the 'message in a bottle' (Kingsbury, 1993) – as most episodes of self-harm have a trigger, the majority of which involve an episode of interpersonal conflict. This is often described by the young person as 'the last straw', which although 'it breaks the camel's back' is neither necessarily the heaviest nor most important. A full psychosocial assessment will help to identify underlying more chronic difficulties.

An assessment must be mindful of confidentiality issues and include consideration of the capacity of the young person in this area. Care must also be taken to consider possible child protection concerns and involvement of the relevant statutory services should be considered.

Some services use a formal risk assessment, tools either specific (Kreitman & Foster, 1991) or more general (www.facecode.com). These tools are not adequately positively discriminating, however, and the concept of risk as a continuum (Rose, 1992) is a useful one, encouraging consideration of all relevant factors as outlined above. Most services will have organisation-wide risk assessment tools which should be used.

Strategies for the prevention of recurrence

Intervention and follow-up

Plans for discharge should involve family or carers wherever possible and include initial plans for managing safety. It is often useful to supply the family with emergency contact numbers for CAMHS plus other organisations such as Samaritans and Childline if necessary.

An early follow-up appointment is important and it is now enshrined within NICE guidelines that this should be within 7 days of the episode. Non-attendance rates for routine out-patient clinic attendances are high for this population but can be improved by community-based contact delivered where possible by the initial assessor. Although there is an increasing amount of research into interventions for young people, few studies demonstrate a robust efficacy of enhanced psychosocial intervention (Crawford *et al* 2007). Some smaller studies do show evidence of possible benefit.

- Developmental group psychotherapy (Wood *et al*, 2001) using principles of dialectics.
- Cognitive–behavioural therapy aimed at reducing self-harming behaviours (Slee *et al*, 2008).
- Cognitive analytic therapeutic assessment and treatment model (Ougrin *et al*, 2008).
- Improving social skills, problem-solving skills and care-seeking behaviours (Schotte & Clum, 1987; Lerner & Clum, 1990; Salkovskis *et al*, 1990; McLeavey *et al*, 1994).
- Family interventions (Kerfoot *et al*, 1995; Harrington *et al*, 1998).
- Multisystemic therapy (Huey *et al*, 2004), a community-based treatment using an intensive home-based model of service delivery.
- Networking and advice to other agencies that plan or run crisis hotlines (Evans *et al*, 1999), educational programmes (e.g. school or media-based).
- Opportunity restriction strategies.

Suggestions for enhancing service provision more generally are given in Box 17.3.

Child and adolescent mental health services are sometimes asked to become involved when parents or carers have self-harmed, and this requires CAMHS to work closely with colleagues in adult mental health services and Social Services. Similarly, the consequences of parental suicide may require CAMHS involvement (Wright & Partridge, 1999).

Recording

Episodes of self-harm should all be recorded by all involved departments, partly in order to monitor practice. Such data may be collected in the emergency department or by a paediatric liaison health visitor. Paediatric wards and night admission wards attached to the emergency department should also keep figures of admissions for self-harm. These figures should correlate with the referrals to CAMHS owing to self-harming behaviour. A regular audit should be conducted into the flow of young people through

---

Box 17.3 Enhancing service provision

- Development of a Tier 3 self-harm team, which can take responsibility for assessment and the delivery of comprehensive management packages
- Consultation and training for other professionals concerned in the care of children who may self-harm
- Advice on the prevention of suicide or further self-harm
- Input into the planning of services for those who self-harm
- Planning organisational change to maximise effectiveness
- Auditing the care and experience of young people who self-harm

the system to ensure they all receive a service, as, historically, not all children who self-harm are referred to a CAMHS for assessment (Davies & Ames, 1998; Hurry & Storey, 2000).

Teaching and training on the management of self-harm

Members of CAMHS assessing young people who have self-harmed will require initial training to recognise the factors associated with self-harm (Kerfoot et al, 1996) and in risk assessment. They will subsequently need supervision to discuss their findings and management plans. Child and adolescent mental health service members may be part of paediatric liaison teams and this will allow for discussion of young people who have self-harmed with colleagues working in general hospital settings, which will also extend the psychological training of those working in such settings.

Conclusion

Sadly, we have no hard evidence that mental health assessments and monitoring by mental health professionals of those who self-harm by overdosing, cutting or other physical damage produce a better prognosis, and few have a mental disorder. Child and adolescent mental health services are therefore primarily used for their anxiety-relieving capacities for parents, carers and other involved professionals. However, self-harm is often the only way out for young people who find themselves in intolerable situations, and a mental health professional is likely to be the best informed and skilled person to help them cope and deal with their predicament.

References

Crawford, M. J., Thomas, O., Khan, N., et al (2007) Psychosocial interventions following self-harm. Systematic review of their efficacy in preventing suicide. British Journal of Psychiatry, 190, 11–17.

Davies, G. & Ames, S. (1998) Adolescents referred following overdose. Support for Hawton's classification and the role of a primary child and adolescent mental health worker. Psychiatric Bulletin, 22, 359–361.

Department of Health (2002) National Suicide Prevention Strategy for England: Consultation Document. Department of Health.

Durkheim, E. (1970) Suicide – A Study in Sociology. Routledge & Keegan Paul.

Evans, M. O., Morgan, H. G., Hayward, A., et al (1999) Crisis telephone consultation for deliberate self-harm patients: effects on repetition. British Journal of Psychiatry, 175, 23–27.

Fox, C. & Hawton, K. (2004) Deliberate Self-Harm in Adolescence. Jessica Kingsley.

Gould, M., Greenberg, T., Velting, D. M., et al (2003) Youth suicide risk and preventive interventions: a review of the past ten years. Journal of the American Academy of Child and Adolescent Psychiatry, 42, 386–405.

Harrington, R., Kerfoot, M., Dyer, E., et al (1998) Randomised trial of a home based family intervention for children who have deliberately poisoned themselves. Journal of the American Academy of Child and Adolescent Psychiatry, 37, 512–518.

Hawton, K. & Rodham, K. (2006) By Their Own Young Hand. Deliberate Self Harm and Suicidal Ideas in Adolescemts. Jessica Kingsley.

Huey, S., Hengeller, S., Rowland, M., *et al* (2004) Multi systemic therapy effects on attempted suicide by youths presenting with psychiatric emergencies. *Journal of the American Academy of Child and Adolescent Psychiatry*, **43**, 183–190.

Hurry, J. & Storey, P. (2000) Assessing young people who deliberately harm themselves. *British Journal of Psychiatry*, **176**, 126–131.

Kerfoot, M., Harrington, R. & Dyer, E. (1995) Brief home-based intervention with young suicide attempters and their families. *Journal of Adolescence*, **18**, 557–568.

Kerfoot, M., Dyer, E., Harrington, V., *et al* (1996) Correlates and short-term course of self-poisoning in adolescents. *British Journal of Psychiatry*, **168**, 38–42.

Kingsbury, S. J. (1993) Parasuicide in adolescence: a message in a bottle. *Association for Child Psychology and Psychiatry Review and Newsletter*, **15**, 253–259.

Kreitman, N. & Foster, J. (1991) The construction and selection of predictive scales, with special reference to parasuicide. *British Journal of Psychiatry*, **15**, 185–192.

Lerner, M. S. & Clum, G. A. (1990) Treatment of suicide ideators: a problem-solving approach. *Behavioral Therapy*, **21**, 403–411.

Madge, N., Hewitt, A., Hawton, K., *et al* (2008) Deliberate self-harm within an international community sample of young people: comparative findings from Child and Adolescent Self-Harm in Europe (CASE) Study. *Journal of Child Psychology and Psychiatry*, **49**, 66–77.

McLeavey, B. C., Daly, R. J., Ludgate, J. W., *et al* (1994) Interpersonal problem-solving skills training in the treatment of self-poisoning patients. *Suicide and Life-Threatening Behaviour*, **24**, 382–394.

Meltzer, H., Harrington, R., Goodman, R., et al (2001) *Children and Adolescents who try to Harm, Hurt or Kill Themselves*. Office for National Statistics.

Nadkarni, A., Parkin, A., Dogra, N., *et al* (2000) Characteristics of children and adolescents presenting to accident and emergency departments with deliberate self harm. *Emergency Medical Journal*, **17**, 98–102.

National Collaborating Centre for Mental Health (2004) *The Short-Term Physical and Psychological Management and Secondary Prevention of Self-Harm In Primary and Secondary Care. Clinical Guideline CG16*. National Institute for Health and Clinical Excellence.

O'Connor, R., Rasmussen, S., Miles, J., *et al* (2009) Self-harm in adolescents: self-report survey in schools in Scotland. *British Journal of Psychiatry*, **194**, 68–72.

Ougrin, D., Ng, A. V. & Low, J. (2008) Therapeutic assessment based on cognitive–analytic therapy for young people presenting with self-harm: pilot study. *Psychiatric Bulletin*, **32**, 423–426.

Rose, G. (1992) *The Strategy of Preventative Medicine*. Oxford Medical Publications.

Royal College of Psychiatrists (1998) *Managing Deliberate Self Harm in Young People. Council Report CR64*. Royal College of Psychiatrists.

Rutter, M. (1990) Psychosocial resilience and protective factors. In *Risk and Protective Factors in the Development of Psychopathology* (eds J. Rolf, A. S. Masten, D. Cichetti, *et al*), pp. 181–214. Cambridge University Press.

Salkovskis, P. M., Atha, C. & Storer, D. (1990) Cognitive–behavioural problem solving in the treatment of patients who repeatedly attempt suicide. A controlled trial. *British Journal of Psychiatry*, **157**, 871–876.

Schotte, D. E. & Clum, G. A. (1987) Problem-solving skills in suicidal psychiatric patients. *Journal of Consulting and Clinical Psychology*, **55**, 49–54.

Slee, N., Garnefski, N., van der Leeden, R., *et al* (2008) Cognitive–behavioural intervention for self-harm: randomised controlled trial. *British Journal of Psychiatry*, **192**, 202–211.

Wood, A., Trainor, G., Rothwell, J., *et al* (2001) Randomized trial of group therapy for repeated deliberate self-harm in adolescents. *Journal of the American Academy of Child and Adolescent Psychiatry*, **40**, 1246–1253.

Wright, B. & Partridge, I. (1999) Speaking ill of the dead. *Clinical Child Psychology and Psychiatry*, **4**, 225–231.

Young, R., van Beinum, M., Sweeting, H., *et al* (2007) Young people who self-harm. *British Journal of Psychiatry*, **191**, 44–49.

CHAPTER 18

Learning disability services

Christine Williams and Barry Wright

'For the world's more full of weeping than we can understand.'
William Butler Yeats (1865–1939)

Introduction

Approximately 2–3% of the general population has some form of intellectual disability (Department of Health, 2001). The prevalence of severe intellectual disability (IQ <50) is 3–4 per 1000, and that of moderate intellectual disability (IQ 50–70) is 30–40 per 1000 (Felce *et al*, 1994).

There is abundant evidence that children with intellectual disabilities are at significantly increased risk of developing mental health problems (Dykens, 2000; Stromme & Diseth, 2000; Tonge & Einfield, 2000; Emerson, 2003; Whitaker & Read, 2006) and that this affects between 40 and 75% (Corbett, 1985; Gillberg *et al*, 1986; Wallace *et al*, 1995). Emerson & Hatton (2007) estimate that children with intellectual disabilities are six times more likely to have a diagnosable psychiatric condition than other children in Britain. They are also at increased risk of having specific disorders such as autism-spectrum disorders (Fombonne, 1998; Emerson & Hatton, 2007) and ADHD (Dykens, 2000). Mental health services for children and young people with an intellectual disability and their families should therefore be readily available and of a high quality. In the UK, the government (Department of Health, 1992) and the Royal College of Psychiatrists (1992) have long recognised this. Despite this and the fact that Standard 8 of the NSF for children states that Local Authorities, primary care trusts and CAMHS must work together to 'ensure that disabled children have equal access to CAMHS' (Department for Education and Skills & Department of Health, 2004), only 60% of primary care trusts had commissioned CAMHS for young people with intellectual disabilities in June 2006 (Department for Education and Skills & Department of Health, 2006). This chapter may therefore have a practical role to play as commissioners and services seek to address this gap in service provision.

Organisation of services

It is first necessary to decide where mental health services for children and young people with intellectual disabilities will sit organisationally.

169

Historical models often placed such services within all age services for people with intellectual disabilities. It was argued that this gave rise to good continuity of care. In recent times, dedicated children's services have become accepted as more appropriate.

How such services are managed today varies in the UK. They are variously managed within primary care trusts, mental health trusts, children's or community trusts, and acute or paediatric trusts. The crucial factor here is whether they are valued, supported and developed by their host trust and its managers. In making these decisions, each locality must address the service principles outlined in Box 18.1.

Regardless of which trust structure these services exist within, there is also a decision to be made about where within the landscape of CAMHS they should best be placed. Some have argued for Tier 3 teams within existing CAMHS (Wright *et al*, 2008) that provide local accessible services, while others prefer a supra-regional specialist provision. These two are of course not mutually exclusive with potential for having local and more specialist provision: the main obstacle likely to be adequately resourced commissioning.

Service considerations

In developing a service based on the principles set out in Box 18.1, consideration will have to be given to the following.

- The historical situation. Has the service been, traditionally, provided in one setting (e.g. a lifespan service) or does the retirement of a leading professional, such as a consultant, mean that the situation can be reviewed?
- The allocation of resources. Is one service rather than another funded to deliver the service and is it feasible to move those resources? Children with intellectual disability who have no resources to meet their mental health needs require their needs to be made known to those responsible for commissioning health services for them.

Box 18.1 Service principles

- Children with disabilities 'should be provided for as children first and people with a disability second' (McKay & Hall, 1994)
- Services for children with intellectual disabilities must fit into an organised and structured framework
- Service delivery must be sufficiently flexible to ensure multi-agency working, liaison and consultation
- Links with other agencies providing services for these children and their families must be maintained

---

- The management structure of the provider. Services for these children may be provided from different departments or directorates within one trust or from different trusts. The relationships and working practices of the different departments and trusts will have a considerable bearing on how the service is delivered. How can service provision be sensibly coordinated and integrated?
- Is commissioning able to deliver real resources?
- Staff expertise may be based in one department and not in another. Negotiations may then be necessary if staff are to move to another department, or provide training or co-work cases in order to increase expertise.
- Staff working in different areas have different working practices and those practices may have to be addressed if new ways of working in different organisational settings are to be achieved.
- If existing service configurations are to be changed, the arguments for the change must be clear, with tangible benefits for children and their families.
- National guidance and local strategic thinking may well indicate the most useful management organisation.
- As with all CAMHS, accessibility to services for all those requiring them must be a paramount consideration.
- Is staff training, development and retention adequate? Are any professionals dual-trained? How does this impact upon the team and its functioning?

In the light of these considerations, each locality will have to look at the specific advantages and disadvantages of placing the service within CAMHS or learning disability services (Box 18.2).

There are two recent initiatives (Dugmore & Hurcombe, 2007; Pote & Goodban, 2007) which are excellent resources and make sound recommendations for improving services for multi-agency working. They include referral, assessment, intervention and transitional processes.

Work with children with disabilities involves long-term interventions and inter-agency work with large numbers of other professionals. The children frequently have complex needs; interventions can be intricate and time consuming, and families may be difficult to discharge because they have changing ongoing needs (Green et al, 2001). Many parents require time and support in coming to terms with the losses associated with having a child with a permanent disability. Some parents, including those who have intellectual disabilities themselves, need advice throughout the child's developmental stages. In addition, intervention programmes take time to produce relatively small changes.

In order to cope with the huge demands placed on services, strategies for managing workload will have to be considered. These may include:

- keeping to problem-focused, goal-directed work as far as possible

Box 18.2 The placement of a service for children with an intellectual disability and a mental health problem

Advantages of being within learning disability services
- Staff are trained and experienced in dealing with people with intellectual disabilities across all ages and are familiar with the disorders from which they suffer
- There is continuity of care for young people as they become adults and they do not have to cope with a change of service and support personnel
- Staff are familiar with the agencies, statutory and voluntary, that deal with people with intellectual disabilities and can access them on behalf of their patients

Disadvantages of being within learning disability services
- Training staff to treat people across a broad age range – through understanding their developing needs and the different requirements of the different ages – is very demanding
- Maintaining links with child agencies such as CAMHS and child development centres cannot be a priority when links with adult agencies must also be maintained

Advantages of being within CAMHS
- The clientele have access to full tiered service provision
- Links with other agencies such as Social Services, education, child development centres and voluntary agencies, working primarily with children, are already established
- Premises are centred on services for children and young people
- Children are seen as children first rather than as individuals with disabilities

Disadvantages of being within CAMHS
- It may be difficult to find trained staff where, historically, service provision (and therefore training) has been part of a separate 'lifespan' service

- seeking to utilise empowering interventions that avoid service dependency and that help families to develop the skills to deal effectively with future difficulties as they arise
- targeting and rationing any long-term work to high-risk families
- establishing sharing of work between agencies, particularly with high-risk families.

In this way, parents and staff are encouraged to develop skills and strategies that can be generalised to new problems.

There is an argument that children who have specific diagnostic requirements, complex needs and who may require expert interventions may benefit from seeing members of the team who have experience in the area. It is unlikely that all members of a CAMHS would be in a position to develop this expertise. Much of this thinking leads to the conclusion that certain members of the team may be better placed to take such referrals. They may then form themselves into a Tier 3 team, a 'CAMHS learning disability team', that has a specific role in developing relationships with other clinicians seeing these children, developing liaison and keeping themselves up to date on clinical practice in the area. This gives a focus for consultation, liaison, referral and multi-agency working. However, not all children with an intellectual disability who are referred to CAMHS need be taken by the Tier 3 team. There would be flexibility in how wider team members may rotate in and out of the team, in either the short or longer term, to meet the needs of particular children and their families. For these reasons, learning disability services are best integrated with generic CAMHS.

A Tier 3 learning disabilities team can help to create a specialist facility within a system, which is able to provide access to a wide variety of other services, to the benefit of families. A service integrated into a CAMHS avoids stigmatisation or isolation from other services.

Differentiated funding and managerial commitment can protect a service that historically has had a tendency to be eroded by competing needs within host organisations.

Establishing a new service

Where a new service is being created, the generation of a new team creates exciting opportunities for the development of inter-agency relationships. It is an ideal time to bring together representatives from parents' groups and all of the professionals with whom the team would like to establish links, in order to brainstorm with them potential options for the configuration of the service (Green *et al*, 2001). Once a list of potential services has been generated, the group can be asked to reach a decision about the level of priority they feel should be given to each element of the service.

The process as well as the product of such meetings can be valuable in laying the foundation of a service aimed at creating strong links with parents and professionals. It also creates a joint understanding of the demands and limitations of the service.

Once a service has been developed, it will need to address the issues raised in Box 18.3.

Box 18.3 Service considerations

- How will new services relate to existing services?
- How will the new service work in practice and develop its operational policy?
- How will training needs be met?
- Who will be the users?
- How will discrimination be avoided?
- How will the service be audited and monitored?
- How will users' and carers' views incorporated into its practice?

Team structure

The team composition should reflect the multiple needs of children with intellectual disabilities (Hollins *et al*, 1989; Department of Health, 2001). Most CAMHS do not have the luxury of a large multidisciplinary team, and some harsh decisions need to be made when constructing a team. There will be a tension between a need to have a range of services and a need to get through the large volume of work. The team will need to consider the range of treatments available, as well as team morale and an evidence-based comparison of the effectiveness of the various treatment approaches, efficiency and user/carer experiences. There should also be strong links with professionals who are not part of the core team, including:

- community paediatricians
- paediatricians with an interest in neurology
- school doctors/nurses
- social workers and family workers within Social Services 'health and disability' directorates
- voluntary agencies
- respite care facilities
- educational psychologists and behaviour support services within mainstream and special education
- health visitors.

It may be that some large trusts that have different CAMHS locality teams could identify staff from each that could work together to form a cross-locality team.

Referral process

Referrals can be taken from a number of sources, including GPs, hospital doctors, school doctors, health visitors, educational psychologists, behavioural support teachers and social workers, who all should be clear about the purpose and functioning of the team. This may require considerable educational input. Several services operate a system whereby primary mental health workers assess all children and young people referred to CAMHS initially, including those with intellectual disabilities. They then either signpost families appropriately to other services, into CAMHS Tier 2 or Tier 3 services, or complete short pieces of work themselves as required. Criteria for allocation to the learning disabilities team of referrals into CAMHS should be clear from the operational policy of the team. Different services have used differing criteria with varying degrees of flexibility, as outlined in Box 18.4.

A proportion of children with autism-spectrum disorders do not have low IQs or attend special schools. However, professionals working with children with intellectual disabilities often work with less able children with autism and have developed skills in assessment and management

---

Box 18.4 Referral criteria

- Attendance at a special school
- Autism-spectrum disorder
- IQ below 70 or severe developmental delay
- Statement under the Education Act 1981 of special educational need relating to intellectual disability
- Developmental delay as judged by paediatric/child development centre teams

---

that are valuable throughout the full range of autism-spectrum disorders. Hence, it may be useful to include autism within the referral criteria. However, increasing awareness and understanding of autism-spectrum disorders has recently led to marked increases in referral rates and this must be given careful consideration in the planning of service provision (see Chapter 19). This situation also affords opportunities for learning and training between generic CAMHS professionals and those with intellectual disability experience.

Between 1 and 2% of children have a long-term need for special help at school, although not all of these relate to intellectual disability. However, the team will have to make calculations to determine the number of children with needs because of their intellectual disability and how their needs will fit with available resources. This is particularly pertinent because many local education authorities have implemented inclusion policies making liaison necessary in primary and secondary schools and not exclusively with special schools. In practice, the first two criteria listed in Box 18.4 create a great deal of work and are more likely to identify children with complex needs, where a specialist service can be most usefully targeted.

Role of the learning disabilities team

Standard 8 of the NSF for children states that Local Authorities, primary care trusts and CAMHS must work together to 'ensure that disabled children have equal access' to a full range of CAMH services (Department for Education and Skills & Department of Health, 2004). This includes early identification of impairments and early interventions, coordinated services, family support and continuity of care in the transition to adult services as laid out in *Valuing People* (Department of Health, 2001). A CAMHS learning disabilities team might be expected to perform the following functions.

- Assessment and treatment of child mental health problems in children with intellectual disabilities.
- Involvement in the assessment and treatment of the mental health problems and disorders of children attending the child development

centre, through close links with paediatric and child health teams and the provision of consultation to them.

- Offering behaviour management advice to families with children whose intellectual disability is complicated by behavioural difficulties.
- Teaching, training and consultation with staff working in special schools catering for children with intellectual disability.
- Input into the assessment and management of children with autism-spectrum disorders.
- Consultation with Social Services personnel concerning their provision for families of children with an intellectual disability who also have mental health problems.
- Involvement in multi-agency learning disabilities services by liaison with staff such as paediatricians, educational psychologists, social workers and school doctors.
- Teaching and training to other agencies involved with children with an intellectual disability.
- The development of close links with adult learning disability services; transitional planning for young people moving to adult services.
- Presentations, discussions and liaison with parent support groups.
- Family therapy.
- Audit of team performance.
- Organisation and running of groups for children (e.g. social skills groups).
- Intervention and support groups for parents and carers.

Assessment process

Families of children with intellectual disabilities present with a wide range of complex problems. Comprehensive assessment, including of the school and home environment, is vital before a formulation and intervention plan can be made. The American Association on Mental Retardation (1992) provides a useful framework for assessment. This includes an assessment of intellectual functioning (e.g. British Ability Scales; Elliot, 1996); Wechsler Intelligence Scale for Children (4th edn) (WISC–IV; Wechsler, 2003) and adaptive behaviour scales (e.g. Vineland Adaptive Behavior Scales; Sparrow *et al*, 1984); psychological and emotional assessment by clinical interview, observation and behaviour scales (e.g. Child Behaviour Checklist; Achenbach, 1991); physical health; and aetiological and environmental factors. Pote & Goodban (2007) share detailed ideas about assessment frameworks.

Joint assessments with professionals at child development centres should be considered for children with complex problems where there is a mental health component.

Intervention

A mental health service for children with an intellectual disability and their families should be able to offer a full range of services similar to generic CAMHS. Specialist knowledge will be necessary for autism-spectrum disorders, epilepsy, physical comorbidities, neurodegenerative and metabolic disorders, and specialist knowledge, understanding and skills when facing challenging behaviour and child protection issues (Williams & Wright, 2003). This will include the following.

- Information – giving parents clear, unambiguous information about the child's disability and the implications of the diagnosis.
- Counselling – helping the family to deal with their emotional distress on diagnosis and at transitional periods in the child's life.
- Support – providing clear information about available support systems such as respite services, portage and parents' support groups.
- Referral to other services such as paediatrics, speech therapists, preschool teaching services and Social Services where indicated.
- Behavioural management – functional analysis and assessment of patterns of behaviours (Oliver, 1995), and the development of effective strategies and support with and for parents.
- Individual or group sessions to help children to develop a variety of life skills.
- Therapeutic work for psychological morbidity and mental illness.
- Family therapy.
- Medication.

Consultation and liaison

Consultation and liaison with professionals working directly with children with intellectual disabilities and their families is an integral part of the work of a CAMHS learning disabilities team. Children will often be known to several agencies. Regular discussion between professionals is essential in coordinating services, avoiding duplication of work and establishing consistency of approaches. Formal meetings or forums are often generated by commonality of symptomatology or intervention programmes for disorders such as autism or attentional problems. Similarly, it may be helpful to form a multi-agency learning disabilities team, which could meet monthly or bi-monthly to discuss children with complex needs. One of the team members should take responsibility for compiling a list of children to be discussed, at the request of other team members, and circulating this before meetings.

Establishing relationships with staff in special schools and respite care services should be considered as a major role for a CAMHS learning disabilities team. A regular presence, possibly once each term, allows the opportunity for informal discussion and early intervention.

Transition from child to adult services

The transition from child to adult services is a particularly significant time for young people with intellectual disabilities. Many changes happen simultaneously, making this time especially stressful for them and their families. This transitional period should be carefully managed. However, some of the literature suggests that this does not always happen as hoped (Tutt, 1995). Families report a host of dilemmas (Thorin *et al*, 1996) with which they would value help and support. Examples include learning to cope with the changes and losses, and wanting to create opportunities for independence while assuring that health and safety needs are met. Career, training and housing needs of young people with intellectual disabilities frequently raise issues. Ideally, the planning process should be part of ongoing therapeutic interventions, with a more formal process occurring when the young person is around 14 years of age. Some areas have a policy of organising multi-agency meetings with families as part of the school review. The personal and sensitive transfer of care should ease the transition from child to adult services. This should include ensuring that parents and young people are fully involved throughout the process and that they are given information to help them to inform their choices and to know how to re-access services when required.

Teaching and training

When working in a specialist area it is important to disseminate information at all opportunities. Information about different types of syndromes and intellectual disabilities can be shared with staff in schools and colleges, Social Services and voluntary agencies, as well as with parent support groups, in order to encourage understanding, early detection and intervention strategies. Staff in special schools often value workshops related to the management of challenging behaviours.

Evaluation

To ensure the service is effective, it must have clear objectives and an operational policy that is directed to meeting those objectives. Outcome measurement, audit and the collection of user perspectives are the methods by which the service is monitored and developed.

Audit

The service should be audited at least yearly in order to monitor referral rates, presenting problems, assessment protocols and interventions. Such audits (Green *et al*, 2001) establish whether the standards set for the service are being maintained, but also demonstrate where future challenges for the service may lie, for example if referral rates far exceed discharge rates.

User perspectives

The service offered should not only meet the needs of children with intellectual disabilities and their families, but also be provided in a manner they find acceptable and supportive. Attendance at parent support groups can help to provide insight into perceptions and offer a foundation for the development of user surveys. Professionals should listen carefully to parents' comments and suggestions and avoid being overly defensive. Awareness of the strengths and weaknesses of the service allows for re-evaluation and change. Similarly, professionals working with and using the service can offer important insights into the development of the team.

Where studies have sought user opinions about the shape of services there is often a desire for key workers, access to multidisciplinary services and for good-quality information to be readily available (Beresford & Sloper, 2004). High-quality family support, leisure facilities and substitute care are also priorities for families.

Aiming High for Disabled Children (HM Treasury & Department for Education and Skills, 2007) set out the development of a 'core offer' to improve the responsiveness of local services to the needs of disabled children and their families. These are:

- clear information
- multi-agency assessment
- transparent eligibility criteria
- accessible feedback and complaints procedures
- participation in shaping local polices and services.

The Department of Health (HM Government, 2007) plans to evaluate parents' experience of services for disabled children, focusing on the delivery of these five aspects. They plan to do this through surveys at Local Authority level annually from 2008.

The requirement for Local Authorities to publish information based on this 'core offer' has the potential to help improve services, as there will be greater clarity about where services need development.

Conclusion

Children with intellectual disabilities who also have mental disorders and mental health problems have specific needs, as do their families. If services are expected to be delivered without additional resources or training in generic CAMHS or 'lifespan' learning disabilities services, these specific needs are likely to be ill understood and poorly met. If the objectives of the NSF (Department for Education and Skills & Department of Health, 2004) and *Valuing People* (Department of Health, 2001) are truly to be met in children and young people, specialised services with specially trained staff are required.

At present, the Department of Health and Department of Children, Schools & Families are working together to support the Aiming High for Disabled Children initiative to bring together high levels of expertise from specialist services such as from Local Authorities and health agencies (HM Treasury & Department for Education and Skills, 2007). It is important that CAMHS maintain specific expertise in Tier 3 learning disability teams in order to make best use of their skills, knowledge and their relationships with local services to ensure that mental health remains an integral part of services for disabled children as recommended by the Department of Health and Department of Children, Schools & Families.

References

Achenbach, T. (1991) *Integrative Guide for the 1991 CBCL/4–18, YSR, and TRF Profiles.* Department of Psychiatry, University of Vermont.

American Association on Mental Retardation (1992) *Mental Retardation: Definition, Classifications and Systems of Support* (9th edn). AAMR.

Beresford, B. & Sloper, P. (2004) *Integrating Services for Disabled Children, Young People and their Families: Consultation Project.* Social Policy Research Unit, University of York.

Corbett, J. A. (1985) Mental retardation: psychiatric aspects. In *Child and Adolescent Psychiatry* (eds M. Rutter & L. Hersov), pp. 661–678. Blackwell Scientific.

Department for Education and Skills & Department of Health (2004) *National Service Framework for Children, Young People and Maternity Services. Standard 8. Disabled Children and Young People and those with Complex Health Needs.* DH Publications.

Department for Education and Skills & Department of Health (2006) *Promoting the Mental Health and Psychological Well-being of Children and Young People: Report on the Implementation of Standard 9 of the National Service Framework for Children and Young People and Maternity Services.* TSO (The Stationery Office).

Department of Health (1992) *Health Services for People with Learning Disabilities. HSB (92)42.* Department of Health.

Department of Health (2001) *Valuing People. A New Strategy for Learning Disability for the 21st Century.* Department of Health.

Dugmore, O. & Hurcombe, R. (2007) *QINMAC. Quality Improvement Network for Multi-Agency CAMHS: Learning Disability Standards.* Royal College of Psychiatrists.

Dykens, E. M. (2000) Psychopathology in children with intellectual disability. *Journal of Child Psychology and Psychiatry and Allied Disciplines, 41,* 407–417.

Elliot, C. (1996) *British Ability Scales (2nd edn) (BAS II).* nferNelson.

Emerson, E. (2003) Prevalence of psychiatric disorders in children and adolescents with and without intellectual disability. *Journal of Intellectual Disability Research, 47,* 51–59.

Emerson, E. & Hatton, C. (2007) *Mental Health of Children and Adolescents with Learning Disabilities in Britain.* Institute for Health Research, Lancaster University & Foundation for People with Learning Disabilities.

Felce, D., Taylor, D. & Wright, K. (1994) People with learning disabilities. In *Healthcare Needs Assessment – The Epidemiology Based Needs Assessment Reviews, Vol. 2* (eds A. Stevens & J. Raffery), pp. 414–450. Radcliffe Medical Press.

Fombonne, E. (1998) Epidemiological surveys of autism. In *Autism and Pervasive Developmental Disorders,* p. 32–68. Cambridge University Press.

Gillberg, C., Persson, E., Grufman, M., *et al* (1986) Psychiatric disorders in mildly and severely mentally retarded urban children and adolescents: epidemiological aspects. *British Journal of Psychiatry, 149,* 68–74.

Green, J., Kroll, L., Imrie, D., *et al* (2001) Health gain and predictors of outcome in inpatient and related day patient child and adolescent psychiatry treatment. *Journal of the American Academy of Child and Adolescent Psychiatry, 40,* 325–332.

HM Government (2007) *PSA Delivery Agreement 12: Improve the Health and Wellbeing of Children and Young People.* TSO (The Stationery Office).

HM Treasury & Department for Education and Skills (2007) *Aiming High for Disabled Children: Better Support for Families.* TSO (The Stationery Office).

Hollins, S., Nicol, R., Sacks, B., *et al* (1989) The training required to provide a psychiatric service for children and adolescents with mental handicap. *Psychiatric Bulletin*, **13**, 326–328.

McKay, I. & Hall, D. (1994) *Services for Children and Adolescents with Learning Disability (Mental Handicap)*. British Paediatric Association.

Oliver, C. (1995) Annotation. Self-injurious behaviour in children with learning disabilities: Recent advances in assessment and intervention. *Journal of Child Psychology and Psychiatry*, **30**, 900–927.

Pote, H. & Goodban, D. (2007) *A Mental Health Care Pathway for Children and Young People with Learning Disabilities: A Resource Pack for Service Planners and Practitioners*. CAMHS Evidence Based Practice Unit, University College London & Anna Freud Centre.

Royal College of Psychiatrists (1992) *Psychiatric Services for Children and Adolescents with Mental Handicap. Council Report CR17*. Royal College of Psychiatrists.

Sparrow, S., Balla, D. & Cicchetti, D. (1984) *Vineland Adaptive Behavior Scales*. American Guidance Service.

Stromme, P. & Diseth, T. H. (2000) Prevalence of psychiatric diagnoses in children with mental retardation: data from a population based study. *Developmental Medicine and Child Neurology*, **42**, 266–270.

Thorin, E., Yovanoff, P. & Irvin, L. (1996) Dilemmas faced by families during their young adults transitions to adulthood: a brief report. *Mental Retardation*, **34**, 117–120.

Tonge, B. & Einfield, S. (2000) The trajectory of psychiatric disorders in young people with intellectual disabilities. *Australian and New Zealand Journal of Psychiatry*, **34**, 80–84.

Tutt, N. (1995) Transitions – children with disabilities and their passage into adulthood. *Social Information Systems Management Update*, **1**, 44–56.

Wallace, S. A., Crown, J. M., Berger, M., *et al* (1995) Child and adolescent mental health. In *Health Care Needs Assessment: The Epidemiologically Based Needs Assessment Reviews* (eds A. Stevens & J. Raftery) , pp. 55–74. Radcliffe Medical Press.

Wechsler, D. (2003) *Wechsler Intelligence Scale for Children – Fourth Edition (WISC–IV)*. Pearson Publications.

Whitaker, S. & Read, S. (2006) The prevalence of psychiatric disorders among people with intellectual disabilities: an analysis of the literature. *Journal of Applied Research in Intellectual Disabilities*, **19**, 330–345.

Williams, C. & Wright, B. (2003) *How to Live with Autism and Asperger Syndrome: Practical Strategies for Parents and Professionals*. Jessica Kingsley Publishers.

Wright, B., Williams, C. & Richardson, G. (2008) Services for children with learning disabilities. *Psychiatric Bulletin*, **32**, 81–84.

CHAPTER 19

Services for autism-spectrum disorders

Christine Williams and Barry Wright

'I can't stress enough the importance of early diagnosis because without a diagnosis, without explanation of the way the child is behaving there is nothing you can do, there's no way you can move on...Once a diagnosis has been given, an explanation of why this child is frustrated and behaving this way, then we can begin to put in appropriate strategies for the family and for the child. It makes one huge amount of difference to their lives.'

Dr Judith Gould

Introduction

Autism-spectrum disorders are thought to affect many more people than is generally recognised. It is very difficult to give precise figures about the prevalence of these disorders because of difficulties with diagnosis, use of diagnostic terms and prevalence study methodology. Reviews indicate approximately 60 per 10000 children under the age of 8 years (Medical Research Council, 2001), but other estimates are around 1 in a 100 children in the UK (Green *et al*, 2005; Baird *et al*, 2006).

Children and adolescents with autism show abnormalities in:

- communication and language development
- reciprocal social interaction
- symbolic play
- patterns of interests (the range of interests is restricted, and they centre on repetitive or stereotyped activities).

A number of different disorders appear to overlap, each overlapping area having different characteristics (Fig. 19.1).

Difficulties in each of these areas vary considerably with the age of the child, severity of symptoms and individual differences in the child. The autism spectrum includes the syndromes described by Kanner (1943) and by Asperger (1944), but is wider than these two subgroups (Wing & Gould, 1979). Child and adolescent mental health services are frequently asked to assess children who may have autism; such assessment is complex, as described in Box 19.1.

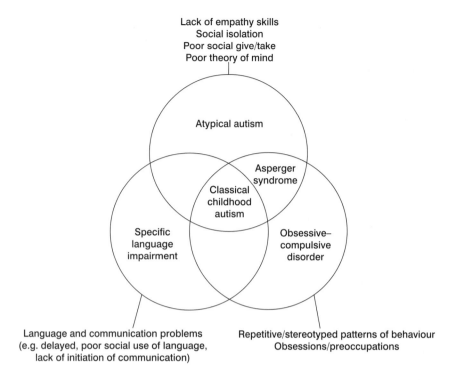

Fig. 19.1 Overlap of disorders in connection with autism.

Box 19.1 Difficulties in assessment

Children and young people with autism-spectrum disorders may present in very different ways at different times.

- The range of intellectual ability extends from severely intellectually disabled to those who are of average or above average intelligence. Similarly, language skills range from those with no language to those who display complex, grammatically correct speech.
- Changes occur with age, especially in those with higher levels of ability; different aspects of the behaviour patterns are more obvious at some ages than at others.
- The social environment can have marked effects on overt behaviour; for example, in a very structured setting, with one-to-one attention, autistic behaviour may be reduced.
- When considering autism-spectrum disorders it is important to exclude other neurodevelopmental, neurological, organic or psychosocial disorders that might either cause or mimic autism (e.g. attachment difficulties; Flood & Perry, 2008).
- Temperaments ranging from very placid to very strong-willed.

Establishing a service for children with autism

There is increasing demand for CAMHS to be instrumental in the organisation of services for children and adolescents with autism-spectrum disorders, including early identification, assessment, diagnosis and intervention. In some CAMHS, autism falls within the remit of a learning disabilities team, in view of the considerable overlap of the two populations. In some teams (particularly in larger areas), the size of the clientele may justify a Tier 3 team within CAMHS or a neurodevelopmental Tier 3 team. Such specialist provision has the following advantages:

- clarity of purpose;
- networking of professionals working collaboratively to the benefit of children and families;
- the opportunity to generate an identity (e.g. with a name such as autism-spectrum disorders forum) that encourages the development of expertise and cooperative working;
- facilitating the development of a policy and protocol for working, based around procedures for assessing, making diagnoses and formulating/coordinating management plans;
- developing a common language and nomenclature across agencies and disciplines;
- operating common diagnostic procedures;
- joined-up thinking in the planning of interventions;
- clear inter-agency planning of services for children and young people with autism;
- efficiency;
- improved user and carer experiences.

The establishment of such a team then provides a focus for the development of a strategy to deliver services to children with autism and their families.

However, it is important to ensure that there are no service gaps between the teams that are established. Ideally, Tier 3 teams should be embedded within a wider generic CAMHS. If not, there needs to be careful discussion between interlinking CAMHS or tiers of CAMHS to make sure that there are no gaps created by referral criteria boundaries. This can lead to unmet need (e.g. for children and adolescents with Asperger syndrome). The services need to be planned, agreed locally and provide services for all children with autism-spectrum disorders.

Early identification

Screening

The possibility of systematising screening for autism into health visitor or GP developmental checks should be encouraged by CAMHS. For example, the Checklist for Autism in Toddlers (CHAT; Baron-Cohen *et al*, 1992) is an early screening tool that may be used at the 18-month check; it has been found useful for primary care professionals, particularly health visitors, who have regular access to the under-5 age group. The service should then allow those working at Tier 1 access to Tier 2 professionals, who are experienced at working with these children and families, and to Tier 3 teams such as an autism-spectrum disorders team. Many professionals such as teachers may have concerns about a child's socialisation or communication skills, for instance, without necessarily being aware of some of the features of autism, particularly at the milder end of the spectrum. They need to have access to consultation and referral. In some CAMHS this may be systematised, for example, through a primary mental health worker who can offer screening, or there may be regular, formal consultation sessions with health visitors, school nurses or paediatric liaison teams (see Chapter 16).

Training

The National Autistic Society estimates that autism-spectrum disorders are greatly underdiagnosed. It recommends that health professionals be trained in developing awareness of symptoms. Paediatricians and CAMHS with expertise in these areas are encouraged to help build understanding of autism-spectrum disorders within Tier 1 by supplying information and running workshops.

Training must also emphasise basic topics such as confidentiality, parental consent and ways of sharing concerns about young people with parents. These are issues that can be forgotten when dealing with children with poor communication skills.

Professionals engaged in the assessment and diagnosis of children with autism should also ensure that their own skills are up to date by attendance at one of the courses available to them. Such courses include training in the use of the Diagnostic Interview for Social and Communication Disorders (DISCO) (Leekam *et al*, 2002; Wing *et al*, 2002), the Autism Diagnostic Interview – Revised (ADI–R; Lord *et al*, 1994) and the Autism Diagnostic Observation Schedule – Generic (ADOS–G; Lord *et al*, 2000).

Assessment

There are various models for assessment, and the development of services will often be contingent on local issues and areas of expertise. Whatever the model or assessment process, there should be a strong emphasis on the partnership between parents and professionals throughout. Information about the content and process of assessment and diagnosis should be shared and discussed openly. There should be no surprises when a final diagnosis is made, as parents should be given a clear rationale and justification for the clinician's formulation throughout the procedure. This allows for the building of a trusting relationship, which is vital in helping parents to make sense of their child's difficulties, their own emotional distress and intervention strategies. The family should be assured that regardless of diagnostic outcome, they will still receive help and that their concerns about their child will be addressed.

The National Autism Plan for Children (National Autistic Society, 2003) has produced guidelines relating to assessment, diagnosis and interventions for preschool children and primary school-aged children. It recommends a three-stage approach to assessment, which can be adapted for local service. Stage 1 is a general multidisciplinary assessment for children where parents or professionals have highlighted a possible developmental difficulty. Stage 2 is a more detailed multi-agency, multidisciplinary assessment to be applied where autism is suspected. Stage 3 is a tertiary assessment which may be necessary where there is still uncertainty about diagnosis, complexity or a where a second opinion is required.

These guidelines provide a sound framework and can be used creatively where resources are low. For example, some services have developed a very successful multidisciplinary, multi-agency autism-spectrum disorders forum system. This type of forum is helpful in maintaining quality and consistency in diagnosis and intervention strategies. A protocol for the organisation of referral for assessment and the usage of such a forum is outlined in Figs 19.2. and 19.3. In this case, the under-5s have a multidisciplinary developmental assessment initially and where autism is suspected they are referred for any additional assessments which may not have been completed (e.g. nursery or home observations, speech and language assessment). Sometimes the child is referred to CAMHS, particularly if they are older. Many CAMHS now have primary mental health workers who are able to conduct screening assessments and refer

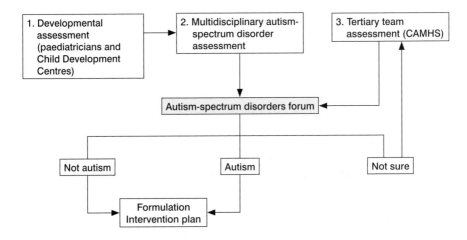

Fig. 19.2 Autism-spectrum disorder assessment process for under-5-year-olds.

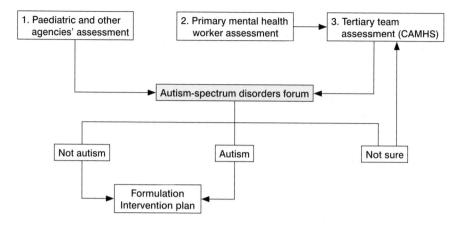

Fig. 19.3 Autism-spectrum disorder assessment process for 6- to 9-year-olds.

families on to CAMHS Tier 3 teams when necessary. With parental consent, the child is then discussed in detail at the forum. Professionals contribute information from their assessments within psychosocial and diagnostic frameworks. Formulation and intervention plans are then agreed with the multi-agency team. Where there is uncertainty or complexity (e.g. hearing loss, severe language impairment, global developmental delay), the child is referred to a tertiary CAMHS team for further assessment. These children are discussed at the forum following further assessment. Children should only be discussed with parents' full consent. In all cases, a full multi-agency assessment should include:

- developmental history
- family history
- systematic autism symptomatology enquiry
- observation of the child in different settings including nursery or school and home
- a play assessment or formal diagnostic assessment such as the Autism Diagnostic Observation Schedule (ADOS; Lord *et al*, 2000)
- paediatric assessment
- cognitive/developmental assessment
- speech and language assessment
- Social Services assessment for service provision
- consideration of alternative diagnoses such as hearing impairment, intellectual disability, developmental language delay or severe psychosocial deprivation
- if necessary, occupational therapy assessment including fine and gross motor skills
- physiotherapy assessment including self-help skills and physical functioning.

Whichever model is used, assessment should be multidisciplinary (Sparrow, 1997) and systematised to a protocol agreed between the different professionals involved. There should be a core diagnostic team of paediatrician, child psychiatrist, clinical psychologist and speech therapist with access to additional professionals, including the child's teacher, educational psychologist, learning support teacher or special educational needs coordinator. Other professionals who may be called upon to be involved include social workers, family workers, occupational therapists, physiotherapists, school doctors/nurses, autism specialist workers, community psychiatric nurses, portage workers and respite care workers. Parents should be fully involved throughout the assessment.

The focus should extend beyond assessment. Time and thought should be devoted to the provision of interventions provided both from the CAMHS and by multi-agency colleagues. Interventions should be detailed in the final report on the child and offered to the child's parents, with an opportunity for discussion so that they can correct any points of fact and ask any further questions. The final copy should then be sent back to the parents and other professionals to whom it is relevant.

Interventions

There is no known cure for autism (Cohen & Volkmar, 1997). Intervention is based on helping children to develop strategies to compensate for their difficulties with communication, preventing secondary emotional and social dysfunction, and helping parents to manage their children's behaviour in order that they may all lead as healthy a life as possible. It is good practice for intervention to begin at first contact with parents; shared goals should be agreed and a partnership established. This should continue throughout the assessment and treatment process. The care plan should be carefully coordinated with all agencies. A comprehensive intervention programme involves the following.

- Information about autism – providing the family with information about assessment, diagnosis and prognosis. This can occur throughout the assessment process through general discussion and by giving information sheets and books (e.g. *How to Live with Autism and Asperger Syndrome: Practical Strategies for Parents and Professionals;* Williams & Wright, 2003). The National Autistic Society provides a wide range of literature. Jessica Kingsley Publishers have a wide range of excellent books for parents, young people and siblings.
- Information about local services, including:
  - parent support groups
  - groups for young people with autism
  - individual therapeutic work for children with autism
  - computer-based instruction (Williams *et al*, 2002)
  - respite services

- family support (e.g. Crossroads Association)
- preschool parenting support (e.g. Portage)
- Social Services facilities
- education services
- Sure Start
- autism workers.
- Educational placement – the educational psychologist should take responsibility for guiding parents through the options available locally.
- Family support – many families benefit from the availability of support to help them to understand and cope with the adjustment process that often follows diagnosis.
- Strategies for managing behaviour.
- TEACHH (Schopler, 1997) – a structured learning programme aimed at utilising the strengths of children with autism.
- Behaviour-based treatment strategies.
- Medication.
- Parent training intervention courses, for example:
  - Early Bird (National Autistic Society, www.nas.org.uk/earlybird)
  - ASCEND (Wright & Williams, 2007)
  - Adapted Hanen Programme.
- Social stories workshops (Gray, 2007).
- Help with the transition from child and adolescent services to adult services. This can be a particularly stressful period for families and requires careful liaison between the professionals working in the two services.

Conclusion

Children with autism-spectrum disorders are recognised at different stages of their lives. Autism is often recognised early, whereas Asperger syndrome may not be recognised until adolescence. Sensitivity to the possibility of the diagnosis must be present in all those who work with children and young people at all developmental stages so that assessment of their complex needs is competently undertaken and management strategies instituted in all areas of the child's functioning.

References

Asperger, H. (1944) Die autistischen psychopathen im kindesalter [Autistic psychopathy of childhood]. *Archiv für Psychiatrie und Nervenkrankheiten*, **117**, 76–136.

Baird, G., Simonoff, E., Pickles, A., *et al* (2006) Prevalence of disorders of the autism spectrum in a population cohort of children in South Thames: the Special Needs and Autism Project (SNAP). *Lancet*, **368**, 210–215.

Baron-Cohen, S., Allen, J. & Gillberg, C. (1992) Can autism be detected at 18 months? The needle, the haystack, and the CHAT. *British Journal of Psychiatry*, **161**, 839–843.

Cohen, D. & Volkmar, F. (1997) *Handbook of Autism and Pervasive Developmental Disorders.* Wiley.

Flood, A. & Perry, P. (2008). Autistic spectrum disorder and attachment. Where are we now? *Clinical Psychology Forum,* **185**, 20–24.

Gray, C. (2007) *Writing Social Stories with Carol Gray – DVD and Booklet.* The Gray Center (http://www.thegraycenter.org).

Green, H., McGinnity, Á., Meltzer, H., *et al* (2005) *Mental Health of Children and Young People in Great Britain, 2004.* Palgrave Macmillan (http://www.statistics.gov.uk/downloads/theme_health/GB2004.pdf).

Kanner, L. (1943) Autistic disturbances of affective contact. *Nervous Child,* **2**, 217–250.

Leekam, S. R., Libby, S. J., Wing, L., *et al* (2002) The Diagnostic Interview for Social and Communication Disorders: algorithms for ICD–10 childhood autism and Wing and Gould autistic spectrum disorder. *Journal of Child Psychology and Psychiatry,* **43**, 327–342.

Lord, C., Rutter, M. & Le Couteur, A. (1994) Autism Diagnostic Interview – Revised: a revised version of a diagnostic interview for caregivers of individuals with possible pervasive developmental disorders. *Journal of Autism and Developmental Disorders,* **24**, 659–685.

Lord, C., Risi, S., Lambrecht, L., *et al* (2000) The Autism Diagnostic Observation Schedule – Generic. A standard measure of social and communication deficits associated with the spectrum of autism. *Journal of Autism and Developmental Disorders,* **30**, 205–223.

Medical Research Council (2001) *MRC Review of Autism Research: Epidemiology and Causes.* MRC.

National Autistic Society (2003) *National Autism Plan for Children.* National Autistic Society.

Schopler, E. (1997) Implementation of TEACHH philosophy. In *Handbook of Autism and Pervasive Developmental Disorders* (eds D. Cohen & F. Volkmar), pp. 767–795. John Wiley & Sons.

Sparrow, S. (1997) Developmentally based assessment. In *Handbook of Autism and Pervasive Developmental Disorders* (eds D. Cohen & F. Volkmar), pp. 411–477. John Wiley & Sons.

Williams, C. & Wright, B. (2003) *How to Live with Autism and Asperger Syndrome: Practical Strategies for Parents and Professionals.* Jessica Kingsley Publishers.

Williams, C., Wright, B., Callaghan, G., *et al* (2002) Do children with autism learn to read more readily by computer assisted instruction or traditional book methods? A pilot study. *Autism,* **6**, 71–91.

Wing, L. & Gould, J. (1979) Severe impairments of social interaction and associated abnormalities in children: epidemiology and classification. *Journal of Autism and Childhood Schizophrenia,* **9**, 11–29.

Wing, L., Leekam, S. R., Libby, S. J., *et al* (2002) The Diagnostic Interview for Social and Communication Disorders: background inter-rater reliability and clinical use. *Journal of Child Psychology and Psychiatry,* **43**, 307–325.

Wright, B. & Williams, C. (2007) *Intervention and Support Programme for Parents and Carers of Children with Autism and Asperger Syndrome: A Resource for Trainers.* Jessica Kingsley Publishers.

CHAPTER 20

Attentional problems services

Sarah Bryan, Barry Wright and Christine Williams

'No fine work can be done without concentration, and self-sacrifice and toil and doubt.'

Max Beerbohm

Introduction

In the UK, ADHD has been shown to be the most common reason for follow-up appointments to be offered by CAMHS (Meltzer et al, 2000). Child and adolescent mental health services are regularly called upon to assess children who have problems with attention, concentration, distractibility, impulsivity, overactivity, regulatory difficulties, or a combination of these. These difficulties may be part of ADHD or may be symptoms of other disorders that mimic the clinical features of ADHD (Hill & Cameron, 1999). Attention-deficit hyperactivity disorder is a condition where the symptom profile and aetiology are regularly being redefined. Comprehensive guidelines from NICE (National Institute for Health and Clinical Excellence, 2006; National Collaborating Centre for Mental Health, 2008) and a large US study, with its recently published follow-up study (MTA Cooperative Group, 1999; Jensen et al, 2007) have also informed good practice. As additional resources have not often generally been forthcoming to support such good practice, existing services may restructure aspects of their functioning in order to form Tier 3 teams.

One way of rationalising resources effectively is to establish inter-agency links so that multidisciplinary working is not limited by professional boundaries. Some centres have done just this to meet the needs of children with complex problems, including ADHD complicated by comorbid difficulties (Williams et al, 1999). Where there is no coordinated approach to assessment and intervention for children who present with these difficulties, confusion may arise and contradictory advice may be given by different agencies. Parents and carers need to feel confident that professionals are working with them and with other agencies to provide a comprehensive assessment and treatment package for their children. A Tier 3 team within a CAMHS has the advantage of multidisciplinary working, and this facilitates the development of shared learning and understanding, and the evolution of clear protocols (Voeller, 1991). A specific attentional problems clinic can provide assessment, diagnosis, monitoring and a range of ongoing interventions.

The attentional problems team should ideally include a child psychiatrist, a clinical psychologist and a community psychiatric nurse. The service will be enhanced by input from other CAMHS members such as occupational therapists, social workers or Social Services family workers, education support staff, and members of the child health team, for example community paediatricians, school doctors and school nurses. The principles of the team's service provision are set out in Box 20.1.

Attention-deficit hyperactivity disorder behaviours and symptoms can result from genetic, physical, environmental or social/environmental causes and it is important to bear this is mind when assessing (National Collaborating Centre for Mental Health, 2008).

A thorough assessment and formulation of the child's problems must consider all relevant factors and avoid becoming linear. Interventions then seek to address the formulation rather than focusing exclusively on medication.

Nature of the service

In different centres, different professionals or teams carry out assessment. For example, community or hospital paediatricians may be involved in assessment and diagnosis. This works well when integrated with CAMHS. Many paediatric teams work closely with child mental health teams (Dungar *et al*, 1986; Black *et al*, 1999; National Collaborating Centre for Mental Health, 2008) and the paediatrician may be linked to a CAMHS through joint clinics or meetings (Voeller, 1991). In this way, if paediatricians are making the diagnosis, they may be part of a multidisciplinary service that assesses, diagnoses and formulates treatment plans, based on a protocol that reflects shared beliefs about practice worked out in a coordinated fashion.

Box 20.1 Principles of service provision

- Multidisciplinary working
- A clear operational policy
- A responsive service with good feedback to the referrer
- A protocol for assessment and diagnosis that is regularly audited
- A range of interventions that takes on the social, educational, emotional and medical needs of the young person and family
- A cooperative alliance with families
- A protocol for communication with education services
- Information to other services about routes of consultation and referral

---

Cooperative working with CAMHS aside, the service can also be provided by a child development centre or as part of paediatric services, where professionals such as clinical psychologists, occupational therapists and community nurses are employed within the team and can deliver a range of interventions. It is always necessary to make links with education support staff.

If a paediatric unit has stand-alone diagnostic and treatment services, this does not create difficulties if a full range of options is open to children and families. Problems may arise if treatment options are restricted. Some diagnosing paediatricians provide medication and ask CAMHS to provide psychosocial interventions for children with ADHD but without CAMHS having any input to the assessment process. This may be problematic to CAMHS, particularly if assessment standards that it sets for itself are not being met by the diagnosing service. Moreover, interventions are best planned during assessment, as there is a need to influence, before diagnosis, early attributions about the meaning of ADHD for the child and the family. Such attributions have an impact on how parents manage their child, what treatments are acceptable to families and what beliefs are passed on to the child (Wright *et al*, 2000). All these are likely to influence prognosis. In addition, since diagnosis is there to clarify and facilitate management possibilities, it makes no sense to divorce the two. Most CAMHS believe in either unified services, where one team or another has full responsibility for assessment, diagnosis and the full range of interventions, or integrated services where both child health services and child mental health services work closely together. Split services, where one service is expected to make diagnoses and the other to provide the bulk of the management, present incoherent practice to children and their carers. Therefore, CAMHS and child health services must discuss roles and responsibilities with respect to these children and to have clear and agreed ways of working with each other. This is especially the case when second opinions are sought, as a second opinion must be integrated into the local management package (Richardson & Cottrell, 2003).

Assessment

Figure 20.1 outlines a protocol for the assessment of children with attentional problems. The primary mental health worker is in an ideal position to carry out preliminary screening to determine the best form of support for a young person and the necessity for referral to the Tier 3 team. First, a detailed history and thorough assessment are, as always, essential. The time spent during this process not only provides valuable information but also facilitates the building of a relationship with the family. Parents should be consulted throughout the assessment process, and be allowed to ask questions and seek clarification. A semi-structured interview with the child will provide important insight. Questionnaires from home and school

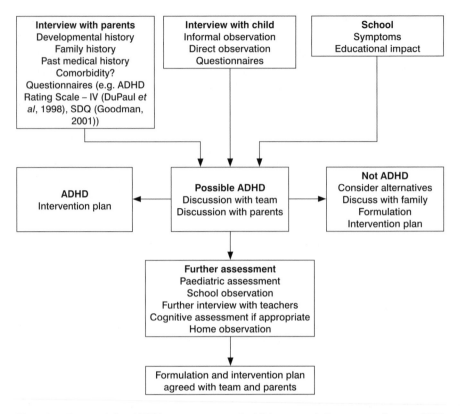

Fig. 20.1 Protocol for ADHD assessment of children aged 5 years and over. SDQ, Strengths and Difficulties Questionnaire.

are recommended (Barkley, 1990; Goodman, 2001). Clinicians should be mindful of the family's attributions about the child's difficulties, as these will have important implications for intervention. For example, if parents believe that the child's attentional and behavioural difficulties are entirely related to a biological problem requiring only medication as the remedy, they may be reluctant to engage in additional treatment programmes aimed at empowering both the child and parents (Wright *et al*, 2000).

If the team is sure that the child does not have ADHD, the family should be given clear information about their reason for this and alternative explanations for the child's behaviour should be discussed in detail. The relationship built during the assessment process will become invaluable in the communication of outcomes with a family, particularly if it is evident that the behaviours reported are associated with repetitive, intra-familial trauma (Hughes, 2007). If ADHD cannot be ruled out at this stage, further investigations should be carried out, including a paediatric assessment, direct observations at school and home, interviews with teachers, and an educational psychology assessment if indicated. If a cognitive assessment has not already been completed and the child is in serious difficulty in school, it may be helpful to make a referral for this purpose. An educational psychologist would usually carry out this work. This often provides important information about the child's intellectual ability, strengths, weaknesses and discrepancies. A multidimensional evaluation approach will determine whether the child has ADHD and how it effects the child's development and performance in different areas of their life. Additionally, associated comorbidities, which affect over half of the children with ADHD, can be identified as these are recognised to cause additional psychiatric, neurological and learning problems (Chu, 2007). These may include developmental coordination disorder, oppositional defiant disorder, specific learning difficulties, depression and anxiety (Jensen *et al*, 2001; Kadesjö & Gillberg, 2001).

Overall, recognising the child's unique constellation of difficulties will facilitate the development of the formulation and a tailored treatment approach, which can be agreed with the team and the family. This should take into account the often complex interactions between physiological, psychological, developmental and psychosocial factors which assessment may have highlighted. Good liaison and communication with all agencies help to facilitate a joint understanding and hence a strong supported intervention plan.

Intervention

Given the varied options for treatment and ongoing research, it is sensible for services to establish standards for the treatment of ADHD that can be regularly audited and reviewed. The NICE guidelines (National Collaborating Centre for Mental Health, 2008) should be carefully consulted and woven into developing services.

- Children should have gone through a clear assessment protocol (Fig. 20.1) before intervention packages are discussed with families, who should be involved in treatment planning.
- Multifaceted (psychosocial and educational) intervention packages should be employed.
- Interventions both at home and at school should be closely monitored, using narratives and questionnaires.
- Criteria for the use of medication should be established based on factors such as age, severity and pervasiveness of symptoms, and response to psychosocial interventions. Clear diagnosis of ADHD (or hyperkinetic disorder) must be established, for example by Research Diagnostic Criteria (World Health Organization, 1993), and the condition should be having a significant impact on social and educational functioning.
- Family attributions about the disorder need to be considered and addressed to avoid attributions that militate against a better prognosis, or hamper healthy beliefs.

- Any comorbid conditions should be identified and discussed in full with parents.

Where medication is recommended (Joughin & Zwi, 1999) there should be the following.

- Adherence with national guidelines (National Institute for Health and Clinical Excellence, 2006; National Collaborating Centre for Mental Health, 2008).
- Liaison with school, having obtained permission from the parent and/ or child to establish a protocol for giving the child the medication in school if required and keeping it safely locked up. It may be helpful to provide a leaflet.
- Checking of cautions and contraindications with the child and family.
- A protocol to establish a trial of medication (e.g. over a 4-week period) with monitoring (e.g. by questionnaire) at home and particularly at school.
- Information during and after the trial that includes weight, height, blood pressure, pulse, as well as narrative information and questionnaires from parents and teachers.
- Information for the child's GP and often a request to continue repeat prescriptions.
- A protocol for drug holidays (e.g. weekdays, school holidays, annually) to avoid the risk of disturbance of growth patterns and to assess symptom pattern changes with and without medication as the young person develops.
- Ongoing monitoring with clear plans agreed, and reviews at agreed time points.
- Ongoing psychosocial and educational interventions.

Intervention should be tailored to the child and family's needs, and strong links between all agencies must be maintained. The research literature suggests that single-treatment approaches (e.g. either medication or behavioural modification) have several shortcomings. Pelham *et al* (1993) found that these could be reduced when approaches are combined, with suggestions that the primary symptoms are most successfully treated by medication and the secondary symptoms by behavioural approaches. The MTA Cooperative study in the USA suggests that improvement in most ADHD symptoms is obtained in the short term by medication alone (MTA Cooperative Group, 1999). However, allied behaviour and conduct problems, social skills, internalising symptoms and reading achievement are all enhanced by psychosocial interventions (MTA Cooperative Group, 1999). More careful analysis of the data shows that childhood outcome from psychosocial interventions is clearest where process outcome is achieved such as a reduction in negative, ineffective parenting (Hinshaw *et al*, 2000). Follow-up at 3 years shows no apparent advantage of treatment with medication over other treatments (Jensen et al, 2007), suggesting a complex picture where many symptoms naturally abate with age, and many other factors such as comorbidities, parental psychopathology and intervention history play important roles in developmental trajectories. Box 20.2 summarises the treatment approaches.

Conclusion

Attention-deficit hyperactivity disorder teams usefully link paediatricians, child mental health professionals and professionals from education support services. The advantages of forming such a team include: the development of expertise and cooperative working; the facilitation of a protocol for

---

Box 20.2 Treatment approaches

- Behaviour therapy and parenting programmes, whether large scale and community based (Cunningham *et al*, 1995) or small scale and focused (Overmeyer & Taylor, 1999), can reduce conduct problems in children with attentional problems. Large-scale studies have confirmed this (MTA Cooperative Group, 1999).
- Individual work can include cognitive therapy (Whalen *et al*, 1985) aimed at helping children internalise external messages of control and social problem-solving skills training.
- Group work can focus on social skills (Pelham & Bender, 1982), social problem-solving skills or anger management skills. The MTA study included a summer treatment programme (Wells *et al*, 2001).
- Educational interventions enhance learning (Cantwell & Baker, 1992; Wells *et al*, 2001). To include adaptation of the classroom environment and routine alongside ADHD-specific behavioural management strategies (Barkley, 1998; Dowdy *et al*, 1998)
- Work on child and family attributions is also important. Unnecessary blame alienates families (Bramble, 1998) and other strategies may help to empower parents to manage the child's behaviour and to view themselves as part of a solution, and to allow the child to believe in the possibilities of positive change and self-control (Wright *et al*, 2000). In this way, managing the attributions also becomes important in order to encourage healthy developmental trajectories for children. Some families may benefit from the team support of family therapy, helping them to recognise the resources existing within their family.
- Referral to other professionals should be considered, for example following the identification of comorbidities.
- Medication improves the concentration and reduces distractibility in most children, and therefore has clear benefits for children with ADHD in the short term (MTA Cooperative Group, 1999). Longer-term outcomes of the use of medication are less clear and have been published in a follow-up of the above study (Jensen *et al*, 2007). A close analysis of the multifaceted outcomes is recommended and should be considered in discussing treatment choices with parents.

197

assessment and diagnosis; and the coordination of management plans. Working with education services in particular helps to build a joint understanding that can be passed on to the teaching staff who have daily direct contact with the children.

References

Barkley, R. A. (1990) *Attention Deficit Hyperactivity Disorder: A Handbook for Diagnosis and Treatment*. Guilford Press.

Barkley, R. A. (1998) *Attention-Deficit Hyperactivity Disorder: A Handbook for Diagnosis and Treatment, Second Edition*. Guildford Press.

Black, D., Wright, B., Williams, C., *et al* (1999) Paediatric liaison service. *Psychiatric Bulletin*, **23**, 528–530.

Bramble, D. (1998) Attention deficit hyperactivity disorder. Child psychiatrists should help parents with difficult children, not blame them. *BMJ*, **317**, 1250–1251.

Cantwell, D. P. & Baker, L. (1992) Association between attention deficit hyperactivity disorder and learning disorders. In *Attention Deficit Disorder Comes of Age: Towards the Twenty-First Century* (eds S. E. Shaywitz & B. A. Shaywitz), pp. 145–164. Pro-Ed.

Chu, S. (2007) Occupational therapy for children with attention deficit hyperactivity disorder (ADHD). Part 1: a delineation model of practice. *British Journal of Occupational Therapy*, **70**, 372–383.

Cunningham, C. E., Bremner, R. & Boyle, M. (1995) Large group community based parenting programs for families of preschoolers at risk for disruptive behaviour disorders: utilization, cost effectiveness and outcome. *Journal of Child Psychology and Psychiatry*, **36**, 1141–1159.

Dowdy, C. A., Patton, J. R., Smith, T. E. C., *et al* (1998) *Attention-Deficit/Hyperactivity Disorder in the Classroom: A Practical Guide for Teachers*. Pro-Ed.

Dungar, D., Pritchard, J., Hensman, S., *et al* (1986) The investigation of atypical psychosomatic illness: a team approach to diagnosis. *Clinical Pediatrics*, **25**, 341–344.

DuPaul, G. J., Power, T. J., Anastopoulos, A. D., *et al* (1998) *ADHD Rating Scale – IV. Checklists, Norms, and Clinical Interpretation*. Guilford Press.

Goodman, R. (2001) The psychiatric properties of the strengths and difficulties questionnaire. *Journal of the American Academy of Child and Adolescent Psychiatry*, **40**, 1337–1345.

Hill, P. & Cameron, N. (1999) Recognising hyperactivity: a guide for the cautious clinician. *Child and Adolescent Mental Health*, **4**, 50–60.

Hinshaw, S. P., Owens, E. B., Wells, K. C., *et al* (2000) Family processes and treatment outcome in the MTA: negative/ineffective parenting practices in relation to multimodal treatment. *Journal of Abnormal Child Psychology*, **28**, 569–583.

Hughes, D. (2007) *Attachment Focused Family Therapy*. WW Norton & Co.

Jensen, P. S., Hinshaw, S. P., Kraemer, H. C., *et al* (2001) ADHD comorbidity findings from the MTA study: comparing comorbid subgroups. *Journal of the American Academy of Child and Adolescent Psychiatry*, **40**, 147–158.

Jensen, P. S., Arnold, L. E., Swanson, J. M., *et al* (2007) 3 year follow up of the NIMH MTA study. *Journal of the American Academy of Child and Adolescent Psychiatry*, **46**, 989–1002.

Joughin, C. & Zwi, M. (1999) *FOCUS on the Use of Stimulants in Children with Attention Deficit Hyperactivity Disorder: Evidence-Based Briefing*. Royal College of Psychiatrists Research Unit.

Kadesjö, B. & Gillberg, C. (2001) The comorbidity of ADHD in the general population of Swedish school-age children. *Child Psychology and Psychiatry*, **42**, 487–492.

Meltzer, H., Gatward, R., Goodman, R., *et al* (2000) *Mental Health of Children and Adolescents in Great Britain*. TSO (The Stationery Office).

MTA Cooperative Group (1999) Moderators and mediators of treatment response for children with attention-deficit/hyperactivity disorder: the Multimodal Treatment Study of children with Attention-deficit/hyperactivity disorder. *Archives of General Psychiatry*, **56**, 1088–1096.

National Collaborating Centre for Mental Health (2008) *Attention-Deficit Hyperactivity Disorder. The NICE Guideline on Diagnosis and Management of ADHD in Children, Young People and Adults.* British Psychological Society & Royal College of Psychiatrists (http://www.nice.org.uk/nicemedia/pdf/ADHDFullGuideline.pdf).

National Institute for Health and Clinical Excellence (2006) *Methylphenidate, Atomoxetine and Dexamfetamine for Attention Deficit Hyperactivity Disorder (ADHD) in Children and Adolescents.* NICE (http://www.nice.org.uk/nicemedia/pdf/TA098guidance.pdf).

Overmeyer, S. & Taylor, E. (1999) Annotation. Principles of treatment for hyperkinetic disorder: practice approaches for the U.K. *Journal of Child Psychology and Psychiatry*, **40**, 1147–1157.

Pelham, W. E. & Bender, M. (1982) Peer interactions of hyperactive children: assessment and treatment. In *Advances in Learning and Behaviour Difficulties* (eds K. Gradow & I. Gialer). JI Press.

Pelham, W. E., Carlson, C., Sams, S. E., *et al* (1993) Separate and combined effects of methylphenidate and behavior modification on boys with attention deficit hyperactivity disorder in the classroom. *Journal of Consulting and Clinical Psychology*, **61**, 506–515.

Richardson, G. & Cottrell, D. (2003) Service innovations: second opinions in child and adolescent psychiatry. *Psychiatric Bulletin*, **27**, 22–24.

Voeller, K. K. (1991) Clinical management of attention deficit hyperactivity disorder. *Journal of Child Neurology*, **6** (suppl.), S51–S67.

Wells, K. C., Pelham, W. E., Kotrein, R. A., *et al* (2001) Psychosocial treatment strategies in the MTA study: rationale, methods and critical issues in design and implementation. *Journal of Abnormal Child Psychology*, **28**, 483–505.

Whalen, C. K., Henker, B. & Hinshaw, S. B. (1985) Cognitive behavioural therapies for hyperactive children: premises, problems and prospects. *Journal of Abnormal Child Psychology*, **13**, 391–410.

Williams, C., Wright, B. & Partridge, I. (1999) Attention deficit hyperactivity disorder – a review. *British Journal of General Practice*, **49**, 563–571.

World Health Organization (1993) *The ICD–10 Classification of Mental and Behavioural Disorders: Diagnostic Criteria for Research.* WHO.

Wright, B., Partridge, I. & Williams, C. (2000) Evidence and attribution: reflections upon the management of attention deficit hyperactivity disorder (ADHD). *Clinical Child Psychology and Psychiatry*, **5**, 626–636.

CHAPTER 21

Eating disorder teams

Ruth Norton, Ian Partridge and Greg Richardson

'How disenchanting in the female character is a manifestation of relish for the pleasures of the table!'

William Charles Macready

Introduction

What causes eating disorders and how they are best treated remains the subject of much debate (Royal College of Psychiatrists, 1992; Ward *et al*, 1995; Shoebridge & Gowers, 2000; Gowers & Shore, 2001; Steinhausen, 2002; Gowers *et al*, 2007). However, referral to CAMHS continues and the need for an effective service remains. The NICE guidelines (National Collaborating Centre for Mental Health, 2004) recommend psychological interventions primarily in an out-patient setting, naming CBT for bulimia nervosa and family involvement including siblings in the treatment of young people with eating disorders. Specialist services for these young people are increasing, particularly in the independent in-patient sector. The establishment of a Tier 3 team within a CAMHS makes effective use of resources, in terms of both personnel and time (Roberts *et al*, 1998). The principles that underpin the workings of such a team are set out in Box 21.1.

Eating disorders can present in a number of forms: anorexia nervosa; bulimia nervosa; atypical variations of both; eating disorders not otherwise specified; and other feeding problems or disorders in childhood, described by Nicholls & Bryant-Waugh (2009) as food avoidance emotional disorder, selective eating, food phobias, functional dysphagia and food refusal.

Box 21.1 Service principles

- A multidisciplinary approach
- A clear operational policy
- Prompt responses
- A range of interventions geared to the individual needs of the young person and family
- A continuum of care between out-patient and in-patient services
- Close liaison with paediatric and medical services
- Input from a dietician

Obesity, ironically, remains the result of the major eating disorder of our time – eating too much and exercising too little, but its management is not usually the province of an eating disorder team.

Anorexia nervosa is characterised by a fear of fatness and a preoccupation with food, in which reduction of caloric intake (vomiting may be used) and increase in energy output via exercise and/or forms of purging results in serious weight loss. It may commence prior to puberty, although this is unusual, and affects up to 1% of 15- to 20-year-olds, of whom 10% are male.

Bulimia nervosa is characterised by a fear of loss of control with regard to eating. It results in episodes of binging and vomiting, and a preoccupation with weight and diet. It is more common than anorexia nervosa but tends to develop later in adolescence.

Eating disorders, at whatever age, should be seen within a developmental context – with an interacting multifactorial aetiology of genetic, individual, biological, familial and sociocultural factors (Steinhausen, 2002). In anorexia, the management of starvation is essential as it has emotional, cognitive and physical consequences. Eating disorders occur in young people who can't/don't tolerate themselves at a healthy weight, feel fat, disgusting and ugly, believe they take up too much space, don't feel good enough, don't think they deserve to eat, loathe themselves, feel guilty, scared, sad, angry, overwhelmed and lonely, and feel better for not eating.

A Tier 3 team integrated with locality CAMHS

A specialist eating disorders team may well be the most cost-effective way of dealing with adolescent eating disorders (Byford et al, 2007). The advantages of having a specialist eating disorders team operating within rather than independent of a generic CAMHS are the following.

- The coordinated utilisation of existing resources of personnel and time to provide a discrete and recognisable service.
- Models of treatment are informed from a multidisciplinary perspective.
- Specialist expertise and experience are not siphoned off and isolated in a separate service.
- Specialist resources within a comprehensive CAMHS encourage the recognition that eating disorders often exist within a wider clinical context and may be comorbid with other psychological or psychiatric disorders or difficulties.
- Team members develop expertise that can be used to meet the training needs of a range of disciplines; training programmes can be offered to allied disciplines and, in consultation, to other agencies.
- The team can offer a range of treatment approaches to individuals as a result of the different professional backgrounds and skills of the team members.

- Clinic time can be varied to match demand, ensuring individuals and their families are seen without delay and as often as is felt necessary.
- Supervision is built into the organisation of the team and can, if and when needed, be live.
- The team may deal with the full age range, managing childhood-onset eating problems (Fox & Joughin, 2002) as well as anorexia and bulimia.
- The problem of differential funding for different disorders, with consequent inequity of access, is avoided.
- There is a focused, skilled alternative to in-patient admission.
- A specific clinic whose purpose is well explained appears to reduce non-attendance rates, which can otherwise prove costly in terms of the allocation of team time; this improves efficiency. This could also encourage the commitment of the young person and their family to the long battle that lies ahead in treating the eating disorder.

Specialist provision within an existing CAMHS is labour intensive and removes resources from existing service provision; however, these young people would still have to be treated by the service. Pressure upon such a small service could lead to the lengthening of waiting lists, but if the team is of sufficient size and clinics operate for sufficient sessions per week to meet the demands of the catchment population, this should ensure rapid responses. The team provides an initial assessment service as well as a variety of ongoing therapeutic interventions from various permutations of the team working individually and jointly. Flexibility may entail occasionally working outside of the structured sessional timetable; however, it should be remembered that successful treatment of eating disorders necessitates the use of firm boundaries and taking control back from the eating disorder, and this should be reflected in the way the team operates.

Referral and intervention

A specialist eating disorders team may receive referrals direct from the allocation process (Chapter 11), as well as from other members of CAMHS. The eating disorders team can discuss all referrals, prioritise them and allocate them to specific professionals. A team coordinator is recommended. A standardised, explanatory appointment letter should be sent to the young person and family with an offer of an appointment within 4 weeks of referral. There may need to be emergency responses to acute crises, and paediatric assessment is indicated when the body mass index (BMI) is below 12, blood pressure is below 80/60 mmHg or pulse is less than 40 beats per minute to ensure physical stability before psychological interventions can commence or continue. At the initial assessment (Box 21.2), the whole family should be asked to attend so that from the start there is a clear message that the family is the most powerful therapeutic tool currently available for adolescents with anorexia (Russell et al, 1987).

Box 21.2 Assessment protocol

- Set family at their ease, alleviate their guilt
- Interview with parents
- Interview with child to gain history of presenting problem and update on present situation
- Full family, medical and psychiatric histories
- Physical examination and investigation including height, weight, temperature, pulse and blood pressure
- Questionnaires such as the Eating Attitude Test (EAT; Garner *et al*, 1982)

A structured approach

Assessment should be seen as the first stage of management and should assess the developmental, family, environmental and physical contributions to the young person's difficulties and their psychological sequelae, and investigate the family's and the young person's beliefs about food, weight and body image, including any family history of eating disorders or difficulties around food.

An initial management plan is negotiated with the family in the light of the assessment findings. If not already being monitored, a physical examination and blood tests should be carried out and repeated as necessary. Checking results against a system such as a traffic lights system (Treasure, 2004) can help to highlight abnormal and potentially fatal findings, which need to be managed. The physical consequences of eating disorders, including re-feeding syndrome, may dictate medical treatment and therefore the team should establish close working relationships with colleagues in paediatrics, endocrinology and gastroenterological medicine. It may be wise to prescribe vitamins while weight restoration is ongoing.

The range of therapeutic options used include advice on management, (often based on behavioural principles), CBT (Schmidt, 1998), interpersonal therapy (Gowers & Bryant-Waugh, 2004), motivational interviewing (Treasure & Schmidt, 2001), guided reading (Schmidt & Treasure, 1993), family therapy (Russell *et al*, 1987), and psychoeducation. Individual therapy sessions may be used to look at building self-esteem and to explore why the young person developed and has maintained the eating disorder, as well as gaining current and future mastery over their disorder.

The overriding goal of those working with young people with eating disorders and their families is to enthuse them with the concept that the eating disorder can be beaten, and so avoid hopelessness and resistance (Fig. 21.1).

However, it should be remembered that part of this task involves conveying the seriousness of the problem. Minimalisation on behalf of the patient is often absorbed into the family dynamics within a continuum of

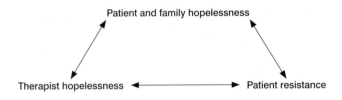

Fig. 21.1 Systemic installation of hopelessness.

under- to overreaction, as is the debate between the eating disorder as an 'illness' (a set of symptoms accompanied by the belief 'there's nothing I/ we can do about it') and a difficult behaviour. It should be noted that such a dialogue is often transmitted to the professionals involved. In eating disorders, the issue of control is often central, therefore it is of the utmost importance to empower the family and, in time, the young person to regain control from the eating disorder; at times of crisis this may involve the professionals temporarily assuming the position of the 'good authority' and gradually re-empowering the family and patient to take appropriate control.

A pattern of eating needs to be established that enables those who are underweight to restore weight (up to 0.5 kg per week as an out-patient, 0.5–1.0 kg per week as an in-patient) and those of normal weight to maintain it, while recognising how difficult this is going to be for all family members. The parents or carers may well have to take responsibility for this initially and, as such, support for them is central to the management of the eating disorder.

Input that is more intensive may be achieved via a specialist outreach service if available; however, admission to an in-patient unit is sometimes necessary. Factors that influence the need for in-patient care include:

- weight loss of more than 25% or a BMI of less than 13
- refusal of all food and drink (dehydration being of major concern)
- rehabilitation after medical admission for physical consequences of the eating disorder
- the young person's specific request for in-patient care
- failure of prolonged out-patient treatment, though the prognosis for this group is particularly bad (Gowers et al, 2007).

The aim of in-patient care of anorexia is to return the young person to developmentally appropriate physical and psychological functioning, weight gain being the initial step. However, the prognosis is worse for young people who are admitted (Gowers et al, 2000), which may reflect the more serious nature of their condition.

There is limited evidence for the use of pharmacological treatment in anorexia apart from those cautiously used to treat comorbid conditions (National Collaborating Centre for Mental Health, 2004). In adults with bulimia or binge eating disorder, selective serotonin reuptake inhibitors, namely fluoxetine, can be tried, but they are not included in the recommendations for treatment in children and adolescents (National Collaborating Centre for Mental Health, 2004).

Conclusion

Eating disorders present complex biopsychosocial difficulties to the patients, their carers and involved professionals. They are likely to be alleviated only by working from many perspectives, including supporting the young person and their family to develop healthier eating behaviours and attitudes to weight and shape. The interventions aim to enable the young person to overcome the lack of self-worth that drives the eating disorder, by facilitating the addressing of developmental and other psychosocial challenges that are causing particular distress for the individual and their family.

References

Byford, S., Barrett, B., Roberts, C., et al (2007) Economic evaluation of a randomised controlled trial for anorexia nervosa in adolescents. British Journal of Psychiatry, 191, 436–440.

Fox, C. & Joughin, C. (2002) Childhood-Onset Eating Problems: Findings from Research. Gaskell.

Garner, D. M., Olmsted, M. P., Bohr, Y., et al (1982) The eating attitudes test: psychometric features and clinical correlates. Psychological Medicine, 12, 871–878.

Gowers, S. & Bryant-Waugh, R. (2004) Management of child and adolescent eating disorders: the current evidence base and future directions. Journal of Child Psychology and Psychiatry, 45, 63–83.

Gowers, S. G. & Shore, A. (2001) Development of weight and shape concerns in the aetiology of eating disorders. British Journal of Psychiatry, 179, 236–242.

Gowers, S. G., Wetman, J., Shore, A., et al (2000) Impact of hospitalisation on the outcome of adolescent anorexia nervosa. British Journal of Psychiatry, 176, 138–141.

Gowers, S. G., Clark, A., Roberts, C., et al (2007) Clinical effectiveness of treatments for anorexia nervosa in adolescents. Randomised controlled trial. British Journal of Psychiatry, 191, 427–435.

National Collaborating Centre for Mental Health (2004) Eating Disorders. Core Interventions in the Treatment and Management of Anorexia Nervosa, Bulimia Nervosa and Related Eating Disorders. Clinical Guideline CG9. National Institute for Health and Clinical Excellence.

Nicholls, D. & Bryant Waugh, R. (2009) Eating disorders of infancy and childhood: definition, symptomatology, epidemiology and comorbidity. Child and Adolescent Psychiatric Clinics of North America, 18, 17–30.

Roberts, S., Foxton, T., Partridge, I., et al (1998) Establishing a specialist eating disorders team. Psychiatric Bulletin, 22, 214–216.

Royal College of Psychiatrists (1992) Eating Disorders. Council Report CR14. Royal College of Psychiatrists.

Russell, G., Szmukler, G. I., Dare, C., et al (1987) An evaluation of family therapy in anorexia nervosa and bulimia nervosa. Archives of General Psychiatry, 44, 1047–1056.

Schmidt, U. (1998) Eating disorders and obesity. In Cognitive–Behaviour Therapy for Children and Families (ed. P. Graham), pp. 262–281. Cambridge University Press.

Schmidt, U. & Treasure, J. (1993) Getting Better Bit(e) by Bit(e). Lawrence Erlbaum.

Shoebridge, P. J. & Gowers, S. G. (2000) Parental high concern and adolescent-onset anorexia nervosa. A case–control study to investigate direction of causality. *British Journal of Psychiatry*, **176**, 132–137.

Steinhausen, H. C. (2002) Anorexia and bulimia nervosa. In *Child and Adolescent Psychiatry* (eds M. Rutter & E. Taylor). Blackwell.

Treasure, J. (2004) *A Guide to the Medical Risk Assessment for Eating Disorders*. Kings College London, South London and Maudsley NHS Trust.

Treasure, J. & Schmidt, V. (2001) Ready, willing and able to change: motivational aspects of the assessment and treatment of eating disorders. *European Eating Disorders Review*, **9**, 4–18.

Ward, A., Ramsay, R. & Treasure, J. (1995) Eating disorders: not such a slim speciality? *Psychiatric Bulletin*, **19**, 723–724.

CHAPTER 22

Bereavement services

Barry Wright, Ian Partridge and Nick Jones

'To the bereaved nothing but the return of the lost person can bring true comfort; should what we provide fall short of that it is felt almost as an insult.'
John Bowlby

Introduction

Bereavement is not a pathological process, but can lead to a significant mortality and morbidity. Some children may suffer significant psychological consequences (Pettle-Michael & Lansdown, 1986) but depression is rare (Pfeffer *et al*, 2000). The evidence for the efficacy or usefulness of therapeutic work is limited (Harrington & Harrison, 1999; Currier *et al*, 2007). Research suggests that positive outcomes from therapeutic work are more likely to be achieved if certain groups of children are selected and provided 'timely' treatment (Currier et al, 2007). The corollary of this is that many children do well with family and community support and never need to see child mental health services (Dyregov, 2008).

Indications for bereavement work

Children may need support at times of family bereavement. There are a number of reasons the impact of bereavement on the development of children might be more pronounced.

- Bereavement may be associated with circumstances in which the normal supportive family influences are severely hampered; such circumstances include parental mental illness (Van Eerdewegh *et al*, 1985), catastrophic parental bereavement responses, and emotionally abusive or neglecting parents (Elizur & Kaffman, 1983; Bifulco *et al*, 1987).
- Severe psychological trauma associated with the death, including parental suicide (Wright & Partridge, 1999; Pfeffer *et al*, 2000; Department of Health, 2008).
- Repeated bereavement.
- Prolonged disruption to the child's life.
- Family system changes (Wasserman, 1988).
- Extreme circumstances such as war (Goldstein *et al*, 1997).

Managing bereavement

Childhood bereavement services look at the effects of bereavement on children in a number of ways.

- Diagnostically: bereavement can lead to emotional or behavioural problems that have social or educational effects and that represent a diagnosable entity.
- Adult mental health: there may be effects on the parenting available to the child before or after the bereavement.
- Child protection: bereavement may upset parents' emotional or physical care of a child.
- Systemically: there may be systemic effects that represent risk factors for the child.
- Developmentally: the circumstances surrounding the bereavement may damage the child's development.
- Attributionally: beliefs and attributions regarding the death, in either the child or the family, may be damaging.

In considering these factors, CAMHS need to have a clear view of its functions (Box 22.1).

There appears to be a spectrum of provision throughout the country ranging from CAMHS that have no involvement with bereavement unless a diagnosable mental disorder is present, to CAMHS that take a lead role in coordinating and integrating a range of bereavement services across a district.

Given a lack of clarity in the research about outcomes for children who have been bereaved (Harrington & Harrison, 1999), there are differences of opinion about when services should be provided. For example, should we provide services for all bereaved children, for those children screened as being at risk after bereavement or only for those children reaching a threshold of emotional and behavioural problems (Worden, 1996). This problem is neatly side-stepped when the four-tier model of CAMHS is evoked (NHS Health Advisory Service, 1995). This recognises that parents and all professionals (Tiers 1–4) have responsibilities for the emotional

---

Box 22.1 Functions of a bereavement team

- Treating mental health problems in the child
- Prevention of child mental ill health by working with children at high risk
- Prevention of future child mental ill health by working with parents, including preventing mental ill health in a parent
- Leadership and consultation in fashioning district-wide services, and coordinating and integrating statutory and voluntary agencies in their provision

welfare and healthy development of children, and this must inevitably include supporting them through bereavement. This does not necessarily mean therapy. It may mean support to the parents, telephone advice, training of teachers and a range of options across the tiers.

In practice, CAMHS can be usefully involved in:

- networking with other professionals to ensure a comprehensive range of services;
- providing consultation to those supporting children and their families (e.g. teachers, general practice counsellors, school nurses, Cruse Bereavement Care counsellors, pupil support staff, social workers, family support workers, GPs and chaplains);
- taking referrals for those bereaved children with emotional and behavioural problems where families and Tier 1 professionals are struggling or where significant mental health problems are present.

Networking

Parents or carers are often best placed to support bereaved children, although they may call on Tier 1 professionals for support. The involvement of Tier 2 professionals may occur subsequently if there are clear indications of a mental health problem. Evidence suggests that existing UK bereavement services vary greatly in different parts of the country (Rolls, 2003), often relying heavily on voluntary services and including a range of provision. National self-help advice is available (Department of Health, 2008).

It is common sense for the various professionals involved in bereavement support to know each other and to have an understanding of the way services relate to each other. It also makes sense for any network to coordinate and agree a range of services, and to liaise with each other to maintain standards and care pathways. There are a number of ways to achieve this, including networking meetings or established mechanisms for liaison. Formal links may be usefully established through:

- palliative care teams
- local adult hospices
- local children's hospices
- Cruse Bereavement Care counsellors
- health visitors
- school nurses
- hospital chaplaincy services
- pupil support services.

Such links serve to highlight existing services and gaps in services that the network may decide to address. The tasks will include offering advice and support in a family-centred provision that dovetails with services from other agencies; key aims must be to avoid both pathologising and disempowering families.

Child and adolescent mental health services have an advice and consultation role, and may be able to draw upon a range of models to inform, advise and support. Team members will be able to draw on their understanding of the following.

- Attachment issues (Bowlby, 1980) that acknowledge a young person's fear of rejection, isolation, not being understood or fears for the future (Balk, 1990; Silverman *et al*, 1992).
- Systemic issues, including changes in roles within the family and changes in affective functioning within the family (Wasserman, 1988).
- How children may experience significant psychological and behavioural difficulties in bereavement (Pettle-Michael & Lansdown, 1986; Noonan & Douglas, 2002).
- Communication and how adult anxiety may affect healthy coping (Baulkwill & Wood, 1994).
- The importance of maintaining family integrity and self-efficacy (Bandura *et al*, 1980; Silverman & Worden, 1992).
- The child's age and developmental stage (Kane, 1979).
- The importance of establishing the meaning of events to the child (Pollock, 1986).
- Adjustment as family members simultaneously negotiate change (Silverman *et al*, 1992).
- Resilience – the capacity to minimise or overcome the damaging effects of adversity (Newman, 2004).
- The factors other than bereavement that may affect a child, and the need to arrive at a formulation that takes account of emotional, psychosocial, intellectual, educational, developmental, family and environmental factors.
- That bereavement in itself is not a pathological process, although a range of vulnerability factors and resilience factors may be operating at both the parental (e.g. poor parenting after the death of one parent, parental mental illness) and the child level (e.g. social and peer support, intelligence) that can have an effect on both present and future child mental health.

Team membership

Although all CAMHS members would normally be expected to have a grasp of issues relating to bereavement and to be able to provide consultation and take referrals where necessary, there may be a number of reasons to identify certain professionals within the team to take a lead role with bereavement:

- to enable them to develop more expertise in particularly difficult scenarios such as suicide;
- to provide a focus for consultation and liaison with other teams (e.g. palliative care, hospices, paediatric liaison);

- to take a lead role in networking;
- to take a lead role in the development of services.

Any of the professionals within CAMHS would be able to do this. In larger areas, two or more professionals may share this work. Formal referrals can be processed through the referral management process.

Planning and training

Child and adolescent mental health service members may need training from time to time in this area, since such referrals are not uncommon. By the same token, CAMHS professionals may be called on to provide training for a variety of other professionals from both voluntary and statutory agencies.

Interventions

Clinicians would usually encourage good emotional and psychological support from the family, with open and honest communication with the child about the death. Fewer specific interventions have been systematically studied (Stokes *et al*, 1997; Harrington, 1998; Currier *et al*, 2007). Children's natural resilience to cope with trauma may be impaired and therefore interventions should focus on rebuilding resilience which is best achieved by the primacy of listening to children uncritically as they 'tell their story'. Consideration needs to be given to the justification of any intervention in terms of the benefits for the child and family. Box 22.2 lists the interventions that a CAMHS may consider providing.

Multi-agency groups

In some districts, the development of groups for children may involve professionals from different agencies (voluntary and statutory) coming

---

Box 22.2 Possible interventions

- Provision of information
- Advice to parents, carers and other supporting adults (Department of Health, 2008)
- Consultation to Tier 1 professionals
- Individual work and the promotion of resilience
- Group work (Pennels *et al*, 1992; Baulkwill & Wood, 1994; Smith & Pennels, 1995; Wright *et al*, 1996, 2002)
- Family work (Gibbons, 1992; Gillance *et al*, 1997)

---

together. Different models and settings for this might include a children's hospice in a voluntary service sector (Wright *et al*, 1996), a programme such as Winston's Wish (Stokes *et al*, 1997) in a private but commissioned capacity or in a multi-agency capacity in a CAMHS setting (Wright *et al*, 2002). This last model involves various agencies bringing children, with whom they may have been working individually, into a group setting. Since this can be set up in such a way as to involve the same number of hours of work, it can be resource neutral to each agency. This allows children to work alongside each other and means that no agency commits more time than it would have committed ordinarily. Groups do not preclude individual or family work before or after group work. This has the advantages of:

- providing a wider range of services for children and families
- improving professional networking
- cross-fertilisation of ideas among local professionals
- improving peer supervision
- avoiding stigmatisation engendered by referral to mental health services.

Once a networked service is established, it is necessary for professionals at Tier 1 to be aware both of its existence and of the range of services available. This can be done by providing relevant information to primary mental health workers, general practice surgeries, customer service departments within Social Services, hospital chaplaincy, palliative care teams and pupil support services. Such information should include a service map that delineates all the various agencies, contact details, their expertise, how they work and how they relate to other professionals.

Audit and evaluation

Regular audit ensures that services have standards and maintain them. More research needs to be done to clarify the role of bereavement support services. Families should be asked for feedback about services and be given evaluation forms. Services need to be accessible to all children and their families, including those with specific needs (e.g. children with physical and learning disabilities or sensory impairments). Improved research into this area of work is necessary to be clearer about the outcomes for children with and without services.

References

Balk, D. E. (1990) The self concept of bereaved adolescents: sibling death and its aftermath. *Journal of Adolescent Research*, **5**, 112–132.

Bandura, A., Adams, N. E., Hardy, A. B., *et al* (1980) Tests of the generality of the self-efficacy theory. *Cognitive Therapy and Research*, **4**, 39–66.

Baulkwill, J. & Wood, C. (1994) Group work with bereaved children. *European Journal of Palliative Care*, **1**, 113–115.

Bifulco, A. T., Brown, G. W. & Harris, T. O. (1987) Childhood loss of a parent, lack of parental care and adult depression: a replication. *Journal of Affective Disorders*, **12**, 115–128.

Bowlby, J. (1980) *Attachment. Vol. III. Loss, Sadness and Depression*. Hogarth Press.

Currier, J. M., Holland, J. M. & Neimeyer, R. A. (2007) The effectiveness of bereavement interventions with children: a meta-analytic review of controlled outcome research. *Journal of Clinical Child and Adolescent Psychology*, **36**, 253–259.

Department of Health (2008) *Help is at Hand*. TSO (The Stationery Office).

Dyregov, A. (2008) *Grief in Children: A Handbook for Adults*. Jessica Kingsley Publishers.

Elizur, E. & Kaffman, M. (1983) Factors influencing the severity of childhood bereavement reactions. *American Journal of Orthopsychiatry*, **53**, 668–676.

Gibbons, M. B. (1992) A child dies, a child survives: the impact of sibling loss. *Journal of Pediatric Health Care*, **6**, 65–72.

Gillance, H., Tucker, A., Aldridge, J., et al (1997) Bereavement: providing support for siblings. *Paediatric Nursing*, **9**, 22–24.

Goldstein, R. D., Wampler, N. S. & Wise, P. H. (1997) War experiences and distress symptoms of Bosnian children. *Pediatrics*, **100**, 873–878.

Harrington, R. (1998) Clinically depressed adolescents. In *Cognitive–Behaviour Therapy for Children and Families* (ed. P. Graham), pp. 156–193. Cambridge University Press.

Harrington, R. & Harrison, L. (1999) Unproven assumptions about the impact of bereavement on children. *Journal of the Royal Society of Medicine*, **92**, 230–233.

Kane, B. (1979) Children's concepts of death. *Journal of Genetic Psychology*, **134**, 141–153.

Newman, T. (2004) *What Works in Building Resilience?* Barnardo's.

NHS Health Advisory Service (1995) *Together We Stand: Commissioning, Role and Management of Child and Adolescent Mental Health Services*. HMSO.

Noonan, K. & Douglas, A. (2002) *Supporting Children After Suicide. Information for Parents and Care-Givers*. New South Wales Department of Health.

Pennels, M., Smith, S. & Poppleton, R. (1992) Bereavement and adolescents: a groupwork approach. *Association of Child Psychiatry and Psychology Newsletter*, **14**, 173–178.

Pettle-Michael, S. A. & Lansdown, R. G. (1986) Adjustment to the death of a sibling. *Archives of Disease in Childhood*, **61**, 278–283.

Pfeffer, C. R., Carus, D., Seigel, K., et al (2000) Child survivors of parental death from cancer or suicide: depressive and behavioural outcomes. *Psychooncology*, **9**, 1–10.

Pollock, G. H. (1986) Childhood sibling loss. A family tragedy. *Pediatric Annals*, **15**, 851–855.

Rolls, L. (2003) Childhood bereavement services: a survey of UK provision. *Palliative Medicine*, **17**, 423–432.

Silverman, P. R. & Worden, J. W. (1992) Children's reactions in the early months after the death of a parent. *American Journal of Orthopsychiatry*, **62**, 93–104.

Silverman, P. R., Nickman, S. & Worden, J. W. (1992) Detachment revisited. The child's reconstruction of a dead parent. *American Journal of Orthopsychiatry*, **62**, 494–503.

Smith, S. C. & Pennels, M. (1995) *Interventions with Bereaved Children*. Jessica Kingsley.

Stokes, J., Wyer, S. & Crossley, D. (1997) The challenge of evaluating a child bereavement programme. *Palliative Medicine*, **11**, 179–190.

Van Eerdewegh, M. M., Clayton, P. J. & Van Eerdewegh, P. (1985) The bereaved child: variables influencing early psychopathology. *British Journal of Psychiatry*, **147**, 188–194.

Wasserman, A. L. (1988) Helping families get through the holidays after the death of a child. *American Journal of Diseases in Childhood*, **142**, 1284–1286.

Worden, J. W. (1996) *Children and Grief: When a Parent Dies*. Guilford Press.

Wright, B. & Partridge, I. (1999) Speaking ill of the dead. *Clinical Child Psychology and Psychiatry*, **4**, 225–231.

Wright, B., Elvans, H., King, P., et al (2002) Developing a multiagency bereavement service. *European Journal of Palliative Care*, **9**, 160–163.

Wright, J. B., Aldridge, J., Gillance, H., et al (1996) Hospice based groups for bereaved siblings. *European Journal of Palliative Care*, **3**, 10–15.

CHAPTER 23

CAMHS for refugees and recent immigrants

Matthew Hodes

'A cold coming we had of it.'

> T. S. Eliot, *Journey of the Magi*

Introduction

The UK has a centuries-old tradition of receiving immigrants (Kushner & Knox, 1999; Winder, 2004). After the 1950s, the number of people coming to the UK predominantly from the Commonwealth countries of the Caribbean and South Asia (India, Pakistan and Bangladesh) increased. Recent migrants have come from all over the world with significant numbers from the European Union, South Asia and Ireland. The ethnicity of the UK is becoming more diverse with 8% belonging to Black and minority ethnic groups, mainly Asian or Asian British and Black or Black British, Mixed, or Chinese (Office of National Statistics, 2007). In 1981, just over 6% of the UK population had been born overseas, but this had risen to just over 8% by 2001 and almost 10% by 2006 (Office of National Statistics, 2007). The age structure of the population shows that ethnic minority groups have much higher proportions of young people (i.e. under 20 years) than White ethnic groups. Those born outside the UK have much higher fertility rates than those born in the UK, suggesting that the population may continue to become more ethnically heterogeneous.

Reasons for migration are varied. Immigrants may leave their countries of origin seeking improved life chances through work and educational opportunities. Since the Second World War, the UK has had high demand for immigrants to satisfy the demand of the labour market (Winder, 2004). Others have come as asylum seekers or refugees, fleeing their countries because of fear or experience of persecution and organised violence (Winder, 2004). Asylum seekers travel to resettlement countries, including the UK, and apply for rights to remain, which confers refugee status (UNHCR, 2006). Refugee status gives entitlement to work and benefits of the welfare state. Over the 15 years until 1998, it was estimated that approximately 300 000 refugees and asylum seekers came to the UK (Bardsley & Storkey, 2000). In 2006, there were 23 610 asylum applications to the UK, of which 6225 resulted in grants of asylum, humanitarian protection or discretionary leave (Home Office, 2007). The top five applicant nationalities in 2006 were: Eritrean, Afghan, Iranian, Chinese and Somali. One special group are unaccompanied asylum-seeking children who are under the age of 18 years on arrival (Watters, 2007). Over the years 2000–2006 there have been about 5500 unaccompanied asylum-seeking children in England and Wales, mostly living in London and Kent.

Migration and mental health

It has long been known that migration affects mental health, and the direction and nature of this association is complex and varied (Bhugra, 2004). Internationally, migrant children do not show a higher level of mental health problems compared with non-migrant peers (Stevens & Vollebergh, 2008). In the UK, the limited evidence available suggests that children from Indian and Black African ethnic groups have fewer mental disorders than White British children, but children from African–Caribbean and Bangladeshi communities have higher rates for some disorders (Meltzer *et al*, 2000; Goodman *et al*, 2008; Hodes *et al*, 2008*a*). However, many existing studies have methodological limitations and have not delineated the range of relevant factors such as reasons for migration, duration of settlement and country of birth, the economic and cultural background of the migrants, and the level of support in the host society.

Many factors interact to increase or reduce the risk of psychopathology and poor social function for migrant children. Planning for migration with realistic expectations, low level of disruption of family relationships, with social networks that can be activated on arrival in the adopted country and good parental employment prospects will be associated with lower risk (McKelvey & Webb, 1996; Simich *et al*, 2006). For asylum seekers and refugees, high level of war exposure, disruption of relationships and loss of family and community with hazardous journeys and resettlement adversities such as legal uncertainties, poverty and social isolation are associated with high risk for children and parents (Sack *et al*, 1996; Fazel *et al*, 2005; Hodes, 2008). Unaccompanied asylum-seeking children may have experienced a high level of family separation and losses, war trauma, arduous journeys, and difficulties in obtaining adequate support on arrival in resettlement countries (Wade *et al*, 2005; Hodes *et al*, 2008*b*). However, psychological distress for refugee children and adults diminishes over time during settlement, in association with legal security and rights to obtain permanent housing and employment for parents. Children become established in schooling and rapidly acquire language fluency, and the family as a whole are able to establish social networks (Almqvist & Broberg, 1999; Sack *et al*, 1999; Vojvoda *et al*, 2008).

Asylum-seeking and refugee children have high prevalence rates of post-traumatic stress symptoms and disorders, depression and adjustment disorders (Fazel *et al*, 2005). Young refugees who came to resettlement countries early in their childhood may have elevated levels of conduct problems (Tousignant *et al*, 1999), but it is not known whether this would also be found among those who came in later childhood or adolescence.

215

They may also have disorders that might have occurred in the absence of experience of war and displacement such as neurodevelopmental problems (e.g. hyperkinetic disorder and pervasive developmental disorders; Howard & Hodes, 2000). Unaccompanied asylum-seeking children have high levels of psychological distress manifest as post-traumatic stress, anxiety and depressive symptoms (Bean *et al*, 2006; Hodes *et al*, 2008*b*). Intellectual disability, specific learning disorders and psychosis might also occur among migrant children (Westermeyer, 1991; Tolmac & Hodes, 2004).

Children and adolescents who have recently migrated may have experienced disruptions of close relationships and other stressful events. These may result in adjustment difficulties, mood or anxiety symptoms which may manifest at home or school. These problems may be related to parental coping with migration, their ability to re-establish routines, and the quality of relationships with children. The ability of family members to settle and adjust to life in their adopted country will vary substantially according to their legal status, ability to prepare for migration, social, cultural and linguistic links, and individual variables such as age, gender, employment potential and mental health (Berry *et al*, 2002). Within the family, relationships may change if children assimilate more rapidly than parents and take on a 'carer' role. The extent to which this is a risk for mental health problems depends on the circumstances including age and ability of the child, and the extent to which the child or adolescent experiences appropriate warmth and support from parents and other older relatives.

Intergenerational tensions may occur as the migrant children settle into school and acquire British culture more rapidly than their parents. Impressions are that this raises difficulties particularly in adolescence when school and peer influence becomes more important. Tensions may arise for migrant youngsters who have divided loyalties between family and peers and other influences, especially if the youngsters are carers or provide a highly supportive role because of parents' poor language fluency in their adopted country or social isolation. These tensions might contribute to various problems such as conduct or mood symptoms.

Presentation of mental disorders

Mental disorders are generally similar to those seen in non-migrant children. However, there is a higher prevalence of some disorders among asylum seekers and refugees such as PTSD, often comorbid with depression. There are also reports of rarer problems such as violent self-harm (Patel & Hodes, 2006) and somatoform disorders associated with depression, in which children become withdrawn and lose the ability to eat and talk (Bodegard, 2005). Young asylum seekers may suffer the physical effects of maltreatment, including physical injuries, sexually transmitted diseases and pregnancy arising from sexual assault. Migrant children may also have mental health problems associated with physical disease such as sickle cell disease or infectious disease including HIV and AIDS (Havens & Mellins, 2008).

There are likely to be problems in assessing the severity and nature of such mental health problems. First, linguistic difficulties may be present and a need for communication through interpreters (see p. 220) may make assessment complex in view of the need to assess the range and severity of symptoms, and understand development within a sociocultural context different to the one with which the assessing clinicians are familiar. Assessment of intellectual disability and psychometric testing may also be problematic. Second, migrant children and families may be highly mobile, which may make assessments difficult (e.g. because of school changes and disrupted peer relationships). Third, migrants including refugees may have come from societies very different to the UK and other affluent resettlement countries, and so early-life experience may have been different. This might include reduced or absent schooling. Children may have been reared in extended families, with separation from parents in the migration process. These factors may make it difficult to elicit the conventional developmental history and assess quality of early care. Fourth, the past disruptions in care and life changes may appear to cause heightened arousal, inattention and behavioural problems. It may be necessary to assess whether the disruptive behaviour symptoms diminish over time after settlement in one home and school. Care is needed because such behaviours may be relatively stable and relate to underlying neurodevelopmental disorders (Bishop & Rutter, 2008) including hyperkinetic symptoms, and occur with specific reading disability and developmental coordination disorder (Gillberg & Kadesjo, 2003).

Tiered services

The tiered model of provision (NHS Health Advisory Sevice, 1995; Hill, 1999) may be adapted for the needs of refugee children (Hodes, 2002), and these principles will be similar for non-refugee migrant children.

Tier 1

In primary care, health visitors and GPs address the normal concerns and minor problems of parents regarding young children's achievement of developmental milestones, sleeping and feeding. Health professionals should be aware of significant cultural variation in household composition, family roles and family routines. Feeding and eating practices vary, as well as attitudes to child growth. For example, in South Asian and Caribbean cultures, mothers regard plumper infants as healthy compared with White British mothers, and South Asian mothers are more likely to bring their concerns about their children not gaining weight and growth to the attention of doctors (Hodes et al, 1996). There is also variation in sleeping arrangements, as in many cultures sharing beds with mothers occurs until a later age than among White British families (Hackett & Hackett, 1994; Liu *et al*, 2003). There are different concerns within schools, where integration of all pupils is an important task. In secondary schools and where teachers and support staff have differentiated roles, induction programmes and sessions to promote the integration of migrant pupils, including those from refugee backgrounds, may be helpful (Ingleby & Watters, 2002; Rutter, 2006).

Tier 2

The many advantages of community-based services are especially relevant for recently arrived immigrants, including refugees. First, recently arrived migrants may lack English language fluency and so negotiating referral to mental health services through primary care, even assuming registration with a GP has taken place, may be a major hurdle. Second, for many ethnic minority people, CAMHS is associated with considerable stigma (Bradby *et al*, 2007) and school-based delivery may reduce this. Third, migrant and ethnic minority parents, for cultural reasons, may have very different understanding of children's difficulties compared with professionals and may find the need for referral to CAMHS perplexing. Fourth, CAMHS professionals may link to specific ethnic minority groups, often through voluntary sector organisations, or target specific groups such as refugee children (O'Shea *et al*, 2000). Finally, evidence is emerging of effectiveness of service delivery in this context. There may be improved outcomes for refugee children with heterogeneous difficulties (O'Shea *et al*, 2000; Hodes, 2002). Furthermore, school-based group psychological interventions have shown benefit for PTSD symptoms (Stein *et al*, 2003) and general anxiety symptoms (Barrett *et al*, 2003) in migrant children. In areas that have a large number of unaccompanied asylum-seeking children, it is beneficial to link directly to Social Services who support the children (Wade *et al*, 2005), in view of the high prevalence of psychiatric symptoms (Hodes *et al*, 2008*b*) and unmet need (Bean *et al*, 2006).

There have been concerns that South Asian youngsters and their families may be less likely to access specialist CAMHS than their White British peers (Goodman *et al*, 2008). Asylum-seeking and refugee youngsters may also encounter barriers to referral, and be more likely to be referred by community professionals such as social workers and teachers rather than GPs compared with economic migrants and White British peers (Howard & Hodes, 2000). Therefore, CAMHS practitioners working in community settings, such as primary care, schools, Social Services and voluntary sector organisations, may well be more accessible. Their role is to provide consultation to Tier 1 community professionals, direct intervention to psychologically distressed children and adolescents, working with their families, and support referral to Tier 3 teams when indicated. They will be able to alert Tier 1 professionals to migration and settlement stressors, and the psychological implications as well as difficulties that are unrelated to specific migration or cultural factors. When in schools, they will be able to liaise with teachers and clarify whether classroom-based interventions or assessment by other professionals such as educational psychologists are required. Initial contact for assessment may be facilitated by introduction by teachers or other school professionals.

Tier 3

Migrant and refugee children referred to Tier 3 teams within CAMHS and who attend with psychiatric or developmental disorders may have a similar level of impairment as White British peers (Howard & Hodes, 2000). Since migrant and refugee children do not have disorders specific to their status, careful planning is required to ensure disorder-specific expertise is made available to this group. For example, in areas with large numbers of asylum-seeking and refugee children, it may be effective for one clinical team to lead on their management. However, impressions are that as migrants and refugees become more settled, developmental disorders and disruptive behaviour problems are more commonly encountered and so access to teams that manage neuropsychiatric disorders including pervasive developmental disorders and also intellectual disabilities is required. Given the ethnic diversity and psychiatric heterogeneity of young people seen in CAMHS, ethnic-specific teams for each ethnic group are not appropriate.

Outside the NHS, charities such as The Medical Foundation for the Care of Victims of Torture (www.torturecare.org.uk/) provide psychological treatment and legal support for young people and families who have experienced torture. Many of these individuals are asylum seekers.

Tier 4

The number of recent migrant and refuge youngsters who require psychiatric admission is small, but they are probably overrepresented in relation to their numbers in the community (Tolmac & Hodes, 2004). These youngsters, who are predominantly adolescents, have high levels of impairment and a high proportion have psychosis. Their experiences of past adversities such as war violence, and often low family and social support and legal difficulties, result in complex management problems (Hodes & Tolmac, 2005).

Challenges in clinical management

Many recently arrived families are highly mobile and this, in addition to language and occasional reluctance of primary care to register new families, may make access to mental health services difficult. Initial contact with CAMHS also needs to be carefully considered to maximise the chance of establishing contact (e.g. whether to telephone or write for the first appointment). The day-to-day difficulties experienced by many recent migrants may result in requests for support to enable access to housing and school, and also support for asylum applications by preparation of psychiatric reports (Tufnell, 2003). Specific problems arise for children and families who are detained in asylum centres or immigration removal centres. They may have poor mental health (Anonymous, 2008; Nielson *et al*, 2008; Pidd, 2008; Lorek *et al*, 2009), inadequate identification of mental health problems and poor access to mental health professionals (Silove *et al*, 2007).

Although large numbers of migrant families have come to the UK from cultures that are similar to that of Britain (e.g. USA, Australia), others come from cultures with which CAMHS clinicians may be unfamiliar. For indigenous clinicians in areas with significant proportions of migrants from one culture, it will be feasible to acquire some understanding of that culture. However, for others who may be working in large metropolitan areas with very culturally diverse communities, this will not be possible. What is required is an awareness of how to work with culturally different families and recognition of the ways in which there may be differences: language and idioms of communication, experience and communications of affect and distress, ideas regarding child development, deviance and misfortune, and understanding of therapies and how to achieve good social function within cultural context (Berry *et al*, 2002). At a practical level, the clinical approach is facilitated by using the 'outsider' perspective, respectfully seeking the families' views and incorporating them into management appropriately (Di Nicola, 1985a,b). Specific help may be obtained in understanding families and young people by working with 'culture brokers' who typically have come from the families' culture but have lived for a long time in the resettlement country, and so act as a bridge between the family and clinician. This may be an extension of the interpreters' role (see Raval (2005) for a full account of the bicultural worker). Recruitment of CAMHS professionals who speak the same language as the families served of course obviates the need for interpreters, but is not practical for areas in which many languages are spoken.

Interpreters

Working with interpreters requires an awareness of how effective communication can be achieved (Raval & Tribe, 2002; Farooq & Fear, 2003). It is useful to meet the interpreter before the interview, and then it is necessary to talk slowly and clearly, addressing the child or family. Ideally, there is a post-session discussion with the interpreter. Involving an interpreter approximately doubles the session duration. Often families who do not have English language fluency do not wish to involve an interpreter but prefer to rely on a child or adolescent in the family, other relatives or a friend. This may make translation of sensitive information difficult, and compromise the relationships between the index patient, the person acting as interpreter and family. For these reasons this situation is best avoided, although sometimes families insist on it.

Treatment provision

There are a number of considerations concerning psychiatric treatment provision. First, treatments need to be offered that can be managed within the constraints of the language fluency of the patient, family and therapist. Thus, some psychological treatments such as group therapies including parenting groups may be impractical. Second, in view of the high mobility of recent migrants, treatments may need to be offered despite the threat of premature termination that may arise because of a change of home or even deportation. Third, it is important to take into account families' culturally shaped views regarding treatments (Aroche & Coello, 2004). Attitudes will vary regarding the usefulness or acceptability of individual psychological and family therapy, and pharmacotherapy. Finally, there are variations in the extent to which children and their families can look back, for example when this is requested by the clinicians for the assessment or exploration of past traumatic events (with a view to using cognitive–behavioural or exposure methods of treatment). In this context, some distressed people want to focus on 'here and now' problems that might relate to migration status such as housing, children's progress in school or legal status and asylum applications. Recent migrants often wish to look forwards as their thinking is organised by their aspirations and hopes for future success in their adopted country. However, it should also be borne in mind that the difficulty in looking into the past may be related to avoidance associated with experience of past traumatic events, and be a feature of PTSD (Van der Veer & van Maning, 2004).

Meeting child and adolescent mental health needs

It is expected that mental health services will meet the needs of migrant and ethnic minority people (Department of Health, 2005). This expectation assumes that there is adequate information available to identify the specific mental health needs of the varied communities in the UK. Inadequate research has been carried out into ethnic variation and the effect of migration on the prevalence of psychiatric disorders, attitudes to mental health problems and treatments, and the optimal context for service delivery for young people. Despite the limitations of the existing evidence base, UK health commissioners are required to identify need on the basis of national epidemiological data, available local demographic data (including ethnicity), and data on service utilisation (Malek, 2004). For some special groups such as unaccompanied asylum-seeking children and other ethnic minority looked-after children, the numbers should be available from the Local Authority Social Services department (Department for Education and Skills, 2006). However, other groups may have migrated to areas since the last census, which obviously makes planning problematic. Commissioners need to provide adequate support to ensure that services are accessible, for example supporting high levels of GP registration and access, appropriate outreach to children and families from ethnic minority communities, funding for interpreters, and adequate time for clinicians working with migrant families, which, as has been indicated, is often more time consuming than working with settled British families. The appropriate mental health providers need to contribute to the dialogue about how to meet mental health needs working imaginatively with other agencies such as Social Services, schools and the voluntary sector.

Attention needs to be given to the training of child and adolescent mental health professionals in cultural psychiatry. Training should cover a range of topics including variations in child development, family organisation and implications for parent–child relationships, variations in psychopathology, epidemiology, and service utilisation (Berry *et al*, 2002; Nikapota, 2008). With regard to treatments, family therapy is probably the psychological treatment that has best addressed the perspective of culture and ethnicity (Di Nicola, 1997; McGoldrick, 1998). Within family therapy training, experiential and didactic and skill-based approaches (e.g. family therapy workshops) to learning can be used (Falicov, 1995; Green, 1998). Other treatment approaches deserving attention include psychopharmacology, as racial–ethnic factors have been the subject of recent investigation (Yu *et al*, 2007) and have implications for child and adolescent populations.

Conclusion

There is still much to be learnt regarding how best to address the mental health needs of young recent migrants including refugees. Although there are plans to restrict general migration to the UK from outside Europe, there will continue to be a flow of migrants who have desired work skills (see UK Home Office, www.ukba.homeoffice.gov.uk/managingborders). In addition, the UK continues to have obligations as a signatory to the United Nations to accept asylum seekers, the flow of which will be unpredictable. The UK's membership of the European Community will ensure continuing mobility and likely inflow of culturally and ethnically diverse people into the country, whose mental health needs it will remain our responsibility to address.

References

Almqvist, K. & Broberg, A. G. (1999) Mental health and social adjustment in young refugee children 3 1/2 years after their arrival in Sweden. *Journal of the American Academy of Child and Adolescent Psychiatry*, **8**, 723–730.

Anonymous (2008) Health care for children in UK detention centres. *Lancet*, **372**, 1783.

Aroche, J. & Coello, M. J. (2004) Ethnocultural considerations in the treatment of refugees and asylum seekers. In *Broken Spirits. The Treatment of Traumatized Asylum Seekers, Refugees, War and Torture Victims* (eds J. P. Wilson & B. Drozdek), pp. 53–80. Bruner-Routledge.

Bardsley, M. & Storkey, M. (2000) Estimating the numbers of refugees in London. *Journal of Public Health Medicine*, **22**, 406–412.

Barrett, P. M., Sonderegger, R. & Xenos, S. (2003) Using FRIENDS to combat anxiety problems among young migrants to Australia: a national trial. *Clinical Child Psychology and Psychiatry*, **8**, 1359–1054.

Bean, T., Eurelings-Bontekoe, E., Mooijaart, A., *et al* (2006) Factors associated with mental health service need and utilization among unaccompanied refugee adolescents. *Administration and Policy in Mental Health and Mental Health Services Research*, **33**, 342–355.

Berry, J. W., Poortinga, Y. H., Segall, M. H., *et al* (2002) *Cross-Cultural Psychology. Research and Applications (2nd edn)*. Cambridge University Press.

Bhugra, D. (2004) Migration and mental health. *Acta Psychiatrica Scandinavica*, **109**, 243–258.

Bishop, D. & Rutter, M. (2008) Neurodevelopmental disorders: conceptual issues. In *Rutter's Child and Adolescent Psychiatry, Fifth Edition* (eds M. Rutter, D. Bishop, D. Pines, *et al*), pp. 32–41. Blackwell.

Bodegard, G. (2005) Life-threatening loss of function in refugee children: another expression of pervasive refusal syndrome? *Clinical Child Psychology and Psychiatry*, **10**, 337–350.

Bradby, H., Varyani, M., Oglethorpe, R., *et al* (2007) British Asian families and the use of child and adolescent mental health services: a qualitative study of a hard to reach group. *Social Science and Medicine*, **65**, 2413–2424.

Department for Education and Skills (2006) *Working Together to Safeguard Children*. TSO (The Stationery Office).

Department of Health (2005) *Delivering Race Equality in Mental Health Care: An Action Plan for Reform Inside and Outside Services and the Government's Response to the Independent Inquiry into the Death of David Bennett*. Department of Health.

Di Nicola, V. F. (1985a) Family therapy and transcultural psychiatry: an emerging synthesis. Part 1: The conceptual basis. *Transcultural Psychiatric Research Review*, **22**, 81–113.

Di Nicola, V. F. (1985b) Family therapy and transcultural psychiatry: an emerging synthesis. Part 2: Portability and culture change. *Transcultural Psychiatric Research Review*, **22**, 151–181.

Di Nicola, V. (1997) *Stranger in the Family. Culture, Families and Therapy*. W. W. Norton & Co.

Falicov, C. J. (1995) Training to think culturally: a multidimensional comparative framework. *Family Process*, **34**, 373–388.

Farooq, S. & Fear, C. (2003) Working through interpreters. *Advances in Psychiatric Treatment*, **9**, 104–109.

Fazel, M., Wheeler, J. & Danesh, J. (2005) Prevalence of serious mental disorder in 7000 refugees resettled in western countries: a systematic review. *Lancet*, **365**, 1309–1314.

Gillberg, C. & Kadesjo, B. (2003) Why bother about clumsiness? The implications of having developmental coordination disorder (DCD). *Neural Plasticity*, **10**, 59–68.

Goodman, A., Patel, V., & Leon, D. A. (2008) Child mental health differences amongst ethnic groups in Britain: a systematic review. *BMC Public Health*, 8, 258.

Green, R. J. (1998) Training programs. Guidelines for multicultural transformation. In *Revisioning Family Therapy. Race, Culture and Gender in Clinical Practice* (ed. M. McGoldrick), pp. 111–117. Guilford Press.

Hackett, L. & Hackett, R. (1994) Child-rearing practices and psychiatric disorder in Gujarati and British children. *British Journal of Social Work*, **24**, 191–202.

Havens, J. E. & Mellins, C. A. (2008) Psychiatric aspects of HIV/AIDS. In *Rutter's Child and Adolescent Psychiatry, Fifth Edition* (eds M. Rutter, D. Bishop, D. Pines, *et al*), pp. 945–955. Blackwell.

Hill, P. (1999) Child psychiatry in Britain. In *Child and Adolescent Psychiatry in Europe: Historical Development Current Situation Future Perspectives* (eds M. Remschmidt & H. Van Engeland), pp. 395–409. Springer.

Hodes, M. (2002) Implications for psychiatric services of chronic civilian strife: young refugees in the UK. *Advances in Psychiatric Treatment*, **8**, 366–374.

Hodes, M. (2008) Psychopathology in refugee and asylum seeking children. In *Rutter's Child and Adolescent Psychiatry, Fifth Edition* (eds M. Rutter, D. Bishop, D. Pines, *et al*), pp. 476–488. Blackwell.

Hodes, M. & Tolmac, J. (2005) Severely impaired young refugees. *Clinical Child Psychology and Psychiatry*, **10**, 251–261.

Hodes, M., Jones, C. & Davis, H. (1996) Cross-cultural differences in maternal evaluation of children's body shapes. *International Journal of Eating Disorders*, **19**, 257–263.

Hodes, M., Dura Vila, G., Kan, C., *et al* (2008a) Psychopathology and adjustment of African Caribbean children in the United Kingdom. In *Culture and Conflict and Child and Adolescent Mental Health* (eds E. Garralda & J. Raynaud), pp. 107–130. Jason Aronson.

Hodes, M., Jagdev, D., Chandra, N., *et al* (2008b) Risk and resilience for psychological distress amongst unaccompanied asylum seeking children. *Journal of Child Psychology and Psychiatry*, **49**, 723–732.

Home Office (2007) *Asylum Statistics: 3rd Quarter 2006 United Kingdom*. National Statistics.

Howard, M. & Hodes, M. (2000) Psychopathology, adversity, and service utilization by young refugees. *Journal of the American Academy of Child and Adolescent Psychiatry*, **39**, 368–377.

Ingleby, D. & Watters, C. (2002) Refugee children at school: good practices in mental health and social care. *Education and Health*, **20**, 43–45.

Kushner, T. & Knox, K. (1999) *Refugees in an Age of Genocide: Global, National and Local Perspectives during the Twentieth Century*. Frank Cass.

Liu, X., Liu, L. & Wang, R. (2003) Bed sharing, sleep habits, and sleep problems among Chinese school-aged children. *Sleep*, **26**, 839–844.

Lorek, A., Ehntholt, K., Nesbitt, A., *et al* (2009) The mental and physical health difficulties of children held within a British immigration detention center: a pilot study. *Child Abuse and Neglect*, **33**, 573–585.

Malek, M. (2004) Meting the needs of ethnic minority groups in the UK. In *Mental Health Services for Minority Ethnic Children* (eds M. Malek & C. Joughin), pp. 81–127. Jessica Kingsley.

McGoldrick, M. (1998) *Revisioning Family Therapy. Race, Culture and Gender in Clinical Practice*. Guilford Press.

McKelvey, R. S. & Webb, J. A. (1996) Premigratory expectations and postmigratory mental health symptoms in Vietnamese Amerasians. *Journal of the American Academy of Child and Adolescent Psychiatry*, **35**, 240–245.

Meltzer, H., Gatwood, R., Godman, R., *et al* (2000) *Mental Health of Children and Adolescents in Great Britain*. TSO (The Stationery Office).

NHS Health Advisory Service (1995) *Together We Stand: Commissioning, Role and Management of Child and Adolescent Mental Health Services*. HMSO.

Nielsen, S. S., Norredam, M., Christiansen, K. L., *et al* (2008) Mental health among children seeking asylum in Denmark – the effect of length of stay and number of relocations: a cross sectional study. *BMC Public Health*, **8**, 293.

Nikapota, A. (2008) Transcultural training in child and adolescent psychiatry. In *Culture and Conflict and Child and Adolescent Mental Health* (eds E. Garralda & J. Raynaud), pp. 205–221. Jason Aronson.

Office of National Statistics (2007) *Population Trends. Winter 2007*. ONS (http://www.statistics.gov.uk/downloads/theme_population/Population_Trends_130_web.pdf).

O'Shea, B., Hodes, M., Down, G., *et al* (2000) A school-based mental health service for refugee children. *Clinical Child Psychology and Psychiatry*, **5**, 1359–1045.

Patel, N. & Hodes, M. (2006) Violent deliberate self harm amongst adolescent refugees. *European Child and Adolescent Psychiatry*, **15**, 367–370.

Pidd, H. (2008) Immigration: High court to rule on incarceration of boy, eight, in detention centre. *Guardian*, Monday 1 September, p. 16.

Raval, H. (2005) Being heard and understood in the context of seeking asylum and refuge: communicating with the help of bilingual co-workers. *Clinical Child Psychology and Psychiatry*, **10**, 197–217.

Raval, H. & Tribe, R. (2002) *Working with Interpreters in Mental Health*. Routledge.

Rutter, J. (2006) *Refugee Children in the UK*. Open University Press.

Sack, W. H., Clarke, G. N. & Seeley, J. R. (1996) Multiple forms of stress in Cambodian adolescent refugees. *Child Development*, **67**, 107–116.

Sack, W. H., Him, C. & Dickason, D. (1999) Twelve-year follow-up study of Khmer youths who suffered massive war trauma as children. *Journal of the American Academy of Child and Adolescent Psychiatry*, **38**, 1173–1179.

Silove, D., Austin, P. & Steel, Z. (2007) No refuge from terror: the impact of detention on the mental health of trauma-affected refugees seeking asylum in Australia. *Transcultural Psychiatry*, **44**, 359–393.

Simich, L., Hamilton, H. & Baya, B. K. (2006) Mental distress, economic hardship and expectations of life in Canada among Sudanese newcomers. *Transcultural Psychiatry*, **43**, 418–444.

Stein, B. D., Jaycox, L. H., Kataoka, S. H., *et al* (2003) A mental health intervention for schoolchildren exposed to violence: a randomized controlled trial. *JAMA*, **290**, 603–611.

Stevens, G. W. & Vollebergh, W. A. (2008) Mental health in migrant children. *Journal of Child Psychology and Psychiatry*, **49**, 276–294.

Tolmac, J. & Hodes, M. (2004) Ethnic variation among adolescent psychiatric in-patients with psychotic disorders. *British Journal of Psychiatry*, **184**, 428–431.

Tousignant, M., Habimana, E., Biron, C., *et al* (1999) The Quebec adolescent refugee project: psychopathology and family variables in a sample from 35 nations. *Journal of the American Academy of Child and Adolescent Psychiatry*, **38**, 1426–1432.

Tufnell, G. (2003) Refugee children, trauma and the law. *Clinical Child Psychology and Psychiatry*, **8**, 431–443.

UNHCR (2006) *The State of the World's Refugees. Human Displacement in the New Millennium.* Oxford University Press.

Van der Veer, G. & van Maning, A. (2004) Creating a safe therapeutic sanctuary. In *Broken Spirits. The Treatment of Traumatized Asylum Seekers, Refugees, War and Torture Victims* (eds J. P. Wilson & B. Drozdek), pp. 187–219. Bruner-Routledge.

Vojvoda, D., Weine, S. M., McGlashan, T., *et al* (2008) Posttraumatic stress disorder symptoms in Bosnian refugees 3 1/2 years after resettlement. *Journal of Rehabilitation Research and Development*, **45**, 421–426.

Wade, J., Mitchell, F. & Baylis, G. (2005) *Unaccompanied Asylum Seeking Children. The Response of the Social Work Services.* British Association of Adoption and Fostering.

Watters, C. (2007) *Refugee Children.* Routledge.

Westermeyer, J. (1991) Psychiatric services for refugee children. In *Refugee Children. Theory, Research and Services* (eds F. Ahearn & J. L. Athey), pp. 127–162. Johns Hopkins University Press.

Winder, R. (2004) *Bloody Foreigners. The Story of Immigration to Britain.* Abacus.

Yu, S. H., Liu, S. K. & Lin, K. M. (2007) Psychopharmacology across cultures. In *Textbook of Cultural Psychiatry* (eds D. Bhugra & K. Bhui), pp. 402–413. Cambridge University Press.

CHAPTER 24

CAMHS and looked-after children

Fiona Gospel, Jackie Johnson and Ian Partridge

'Change is not made without inconvenience, even from worse to better.'
Richard Hooker, *Of The Lawes of Ecclesiastical Politie*

Introduction

There are assorted reasons for children being 'looked after'. A proportion will have suffered physical, sexual or emotional abuse, and parental mental illness. Marital violence, relationship breakdown and parental imprisonment are not uncommon experiences. These children can be seen as enmeshed in a matrix of developmental disadvantage, and have a higher number of risk factors predisposing them to mental health problems. They may already have significant mental health problems as they enter care (Dimigen *et al*, 1999).

The care system presents these young people with further challenges and difficulties, particularly frequent moves and placement breakdowns (Quinton & Rutter, 1984; Minty, 1999), which may influence their already vulnerable state, interacting with and interrelated to social, educational and relationship difficulties. A cycle evolves whereby children with mental health problems are less likely to achieve placement stability, and therefore become more vulnerable (Barber *et al*, 2001).

> 'Upon rereading my old diaries, I realised how hard foster care was and what a detrimental effect it had on me at that time. Before my first foster placement broke down, I thought foster care was a relatively positive experience, apart from the usual problem of occasionally feeling a bit awkward around the family, but when my foster care placement did breakdown, literally overnight, I realised why some young people in care do have the problems they do. I became very defensive and was determined to never let anyone ever hurt me ever again. I developed a very hard exterior to protect me at that time.' (Cuckston, 2004: p. 24)

A study in Oxfordshire, which looked at the mental health needs of looked-after children, found that 97% of children living within residential care and 57% of children living in foster care were found to have significant mental health problems (McCann *et al*, 1996). In their research on the mental health of looked-after children aged 5–17 years of age in England, Meltzer *et al* (2003) discovered that 45% of these children had a mental disorder, 36% a conduct disorder, 12% an emotional disorder and 7% were rated as hyperactive. However, Chaffin *et al* (2006) stated that a history of maltreatment should not necessarily imply any disorder. Many children who are maltreated cope well. Even those experiencing severe maltreatment may exhibit very few or transient behavioural or emotional problems as a consequence of their abuse (Kendall-Tackett *et al*, 2001). Many emerge without any long-term attachment-based disorders (O'Connor & Zeanah, 2003). Resilience, trauma and adversity are not limited to the extremely healthy or robust. Rather, resilience is a common and relatively normal human characteristic (Bonanno, 2004).

CAMHS work with looked-after children

Every Child Matters (Department for Education and Skills, 2004a), the Children Act 2004 (Department for Education and Skills (2004b), the NSF for children (Department of Health, 2004), and *Care Matters* (Department for Education & Skills, 2006) all recognise the need for provision of mental health assessment and therapeutic work for looked-after children (Kurtz *et al*, 1994). Yet despite the evidence, the mental health needs of looked-after children remain largely unmet (Harman *et al*, 2000; Payne, 2000; Richardson & Joughin, 2000) and access to appropriate services is lacking (Geen *et al*, 2005; Viner & Taylor, 2005; Browne *et al*, 2006; Rosenfeld *et al*, 2007). The interventions, disciplines and agencies involved with CAMHS for looked-after children vary substantially around the UK (Minnis & Del Priore, 2001).

Often the children receiving services are not benefiting from a systemically informed understanding of their needs or from interventions tailored to meet their unique circumstances. Although they have many needs similar to the generic CAMHS population, their particular experience often means that they have additional needs. As such, they may require a contextual understanding/provision of enhanced as well as mainstream services (Golding *et al*, 2006).

Historically, problems in accessing CAMHS have included narrow referral criteria, non-detection of mental health problems, referrers' reluctance to pathologise children's behaviour, children's mobility and engagement (Hatfield *et al*, 1996; Nicol *et al*, 2000; Minnis & Del Priore, 2001). Phillips (1997) found that many social workers may have recognised that a particular young person needed mental health intervention, but did not refer. This may be a result of placement instability, dissatisfaction with CAMHS, or lack of Local Authority resources. Minnis *et al* (2006) found that even looked-after children with identified mental health difficulties had a high level of service support from a wide variety of agencies other than CAMHS.

However, it is also important to recognise the danger of over-interpretation of the child's behaviour and the desire for a pathologising referral for 'expert' intervention by a mental health professional. Just as in the majority of cases it is the family who offer the key to improvement in mental health, we must also recognise and be informed by those closest to the looked-after child even if that 'other' is a fellow professional. 'The provision of substitute parents in itself represents the most radical, comprehensive and potent therapeutic change in a child's psychosocial prospects' (Howe, 2006). Normal development can only be understood in terms of the context of that development; if this is ignored, the danger of utopian interventions will result in frustration and further damage to the vulnerable child.

Holland *et al* (2005) reported in their survey about promoting placement stability for looked-after children that there was a high level of concern among Local Authorities and voluntary agencies about the availability of mental health services for children and young people. Interestingly, this was seen as one of the key issues affecting stability and continuity, which highlights the need for CAMHS intervention to be systemic in its approach, and flexible and creative in its delivery.

Developing the service

Specialist mental health provision can be provided from within CAMHS as a structured and resourced Tier 3 team, or from a multi-agency team with input from individual CAMHS professionals. The success of services for looked-after children depends upon their flexibility to adapt models of working to the particular needs of the child.

Not all areas have large multidisciplinary/agency CAMHS, in which case it will be important to think about balancing approaches/interests in order to maximise potential impact.

The team composition should reflect the multiple needs of looked-after young people, ideally a multidisciplinary Tier 3 CAMHS team operating within a multi-agency network and within a context of multi-agency collaboration. The Tier 3 team should not be seen as 'accepting referrals' but rather as working within the multi-agency context offering a range of appropriate interventions and interactions. Referrals for 'therapy' are often meaningless and lead to frustration and misunderstanding, whereas working along a continuum of supportive interventions can allow the 'right' support to be given at the 'right' time.

The model shown in Fig. 24.1 suggests a hierarchy of needs that have to be met if children and young people are to make progress towards emotional health and well-being. Assessing where a young person currently lies on this hierarchy can be helpful in guiding the type and focus of intervention that might be offered. Young people can move up and down this model in response to current circumstances (Golding *et al*, 2006).

CAMHS role in the support of looked-after children

Most CAMHS provision for looked-after children will have limited resources and personnel, so, as with other Tier 3 teams, it is important to have a clear

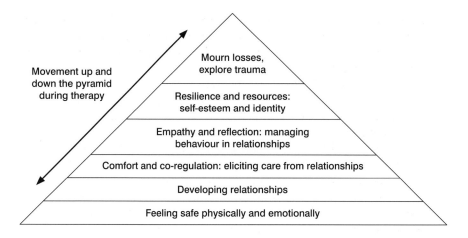

Fig. 24.1 The therapeutic needs of looked-after children (Golding *et al*, 2006).

model of service delivery. A CAMHS team for looked-after children may be expected to perform the following.

- Work in partnership with other key agencies to create a more integrated approach that will:
  - promote the psychological, physical, emotional, social and spiritual health of looked-after children;
  - help identify/establish more stable placements for young people within their home locality with the aim of reducing the number of moves young people can have in their care career.
- Consultation, specialist training and therapeutic input to other agencies involved with the young people.
- Consultation, specialist training and therapeutic input to carers, whether they be foster carers, residential staff, birth family or family carers.
- Direct therapeutic input with young people, with or without significant others.

Consultation

Consultation offers carers or professionals the opportunity to discuss the complexity of their task within a multi-agency context. It should be seen as a means of supporting and empowering others, as well as a means of identifying and increasing understanding of the individual needs of the young person. Establishing good working relationships with colleagues in other local services (e.g. Local Authority, education, health) should be considered a major role for any CAMHS team.

Liaison

Liaison is an essential part of work in this area so that all involved professionals are aware of the referral to CAMHS. Clear lines of communication and confidentiality need to be established for the team and for each individual child, operating within both the law and good practice.

Teaching and training

Specialist training should be developed according to local need. This may involve the development of specific modules for other staff groups or foster carers around various topics linked to the mental health needs of looked-after children (e.g. attachment, self-harm).

Direct therapeutic interventions

Decisions about which therapeutic model would be most helpful should be based on the needs of the child. The development of a single intervention for looked-after children is not realistic (Crittenden, 2000; Crittenden *et al*, 2001).

The relatively recent attachment-based therapies (Delaney, 1998; Blieberg, 2001; Jernberg & Booth, 2001; Brisch, 2002; Hughes, 2006), although case-related in their evidence base, show promising results. More 'traditional' therapies (e.g. CBT) can also be considered if adaptations are made for the needs of the young person. The most beneficial therapeutic approach should be flexible, integrated and based on the needs of the child. It should include the carers either directly in the therapy or indirectly through consultation and/or training.

Evaluation

Measures specific to this population of children are currently being developed under the auspices of clinical psychologists working with looked-after and adopted children (CPLAAC; www.cplaac.org.uk/forum/). However, it would be expected that services are undertaking service-specific evaluations, which should include user perspectives.

Conclusion

Looked-after children have an increased vulnerability to mental health problems. The young people themselves are generally part of a complicated multi-agency system. In order for their needs to be met, their disorders to be overcome and therefore their life chances as outlined in *Every Child Matters* (Department for Education & Skills, 2004*a*) to be increased, specialised CAMHS teams need to be developed, which are accessible and flexible in their approach (Box 24.1). Furthermore, the multi-agency system around looked-after children should have access to consultation from CAMHS to

Box 24.1 Ten characteristics of a successful CAMHS team for looked-after children

1 *Flexibility*
Traditional CAMHS are often difficult to access for children with highly complex needs. Flexibility is the key to providing accessible and acceptable services.

2 *Joint commissioning*
Some services have joint commissioning boards with health education and social care. In others, key senior managers championed the services – both approaches can be effective; commitment is more important than the method used.

3 *Strong leadership*
Individuals with vision and a passion for providing relevant, accessible services to help turn around children's lives and who can enthuse others are a key factor in successful services.

4 *Engagement*
Taking time to engage with children and young people whose past experiences have often caused them to mistrust adults and to battle through life alone must precede any worthwhile intervention. This can take a lot of creative energy and resilience on the part of staff.

5 *Long-term work*
The ability to offer long-term support, when needed, sometimes at an intensive level and at other times in a low-key way, is important. Where services are pressured to close cases quickly, the young person's belief that adults will let them down can be reinforced. Sticking with children during tough periods may demonstrate that some adults can be trusted.

6 *Holistic*
Support for the whole child. Teams with specialist foster carers and education input have good outcomes.

7 *Systemic thinking*
Using systemic thinking when engaging with all those in contact with the child and family – involving them in planning, and helping their understanding of the child's needs and behaviours.

8 *Participative*
Listening to children about what they want from a service, developing formal and informal mechanisms for consulting with children. Involving them in planning services and celebrating their achievements is imperative.

9 *Evidence-based*
Evidence-based practice and regular evaluation is fundamental to producing effective outcomes.

10 *Reflective and responsive*
Successful services rarely have fixed master plans from the outset. The focus tends to be on incremental development. Building in processes of reflection and review and responding to feedback from all stakeholders is implicit in their accomplishment (Bunting, 2007).

address the dynamics and processes that will ultimately have an impact on the child (Sprince, 2000, 2002).

As well as specialised training, creative energy and resilience should be a requirement of staff within these teams. They need to take time to engage with these children and young people whose past experiences have often caused them to mistrust adults and to battle through life alone. Supervision while remaining within the wider CAMHS may require a further multi-agency context if only so that the varied multi-agency organisational imperatives and ideologies can be clarified and understood.

References

Barber, J. G., Delfabbro, P. H. & Cooper, L. L. (2001) The predictors of unsuccessful transition to foster care. *Journal of Child Psychology and Psychiatry*, **42**, 785–790.

Blieberg, E. (2001) *Treating Personality Disorders in Children and Adolescents*. Guilford Press.

Bonanno G. A. (2004) Loss, trauma, and human resilience: have we underestimated the human capacity to thrive after extremely aversive events? *American Psychologist*, **59**, 20–28.

Brisch, K. H. (2002) *Treating Attachment Disorders from Theory to Therapy. English Edition*. Guilford Press.

Browne, K., Hamilton-Glachritisiz, C., Johnson, R., *et al* (2006) Overuse of institutional care for children in Europe. *BMJ*, **322**, 485–487.

Bunting, M. (2007) *Looking After the Mental Health of Looked After Children. Sharing Emerging Practice*. YoungMinds.

Chaffin, M., Hanson, R., Saunders, B. E., *et al* (2006) Report of the APSAC task force on attachment therapy, reactive attachment disorder and attachment problems. *Child Maltreatment*, **11**, 76–89.

Crittenden, P. M. (2000) A dynamic-maturational exploration of the meaning of security and adaptation: empirical, cultural and theoretical considerations. In *The Organization of Attachment Relationships: Maturation, Culture and Context* (eds P. M. Crittenden & A. H. Claussen), pp. 358–384. Cambridge University Press.

Crittenden, P. M., Landini, A. & Claussen, A. H. (2001) A dynamic-maturational approach to treatment of maltreated children. In *Handbook of Psychological Services for Children and Adolescents* (eds J. N. Hughes, A. M. LaGreca & J. C. Conely), pp. 373–398. Oxford University Press.

Cuckston, C. (2004) 'Caroline' British Psychological Society, Division of Clinical Psychology, Faculty for Children and Young People. *Service and Practice Update*, **3**, 24–26.

Delaney, R. J. (1998) *Fostering Changes. Treating Attachment Disordered Foster Children*. Wood and Barnes Publishing.

Department for Education and Skills (2004a) *Every Child Matters: Change for Children*. TSO (The Stationery Office).

Department for Education and Skills (2004b) *Children Act 2004*. TSO (The Stationery Office).

Department for Education and Skills (2006) *Care Matters*. TSO (The Stationery Office).

Department of Health (2004) *National Service Framework for Children, Young People and Maternity Services*. TSO (The Stationery Office).

Dimigen, G., Del Priore, C., Butler, S., *et al* (1999) Psychiatric disorder among children at time of entering local authority care: questionnaire survey. *BMJ*, **319**, 675.

Geen, R., Sommers, A. & Cohen, M. (2005) *Medicaid Spending of Foster Children. Brief No. 2*. Urban Institute (http://www.urban.org/UploadedPDF/311221_medicaid_spending.pdf).

Golding, K. S., Dent, H. R., Nissim, R., *et al* (eds) (2006) *Thinking Psychologically about Children who are Looked After and Adopted. Space for Reflection*. John Wiley and Sons.

Harman, J., Childs, G., Kelleher, K., *et al* (2000) Mental health care utilisation and expenditures by children in foster care. *Archives of Pediatrics & Adolescent Medicine*, **154**, 1114–1117.

Hatfield, B., Harrington, R. & Mohamad, H. (1996) Staff looking after children in local authority residential units: interface with child mental health professionals. *Journal of Adolescence*, **19**, 127–139.

Holland, S., Faulkner, A. & Perez-del-Aguila, R. (2005) Promoting stability and continuity of care for looked after children: a survey and critical review. *Child and Family Social Work*, **10**, 29–41.

Howe, D. (2006) Developmental attachment psychotherapy with fostered and adopted children. *Child and Adolescent Mental Health*, **11**, 128–134.

Hughes, D. A. (2006) *Building the Bonds of Attachment. Awakening Love in the Deeply Troubled Child* (2nd edn). Aronson.

Jernberg, A. & Booth, P. B. (2001) *Theraplay: Helping Parents and Children Build Better Relationships Through Attachment Based Play (2nd edn)*. Jossey Bass.

Kendall-Tackett, K. A., Williams, L. M. & Finkelhor, D. (2001) Impact of sexual abuse on children: a review and synthesis of recent empirical studies. In *Children and the Law: The Essential Readings* (ed. R. Bull), pp. 31–76. Blackwell.

Kurtz, Z., Thornes, R. & Wolkind, S. (1994) *Services for the Mental Health of Children and Young People in England: A National Review*. Department of Public Health.

McCann, J., James, A., Wilson, S., *et al* (1996) Prevalence of psychiatric disorders in young people in the care system. *BMJ*, **313**, 1529–1530.

Meltzer, M., Gatward, R., Corbin, T., *et al* (2003) *The Mental Health of Young People Looked After by Local Authorities in England*. TSO (The Stationery Office).

Minnis, H. & Del Priore, C. (2001) Mental health services for looked after children: implications from two studies. *Adoption and Fostering*, **25**, 27–38.

Minnis, H., Everett, K., Pelosi, A. J., *et al* (2006) Children in foster care: mental health, service use and costs. *European Child and Adolescent Psychiatry*, **15**, 63–70.

Minty, B. (1999) Annotation: outcomes in long-term foster family care. *Journal of Child Psychology and Psychiatry*, **40**, 991–999.

Nicol, R., Stretch, D., Whitney, I., *et al* (2000) Mental health needs and services for severely troubled and troubling young people, including young offenders, in an NHS region. *Journal of Adolescence*, **23**, 243–261.

O'Connor, T. G. & Zeanah, C. H. (2003) Attachment disorders: assessment strategies and treatment approaches. *Attachment and Human Development*, **5**, 223–244.

Payne, H. (2000) The health of children in public care. *Current Opinion in Psychiatry*, **13**, 381–388.

Phillips, J. (1997) Meeting the psychiatric needs of children in foster care. Social workers' views. *Psychiatric Bulletin*, **21**, 609–611.

Quinton, D. & Rutter, M. (1984) Parents with children in care – II. Intergenerational continuities. *Journal of Child Psychology and Psychiatry*, **25**, 231–250.

Richardson, J. & Joughin, C. (2000). *The Mental Health Needs of Looked After Children*. Gaskell.

Rosenfeld, A. A., Pilowsky, D. J., Fine, P., *et al* (2007) Foster care: an update. *Journal of the American Academy of Child and Adolescent Psychiatry*, **36**, 448–457.

Sprince, J. (2000) Towards an integrated network. *Journal of Child Psychotherapy*, **26**, 413–444.

Sprince, J. (2002) Developing containment: psychoanalytic consultancy to a therapeutic community for traumatised children. *Journal of Child Psychotherapy*, **28**, 147–161.

Viner, R. M. & Taylor, B. (2005) Adult health and social outcomes of children who have been in public care: population based study. *Pediatrics*, **115**, 894–899.

CHAPTER 25

Drug and alcohol teams

Norman Malcolm

'Skunk … it only chills you out.'
14-year-old cannabis smoker

Why we need substance misuse services for young people

Drug and alcohol services for young people have developed rapidly over the past decade in the UK (Crome, 1997; Gilvarry, 2000; Gilvarry & McArdle, 2007). In 1997, a task force was commissioned to review services for substance misuse in England (Department of Health, 1997). This work has culminated in national guidelines for the treatment of substance misuse (Department of Health, 2007; National Institute for Health and Clinical Excellence, 2007) and in the formation of the National Treatment Agency for Substance Misuse (NTA) which provides guidance on substance misuse specific to young people (National Treatment Agency for Substance Misuse, 2005, 2007, 2009a).

In the minds of both professionals and the public at large, substance use and subsequent misuse seem to have become ubiquitous. There have been other times when this was the case; however, features that are of contemporary relevance include:

- declining age of initiation into substance use
- multiple drug use
- prevalence of use by girls approaching that of boys
- widespread availability of illicit substances
- proposed link between substance misuse and an increased rate of completed suicide for men aged 15–24 years (Pelkonen & Marttunen 2003)
- widespread use of cannabis, stimulants and LSD within the dance/ rave culture
- the increased strength of current cannabis strains (skunk) through hybridisation and the probable link to the onset of schizophrenia (Arendt et al, 2005; Atakan, 2008)
- the increase in problematic alcohol use
- the decrease in numbers of young people using heroin and crack cocaine (National Treatment Agency for Substance Misuse, 2009b).

Many young people now are aware of psychoactive substances, know people who use them and use them themselves. The likelihood exists, therefore, of greater numbers of young people experiencing problems with substance use. Not surprisingly, young people whose development has already been compromised by a variety of adverse life events may initially find solace in substance use and later find themselves compounding their problems when the negative effects begin to accrue. This has begun to show itself in the high levels of problematic substance use in at-risk groups, including:

- looked-after children
- homeless young people
- children and young people who have experienced abuse
- school excludees
- children and young people from disrupted family backgrounds
- children and young people whose parents misuse substances
- young offenders.

Child and adolescent mental health services are being asked to join with colleagues in Social Services, education and the voluntary sector to provide services for the same young people featured in the list above. As they do so, it is clear that CAMHS will be working with young people who are misusing substances. Current thinking across the board is that services for young substance users must be child focused and take account of primary and secondary prevention as well as treatment. The response needs to be multidisciplinary if it is to succeed in addressing the complex social problems that coexist with substance misuse. The specialist medical and therapeutic skills within CAMHS are an essential element of an effective response.

Strategic planning process

As well as seeing patients, a CAMHS substance misuse team will need to contribute to the strategic planning processes that currently exist (HM Government, 2008; National Treatment Agency for Substance Misuse, 2008a) (Box 25.1). Recent changes to strategic planning structures include the setting up of locality-based primary care trusts and the establishment of the NTA, a special health authority within the NHS charged with increasing the capacity, quality and effectiveness of drug treatment in England, in their own words ensuring the availability of 'more treatment, better treatment and fairer treatment'. The NTA is responsible for integrating the commissioning of specialist treatment for substance misuse in young people with the Children's Plan (Department for Children, Schools and Families, 2007). One component of this strategy is a universal drug education and prevention programme, 'Blueprint', which has been evaluated in schools and communities in England (Baker, 2006) to assess the effectiveness of a

Box 25.1 National strategic planning structure

- Guidance is provided by the 10-year strategy *Drugs: Protecting Families and Communities* (HM Government, 2008).
- The NTA aims to improve the quantity and quality of treatment available for drug misuse in England.
- Nine regional NTA managers are based in the government offices. They provide guidance and support to drug and alcohol teams in spending government funding to best effect and monitor the teams' performance.
- The Memorandum of Understanding between the Department for Children, Schools & Families and the National Treatment Agency for Substance Misuse (2008*b*) sets out their commitment to work in partnership with the aim of impacting positively on specialist drug treatment provision for young people.
- 150 drug action teams and drug and alcohol action teams are established across England – a directory is held by the Home Office (http://drugs.homeoffice. gov.uk/dat/directory). Similar arrangements are in place in Northern Ireland, Scotland and Wales.
- Drug and alcohol reference groups and task groups have roles in consulting with service users in order to refine local service delivery. Local task groups inform services about performance and areas of need. They can help services to set relevant objectives and in performance measurement.

coordinated approach in education, development of skills and knowledge, and young people, parental support and media campaigns. The NTA outlines its plans for commissioning in its annual business plan (National Treatment Agency for Substance Misuse, 2008*a*) and reports annually on substance misuse in young people, which informs the business plan.

Government targets with regard to drug misuse are laid out in the 10-year strategies that began in 1998, and were updated for the period 2008–2018 through the 'Tackling Drugs: Saving Lives' campaign, which espouses a focus on the impact of drug use on families (HM Government, 2008) – drug services for young people remain a national priority.

Although not required by law in England, around 50% of drug action teams have now included alcohol misuse within their planning structures, and so have become drug and alcohol action teams. The key target of the UK drugs strategy is to doube the availability of drug treatment. Drug and alcohol action teams are responsible for coordinating a multi-agency response to meet the government's targets within the broad principles of integration, evidence, joint action, consistency, effective communication, quality standards and accountability. Local planning structures are required to contribute to strategic plans to meet the needs of young substance users and to report to the government via the NTA.

Perhaps the three most relevant targets within the strategy for CAMHS to consider are the following.

- To help young people resist drug misuse in order to achieve their full potential in society.
- Treatment – to enable individuals with drug problems to overcome them and live healthy and crime-free lives.
- To focus more on families, addressing the needs of parents and children as individuals, as well as working with whole families to prevent drug use, reduce risk and get people into treatment.

Local strategic planning structures and membership of relevant bodies will vary geographically, although the majority of such structures are likely to include task groups focusing on the main areas within each target: young people, communities, treatment and availability. Child and adolescent mental health services should be represented on the groups addressing issues regarding young people and treatment. Whatever the local structure, drug and alcohol action teams should not work in isolation from, and neither should they be seen as replacing, existing planning structures for children and young people. There should be close collaboration between these bodies, which may include the integrated Children's Services Plan, the Area Child Protection Committee, the Health Improvement Plan, and structures surrounding education, youth offending and the needs of ethnic minority groups. Child and adolescent mental health services may already be represented on some or all of the groups.

How will the service look?

The setting up of a drug and alcohol team within a CAMHS, and subsequently with those with whom they form working partnerships, depends not only on finding those with an interest in and knowledge of substance misuse, but also on local commissioning. In recent years, this has been the intention of local government offices by attempting to create better working links between CAMHS and substance misuse services. This has obvious training and recruitment implications and there is wide geographical variation in this respect. Team membership therefore may be very varied in terms of professional disciplines and ultimately in the service they can provide.

Furthermore, there is variation in the age range of young people with whom CAMHS work and this, in part, defines the likely substance use problems the team will encounter. The spectrum includes younger children engaging in volatile substance misuse, some will progress to cannabis, stimulant and psychedelic use and later heroin use and dependence, and potentially the use of crack cocaine. Although the main problems associated with alcohol misuse in young people relate to offending behaviour and not to help-seeking behaviour, there is an increasing number of young people with problematic alcohol use who may need appropriate detoxification and rehabilitation.

A CAMHS substance misuse team may therefore focus and advise on a number of conditions such as ADHD, conduct disorder and early formal mental illness complicated by early or recreational substance use. If the expertise is present, the team may also provide a service for a small but usually complex group of young people using crack cocaine, and for those dependent on alcohol or heroin.

Provision

As partnerships with other agencies are likely to continue to evolve, especially those with youth offending teams, around a third of all referrals to specialist services are from youth offending teams (National Treatment Agency for Substance Misuse, 2009a). It therefore behoves CAMHS to develop links with youth offending services and other agencies working with young people with a high risk of substance misuse; the bare minimum that any service will provide, namely consultation, will inevitably include issues around substance misuse. The central question seems to be how the team is able to make an accurate assessment of the degree to which substance use plays a part in the overall problem. This may be overcome if the specialist CAMHS team has a close joint working relationship with either existing adult addiction services or young people's addiction services within the voluntary or statutory sector. Alternatively, the CAMHS team could include members with both substance misuse expertise and expertise in child and adolescent mental health problems such as adult addiction nurses who have transferred to CAMHS after taking relevant courses, or child psychiatrists who have become familiar with substance misuse through their training.

There is a feeling among adult addiction specialists that the whole gamut of interventions delivered to young substance misusers should be in the domain of child and adolescent specialists. The area that is most alien to child and adolescent psychiatrists is dealing with young people addicted to heroin, as it opens up their concerns about the safe prescribing of a number of opiate and non-opiate drugs. This would involve the service having the ability to accurately assess this particular client group in terms of:

- dependency
- current level of use
- mode of use
- injecting practice
- polypharmacy
- stage of motivational change.

Such assessment is necessary in order for the team to be able to deliver:

- effective therapeutic interventions
- prescribing interventions (stabilisation, detoxification)
- detoxification (symptomatic, opiate substitute)
- interpretation of urine toxicology results

- safe dispensing and monitoring (daily collection, supervised consumption by a responsible adult).

Furthermore, in delivering these services, the team must take account of the young person's:

- education
- housing
- physical health
- mental health
- family relationships
- peer relationships
- developmental tasks
- recreation and leisure activities
- offending behaviour.

In order to deliver such a service to a group who have historically been hard to reach, the team may have to develop a more flexible approach and deliver their work in a variety of environments such as 'one-stop shops' or on the premises of new partners. This may raise concerns about note keeping; confidentiality, and reaching mutually agreed definitions of the young person's competence to make informed decisions about opting into treatment plans.

Treatment aims will also have to be considered: whether the goal should be abstinence from substance use or, far more realistically, work within the broader philosophy of harm reduction. If management is shared, conflicting ideologies of service delivery may cause tensions.

Another consideration will be the provision of transitional care and the arrangements for the referral of older adolescents into appropriate adult services if they are still in need of treatment. Where community detoxification has failed or where stabilisation of the environment is required in a more intensive rehabilitation package, Tier 4 services may be required. Many child and adolescent in-patient units may exclude admission based on substance misuse and many older teenagers may fall outside of entry criteria. Local funding arrangements may not be in place to facilitate access to the relatively few units specifically dealing with the detoxification and residential rehabilitation of young people.

Conclusion

Substance use among young people is widespread: further details about the clinical presentation and management of these problems (Crome *et al*, 2004) and more information about policy and best practice are available on the NTA website (www.nta.nhs.uk/).

There are particular groups who are at risk of problematic substance use. These at-risk groups overlap with those for whom CAMHS are already being asked, along with colleagues in other children's services, to provide joined-up interventions. The core, generic skills already present within CAMHS – knowledge of developmental and family functioning, child-centred awareness, assessment of problems in systemic formulations and the delivery of a variety of therapeutic interventions – are essential contributions to service delivery, whether they are exercised through consultation or direct work.

Owing to widespread geographical and interdisciplinary differences in expertise in the field of substance misuse by children and young people, there are many models of service delivery for this group. Innovative partnerships and working styles may have to be developed (National Treatment Agency for Substance Misuse, 2008c). Child and adolescent mental health services need to contribute to strategic planning processes at local, regional and national levels. Training needs, capacity and resources will ultimately shape the response of CAMHS to young substance users. The specialist CAMHS substance misuse team will need to develop smooth pathways for those who require referral to adult services or Tier 4 placements.

Further reading

NHS Health Advisory Service (2001) *Review 2001. The Substance of Young Needs*. Health Advisory Service (http://drugs.homeoffice.gov.uk/publication-search/young-people/Health-advisory-service-report?view=Binary).

References

Arendt, M., Rosenberg, R., Foldager, L., *et al* (2005) Cannabis-induced psychosis and subsequent schizophrenia-spectrum disorders: follow-up study of 535 incident cases. *British Journal of Psychiatry*, **187**, 510–515.

Atakan, Z. (2008) Cannabis use by people with severe mental illness – is it important? *Advances in Psychiatric Treatment*, **14**, 423–431.

Baker, P. J. (2006) Developing a Blueprint for evidence-based drug prevention in England. *Drugs: Education, Prevention and Policy*, **13**, 17–32.

Crome, I. (1997) Young people and substance problems – from image to imagination (editorial). *Drugs: Education, Prevention and Policy*, **4**, 107–116.

Crome, I., Ghodse, H., Gilvarry, E., *et al* (2004) *Young People and Substance Misuse*. RCPsych Publications.

Department for Children, Schools and Families (2007) *The Children's Plan: Building Brighter Futures*. TSO (The Stationery Office).

Department of Health (1997) *The Task Force to Review Services for Drug Misusers. Report of an Independent Review of Drug Treatment Services in England*. Department of Health.

Department of Health (2007) *Drug Misuse and Dependence: UK Guidelines on Clinical Management*. Department of Health.

Gilvarry, E. (2000) Substance abuse in young people. *Journal of Child Psychology and Psychiatry*, **41**, 55–80.

Gilvarry, E. & McArdle, P. (2007) *Alcohol, Drugs and Young People: Clinical Approaches*. MacKeith Press.

HM Government (2008) *Drugs: Protecting Families and Communities. Action Plan 2008–2018*. 'Tackling Drugs: Changing Lives', HM Government.

National Institute for Health and Clinical Excellence (2007) *Community-Based Interventions to Reduce Substance Misuse Among Vulnerable Young People*. NICE.

National Treatment Agency for Substance Misuse (2005) *Young People's Substance Misuse Treatment Services – Essential Elements*. NTA.

National Treatment Agency for Substance Misuse (2007) *Assessing Young People for Substance Misuse*. NTA.

National Treatment Agency for Substance Misuse (2008a) *Business Plan 2008/09*. NTA (http://www.nta.nhs.uk/publications/documents/nta_bus_plan_0809.pdf).

National Treatment Agency for Substance Misuse (2008b) *Memorandum of Understanding between Department for Children, Schools and Families and National Treatment Agency for Substance Misuse on Young People's Specialist Substance Misuse Treatment. September 2008*. NTA (http://www.nta.nhs.uk/areas/young_people/Docs/DCFS_NTA_memorandum_of_understanding_final.pdf).

National Treatment Agency for Substance Misuse (2008c) *The Role of CAMHS and Addiction Psychiatry in Adolescent Substance Misuse Services*. NTA (http://www.nta.nhs.uk/areas/young_people/Docs/yp_camhs280508.pdf).

National Treatment Agency for Substance Misuse (2009a) *Getting to Grips with Substance Misuse Among Young People. The Data for 2007/08*. NTA (http://www.nta.nhs.uk/areas/young_people/Docs/NTA_young_peoples_report_2009.pdf).

National Treatment Agency for Substance Misuse (2009b) *Young People's Specialist Substance Misuse Treatment: Exploring the Evidence*. NTA.

Pelkonen, M. & Marttunen, M. (2003) Child and adolescent suicide: epidemiology, risk factors, and approaches to prevention. *Pediatric Drugs*, **5**, 243–265.

CHAPTER 26

Parenting risk assessment service

Ian Partridge, Geraldine Casswell and Greg Richardson

'We may be excused for not caring much about other people's children, for there are many who care very little about their own.'
>   Samuel Johnson

Introduction

Multi-agency cooperation and multidisciplinary perspectives are two prerequisites of the effective safeguarding of children (as per the Children Act 2004), and this has led to structural and organisational reform in safeguarding children with an emphasis on prevention rather than intervention (HM Government, 2004), but the least detrimental alternative for a child who has suffered significant harm will still need to be determined. The questions now asked of agencies are not about the establishment of the probability or certainty that a particular abusive act has taken place, but about whether the risks of return to parental care or the care of those responsible when the abuse took place outweigh the possible harm of statutory intervention.

Risk depends on the intra-personal characteristics of parents and children and their interpersonal interactions. Mental health input into risk assessment procedures has tended to centre on the psychiatric assessment of the parenting adult and a CAMHS role in the psychological/psychiatric assessment of the child. In addition, there is a role for CAMHS in looking at the parental ability to parent and the risk posed to the child's development, regardless of the absence or presence of psychiatric disturbance.

An independent multidisciplinary team within CAMHS that assesses forensic risks within a systemic and developmental context can contribute to the comprehensive assessment of risk and offer a valuable service to statutory agencies and the courts (Smith *et al*, 2001).

Risk assessment teams that advise the courts are incorporated in the chief medical officer's recommendations for providing reports to the courts in family law cases (Donaldson, 2006). There is a clear requirement to demonstrate the benefit to the child's welfare and well-being of any intervention.

Risk to children depends on the:

- intra-personal characteristics of each parent and carer
- intra-personal characteristics of the alleged abuser

- intra-personal characteristics of the child
- interpersonal relationships between the parents/carers
- interpersonal relationships between the parents/carers and the abuser
- relationship between the parents/carers and potential supportive agencies
- interpersonal relationships between each parent/carer and the child.

Recently, the role of the 'expert' witness in cases concerning both harm and risk to children has become a topic of considerable debate. Health and Social Service professionals have been castigated for an overzealous approach resulting in the conviction of the 'innocent parent', while at the same time being scorned for a lack of intervention in cases where the 'obvious' signs have been missed and a child has been harmed and even killed. Courts are concerned that health professionals in both paediatrics and mental health are becoming reluctant to become involved in preparing reports and appearing in court in relation to safeguarding children because of much of the publicity, not to mention threats from organised groups of aggrieved parents. Professionals should remain above criticism and assist the courts and the children for whom they are responsible if they ensure they address and manage the context of the harm to the child as well as the nature of the harm. Risk assessment is a process whereby risk is minimised rather than eliminated. The professionals involved in risk assessment cannot be reduced to 'warm-blooded lie detectors'; they must present information, evidence and interpretation of that evidence, backed up by professional knowledge to offer an opinion with the arguments for and against that opinion. They must never venture into opinion beyond competence or understanding in order to strengthen the case, even if they consider that it is in the child's interests; 'bad things happen', the guilty escape and the innocent suffer – this cannot be rectified by unrealistic expectations leading to a manipulation of evidence and opinion. Providing information and opinion does not represent the final judgement; that is the responsibility of the court. Nevertheless, the court must be confident that the professional providing an opinion has the competence and training to do so (Royal College of Psychiatrists, 2008).

Structure of the team

To command the respect of referring Social Services departments and the courts, such a team requires a multidisciplinary composition of senior and experienced clinicians, and it is this model that has been recommended by the chief medical officer (Donaldson, 2006). It is unfortunate that, in requiring expert opinion, the courts and Social Services departments often undervalue the contribution of first-line workers, who are usually more familiar with the situation of and the people involved in these cases. Risk assessment in this field is both clinically and emotionally demanding;

working within a team offers a supportive environment as well as a wider range of personal and clinical perspectives. The contribution of an agency outside Social Services ensures the independence of the assessment.

Philosophy of the team

Multidisciplinary perspectives

Multidisciplinary skills and perspectives are a prerequisite of effective working in the field of child protection (HM Government, 2004).

Systems theory

To ensure that abuse is approached not only from the standpoint of the perpetrator–victim dyad but also to seek an understanding of the relational context is controversial (Bentovim et al, 1988; Feminist Review, 1988; Will, 1989). However, a wider perspective is more pertinent in both assessing risk (Elton, 1988) and informing the intervention/non-intervention debate.

Developmental context

A child's welfare is dependent on the parent's or carer's ability to adapt to the child's development. Attachment theory (Rutter, 1981; Bowlby, 1982) provides a structure to explore the childhood experiences of parents and how they contribute to or interfere with the care of their children (Crittenden & Ainsworth, 1989; George, 1996).

Forensic context

The only real indicator of risk is a previous history of abusive behaviour. This fact requires the questioning of the potential for change within developmentally acceptable timescales and the generation of strategies for the management of risk within a system either with or without additional support and monitoring. A multifactorial model of understanding risk is the most helpful (Finkelhor, 1986).

Managing referrals

All referrals to a risk assessment service are necessarily complex and arise from concerns about the protection of children. It is usual that court cases are proceeding or pending. Invariably, the work will be requested in the context of ongoing child protection case conferences; it is therefore probable that the legal department of the Local Authority will be closely involved with the case.

Initial contact with the service will often be by telephone from an involved professional. This allows preliminary discussion of the appropriateness of the referral as well as discussion of timescales for the assessment and report. This must be followed by a more detailed written referral, accompanied by relevant documentation. Where the referral takes place in the context of court proceedings, there should be a letter of instruction from the appropriate legal agencies with a clear articulation of the questions the team is being asked to address.

Following referral, a professional meeting should be arranged at which members of the risk assessment team meet all the professionals and carers involved with the care of the children in the subject family. This meeting has three main objectives.

1   To share background information on the case and to discuss the value of a risk assessment in the context of the current situation and previous assessments by other agencies and teams.
2   To clarify (and to agree and document) the specific questions the risk assessment team is being asked to address, and those issues the team will not be addressing (the team must never act beyond its competence).
3   To agree the input of all agencies into the risk assessment, to ensure a comprehensive, integrated multi-agency assessment.

In addition, timescales for both assessment and presentation of the report will need to be negotiated. A member of the team should be nominated to speak in court if necessary. The communication network and points of contact should be established. The dates of the assessment sessions should be given to the responsible social worker and appointment letters sent to the relevant family members.

This meeting is chaired by a member of the risk assessment team and recorded. A further professionals' meeting will be arranged for feedback of the assessment. There will be occasions when the family and, in particularly contentious cases, their legal representatives will be present at these meetings.

Assessment

The assessment (Box 26.1) will be geared to the concerns of the referring agency and also to the nature of the case referred. However, the team should have a clear focus for its work, which is the assessment of the risk posed by the parents or carers or other adults involved, or potentially involved, with the children. The team offers only a contribution to assessing the least detrimental option for the child – its assessment must be taken in conjunction with other assessments offered by other agencies and professionals.

The areas subject to assessment are considered in relation to risks posed to the child's safety and welfare (Box 26.2). Often there have already been incidents of abuse and neglect; in other cases there is, at the very least, a strong concern that the child's developmental welfare is or will be impaired because of the parenting received.

Box 26.1 Framework of assessment

- The relevance of the psychological and psychiatric state of the child's parents, their partners and other relevant family members to their parenting skills
- The factors relevant to parenting in the relationship between the parents (or parent and partner)
- The availability of supportive factors in the parents' environment
- The parents' willingness to avail themselves of support in parenting

Box 26.2 Factors in assessing risk

- The abusing parent's understanding of the abuse or neglect, or potential abuse or neglect
- The non-abusing parent's understanding of the abuse or neglect, or potential abuse or neglect
- The parents' understanding of the parental task related to an understanding of the child's developmental needs
- The ability and resources to change in order to become a 'good enough' parent
- The additional support or treatment required for the parents to change, and their willingness to use such support

To address the questions of concern, a series of four or five assessment sessions or a whole-day assessment (Wheeler *et al*, 1998) provide the time to work with the parents as a couple, as well as the opportunity to engage in individually focused assessment. To provide gender balance, it may be helpful for two therapists to undertake the assessment, with live supervision provided by the other team members. The family should receive feedback and receive a copy of the assessment report. The report should be sent to the referrer for distribution to all relevant agencies.

Conclusion

Safeguarding children should be the proactive process described in *Every Child Matters* (HM Government, 2004), but unfortunately it remains reactive and only when a child has suffered damage do they come to the notice of statutory authorities. A CAMHS risk assessment team can provide considerable assistance to those agencies that carry the onerous responsibility of trying to ensure that the child's development is no longer impaired.

References

Bentovim, A., Elton, A., Hildebrand, J., *et al* (1988) *Child Sexual Abuse Within the Family: Assessment and Treatment*. Wright.

Bowlby, J. (1982) *Attachment. Vol. I. Attachment and Loss*. Hogarth Press.

Crittenden, P. M. & Ainsworth, M. D. S. (1989) Child maltreatment and attachment theory. In *Child Maltreatment: Theory and Research on the Causes and Consequences of Child Abuse and Neglect* (eds D. Cicchetti & V. Carlson), pp. 432–463. Cambridge University Press.

Donaldson, L. (2006) *Bearing Good Witness*. Department of Health.

Elton, A. (1988) Assessment of families for treatment. In *Child Sexual Abuse in the Family: Assessment and Treatment* (eds A. Bentovim, A. Elton, J. Hildebrand, *et al*), pp. 153–181. Wright.

Feminist Review (1988) *Family Secrets: Child Sexual Abuse*. No. 28, Spring. Routledge.

Finkelhor, D. (1986) *A Sourcebook on Child Sexual Abuse*. Sage.

George, C. (1996) A representational perspective of child abuse and internal working models of attachment and care giving. *Child Abuse and Neglect*, **20**, 411–424.

HM Government (2004) *Every Child Matters: Change for Children*. DfES Publications.

Royal College of Psychiatrists (2008) *Court Work. Final Report of a Scoping Group. College Report CR147*. Royal College of Psychiatrists.

Rutter, M. (1981) *Maternal Deprivation Reassessed*. Penguin.

Smith, J., Wheeler, J. & Bone, D. (2001) Anarchy and assessment of complex families: order not disorder. *Clinical Child Psychology and Psychiatry*, **6**, 605–608.

Wheeler, J., Bone, D. & Smith, J. (1998) Whole day assessments: a team approach to complex multi-problem families. *Clinical Child Psychology and Psychiatry*, **3**, 169–181.

Will, D. (1989) Feminism, child sexual abuse and the (long overdue) demise of systems mysticism. *Context*, **9**, 12–15.

CHAPTER 27

Court work

Greg Richardson and Geraldine Casswell

'No man is exempt from saying silly things. The misfortune is to say them seriously.'

Michel Eyquem de Montaigne (1533–1592)

Introduction

Reports from mental health professionals may be requested in both civil and criminal proceedings. The mental health professional may be asked to prepare a report for the court as a professional witness when the report is on a current or recent patient, or as an expert witness when they are considered to have particular expertise in the field on which the court has to make a decision. As a general rule, therefore, expert work in the criminal courts is best left for those working in the forensic field. The primary responsibility when preparing a report is to the court and it is important that the patient and their family are made aware of that. The primary consideration when preparing a court report is the child's welfare, no matter who has commissioned it or who will pay for it (Department of Health, 1991). This principle must be clear throughout any work for the courts, and the report must not be altered because of pressure from those who have commissioned it. A structure for addressing court work has been described for clinical psychologists (British Psychological Society, 2000), psychiatrists (Tuffnell *et al*, 1996; Black *et al*, 1998) and for all those involved in Children Act cases (Wall, 2007). The problem of quality and supply of expert witnesses in family law cases has been addressed by the chief medical officer, in proposing local teams of experts from different disciplines and specialisms under the aegis of the NHS (Donaldson, 2006). Those who work at the interface between CAMHS and the law have an obligation to provide their patients and legal bodies with clear, focused reports prepared to the highest standards, and give oral testimony with a dignified and confident professional demeanour.

Questions to consider

Does the request come from a solicitor?

Requests for court reports must always come from a solicitor. Requests by parents, carers or social workers should be refused, and the person making the request referred back to their legal representative. There has been a move over recent years for joint instructions to be issued for expert opinion, in an attempt to lessen the adversarial nature of children's proceedings. Questions are being raised as to whether this is just, as contrary opinions are not being examined by the court to determine the court's view on the best interests of the child. Writing a report always involves a possibility of being called to court to explain and elaborate on the opinions expressed in it. The Children and Family Court Advisory Support Service (CAFCASS) acts as a central agency in determining the well-being of children involved with the courts and they may appoint a guardian whose solicitor may seek the opinion of a professional or expert witness.

Does the report concern a young person with whom the professional is currently clinically involved?

Professional witnesses write reports on the work they have undertaken with a young person and family, and answer questions the court may have about that work and what opinions such work is based upon. Such witnesses may be referred to as a 'witness to fact', in that they are giving evidence as to the 'facts' of their involvement with the young person in question and their family. In contrast, an expert witness comes new to the situation to assess the psychiatric state of the child or to give an opinion as to what is in the child's best interests (Box 27.1).

It is important to understand why a report is being requested and what questions are being asked by the court. The child and their involved family must be made aware that a report is being requested and their permission sought to prepare the report. However, the court may override that permission, and not preparing a report may then put the mental health professional in contempt of court.

Box 27.1 Considerations for professional and expert witnesses writing court reports

Professional witness
- Confidentiality
- Effect of the report on the therapeutic relationship
- Effect of the therapeutic relationship on impartiality
- May charge for the report only if the assessment work is not undertaken as part of NHS duties

Expert witness
- Time
- Not primarily a therapeutic relationship
- Impartial
- May charge for all preparatory work as well as the report

Is it a civil or a criminal matter?

Civil matters are those where the court is trying to decide what is the best option for a child's future development. They arise when children have suffered significant harm (Adcock & White, 1998), when their welfare has become a secondary consideration of those responsible for their care, or where a child is seeking to claim compensation (e.g. after an accident or medical error). Children Act proceedings are generally civil matters, and the expert or professional witness is asked what actions would be in the child's best interests (this can include issues of contact or issues of the granting of supervision or care orders).

Criminal matters arise when the young person has committed an offence and the court wishes to know whether the young person is suffering from a mental illness or has some psychological difficulties that represent mitigating factors. Occasionally, but rarely, opinion may be sought in support of a 'not guilty' plea. It should be borne in mind, when recommending treatment of any kind, that the treatment is available and who will provide it has been negotiated. Local CAMHS do not take kindly to being told by the courts what treatment they will undertake because of the recommendations of a distant expert who has taken the money and run; nor do CAMHS have any obligation to take the work on.

Has the request for the report been agreed between all parties?

Increasingly, the courts do not wish to have conflicting evidence from expert witnesses because of the extra expense and court time. It is therefore important to ensure that the solicitor commissioning a report is speaking on behalf of all parties involved in the case. If this is not checked, the professional may be seen as being in one party's camp (e.g. the father's witness), or become involved in the indelicacy of intra-professional confrontations in court.

What are the questions that require answers in the report?

In general, courts request reports for a purpose. They wish to ensure that all relevant matters are taken into consideration when making their decision and require answers to certain questions. It is important to understand the questions in order to address them. It may also be helpful to clarify questions that are beyond the professional's competence (e.g. the prognosis of an illness in a parent, when a child specialist may direct the solicitor to a more appropriate expert). The questions should be clearly laid out in the letter of instruction, and it should be established that the court has given leave to interview all relevant parties and read all relevant documentation; a professional witness may not have access to all the documentation. It is important to have expertise in the areas about which an opinion is being sought – for example, experience with adolescents with an intellectual disability or where there is dispute as to whether a child has been sexually abused (Jones, 1992). If in doubt, withdrawal at this stage is preferable to humiliation later when ignorance is exposed.

What is the timescale for the preparation of the report?

The Children Act 1989 quite rightly lays down that legal matters concerning children should be dealt with as expeditiously as possible (Department of Health, 1991), as children's development is always at risk while they are awaiting court decisions. It is therefore necessary to understand the court's expectations in terms of a report's preparation. If it is not possible to meet a deadline, it is important to say so and to determine a realistic timescale. The timescale must take account of the amount of documentation to be read and the number of interviews to be undertaken. It is better not to be pressured into underestimating the amount of time required. Once a deadline is agreed, it is important to meet it, as elaborate and expensive court processes will be planned around it. It is important to be aware that the pressures on the courts often generate unreasonable expectations in terms of how quickly reports can be prepared.

In which court is the case being heard?

It is helpful to know the level of the court that is requesting the report, as this will influence how much background and explanation the report will require. For example, magistrates may not have as sophisticated an understanding of child development and the roles of CAMHS professionals as will a High Court judge. In addition, the terms of address differ between courts (Table 27.1).

Magistrates' courts are local, county courts are in the nearest large town and High Court sittings are only in large cities. Magistrates' courts deal with juvenile offenders and the 'family panel' with some Children Act issues. County courts deal with Children Act cases passed to them by the magistrates court because of their complexity, so a report prepared for the magistrates' court may be passed to the county court. The Crown Court hears appeals from Children Act proceedings and deals with some juvenile offenders. The family division of the High Court deals with contested Children Act proceedings, contested adoptions and with 'wardship', which has become far less common since the introduction of the Children Act

Table 27.1 Terms of address in court

Type of court	Terms of address
Magistrates	Sir, Ma'am, Your Worship
County and Crown Court judges	Your Honour
High Court judges	My Lord, My Lady, Your Lordship, Your Ladyship

1989. Children Act cases are dealt with at family centres, in which the case is heard 'in chambers', which means the public and press do not have access and the legal professionals do not wear full regalia.

Charging for the report

The solicitor may forget to ask, so it is important for the CAMHS professional to inform the solicitor of the charges the preparation of a report will incur. Differential rates for preparation work, interviews, travel and court appearances may be necessary. It is not reasonable to charge for clinical work undertaken as part of NHS commitments if the information is subsequently used in the preparation of a report. However, it is reasonable to charge for the time involved in the preparation of the report because this would not normally be part of clinical care, extra work is involved in the preparation of the report, and this will be outside the professional's agreed job plan.

How much to charge is probably best discussed with colleagues. If the child and family are in receipt of legal aid, the solicitor should ask for a written estimate of fees and expenses so that they can submit a claim to the Legal Aid Board. If this is not done, there is no assurance that the fees will be paid.

Consultant psychiatrists not on the new consultant contract are entitled to do Category 2 work (work undertaken in NHS time but for which a charge is made to whoever commissioned the report), for which fees may be charged, but which does not count as private practice. For all other members of CAMHS, the issue is much simpler: if they prepare reports on young people or families who are not their patients, this is private work and cannot be undertaken as part of their NHS duties unless they are a member of an NHS expert consortium as described by the chief medical officer (Donaldson, 2006).

It is important to submit an account of detailed charges with the report. Most solicitors will pay the account within a reasonable length of time, although they may first have to submit it to the Legal Aid Board. Occasionally, rogue solicitors are reluctant to settle their accounts, so it is sometimes wise to request payment after the report is prepared but before it is submitted.

Whom to see and what to read

Whom to see and what to read will be determined by the content of the report; seeing people and reading information on the child's development will provide the platform on which the assessment and opinion of what is in the child's best interests are based.

In preparing a professional report on someone seen clinically, most of the information for the report should be in the file. However, if working with a mother and child, to prepare a comprehensive report it may be necessary to see an estranged father. Before doing so, it is important to seek clarification as to issues of parental responsibility and residence. Setting up appointments with family members who have not been involved in treatment can be problematic. An uninvolved expert does not have these problems; this may explain why more guardians are now requesting expert opinions and generally prefer these to those of local services (Brophy *et al*, 1999).

In coming to the case without previous contact, it is useful to discuss with the commissioning solicitor who they think should be seen. A guardian may have been appointed and a discussion with guardians may be helpful as they will have a detailed knowledge of the case and will be able to identify the salient people. Sometimes it is less disruptive to see children in their own home, but awareness of physical and professional safety may necessitate taking a colleague. In residence and contact disputes, it is necessary to see both parents, and in issues involving the Local Authority it is necessary to talk to the social worker and possibly foster parents or residential care workers. In compensation cases, it is not usually necessary to interview the perpetrator of the accident, but copies of the medical notes will be essential for claims of medical negligence.

It is reasonable to ask solicitors to obtain documents that may be helpful in the preparation of the report. Supporting statements by involved parties, case conference minutes and school reports are basic essentials, but other documentation such as previous medical records may also be required to reach an informed view.

Preparation of the report

There are published guidelines on how to write a legal report (Vizard & Harris, 1997; Black *et al*, 1998), the format proposed by Tuffnell (1993) being recommended at the time by the official solicitor to the Supreme Court. *A Handbook for Expert Witnesses in Children Act Cases* (Wall, 2007) is an absolute prerequisite to understand what is required of medical witnesses in Children Act cases.

The front of the report should contain the name of the child and date of birth, the nature of the proceedings, the court reference number(s), the name, qualifications and working address of the person preparing the report, the date of the report and a table of contents. The subsequent sections are outlined in Table 27.2.

The report should be written on A4 paper in a font size of at least 12 points, double-spaced and with wide margins. Sections and paragraphs should be numbered, as should the pages. The report should be written in short, uncomplicated sentences; jargon and technical terminology should be avoided, as should overcomplicated or ambiguous argument. The arguments for and against the opinion given must be clearly stated. Succinct reports that are to the point are appreciated: they allow the giving of evidence in a clear fashion.

Table 27.2 Format for court reports

Section	Content
Introduction	The introduction should cover who has asked for the report to be prepared, the nature of the proceedings, the reasons for the preparation of the report and the questions the report has to address. Sources of information and relevant curriculum vitae should be referred to as appendices.
Background	This section should contain a chronological listing of relevant facts in the development of the child and any background literature or knowledge base that is referred to.
Assessment	This section should contain views, opinions and deductions from the background information. It is often helpful to include a consideration of the welfare checklist (White *et al*, 2004) to clarify to the court that matters identified as important in the Children Act 1989 have been considered. The report is geared to stating what is in the best interests of the child; however, by the time of the report, the best interests of the child have often been damaged by that child's life experience. It is the report writer's task to determine which is the least detrimental option for the child's future and to describe how that option might be enhanced for the child's benefit.
Opinion	This section contains conclusions from the assessment section and is where the questions detailed in the introduction are addressed.
Recommendation	The recommendation section states clearly what action is necessary to ensure the best interests of the child. A report prepared in a compensation case may well not have any recommendations, as it is opinion that is required.
Conclusion	Conclude with the sentence 'I believe that the facts I have stated in this report are true and that the opinions I have expressed are correct' (recommendation by Jordans Solicitors, personal communication, 1999), and a statement should be made clarifying that there has been no conflict of interest in preparing the report (Wall, 2007); then sign the report.
Appendices	Appendices should detail who has been interviewed and what documents were considered in the preparation of the report. Separate appendices may cover the details of specific interviews and curriculum vitae of the author of the report. In civil cases, a copy of the letter of instruction should be appended.

Appearing in court

Most requests for a court report do not result in a court appearance. If the professional is to appear, the date should be established as soon as possible, as the court appearance will disrupt clinical schedules. Some hearings are listed for several days, so it is perfectly reasonable to state availability, after discussion and agreement with the commissioning solicitor. Courts do keep professional and expert witnesses waiting for lengths of time that would not be acceptable for families in clinics. Court hearings often occur some considerable time after the report has been submitted and a lot of clinical material will have flowed under the practice bridge between the two events. It is therefore imperative to read the report and re-establish the salient background factors that led to the conclusions. It is sensible to ask the instructing solicitor to forward any relevant new documents, should they become available.

On the day of the court appearance, the 'court suit' should be clean and pressed – for some reason courts consider that impeccable opinions come only from the impeccably dressed. It is also a display of respect to those involved in the hearing, as well as the court itself. Plenty of time should be allowed to ensure arrival in good time. It is a good idea to know which judge is sitting, as court listings will then establish the location of the hearing.

Occasionally, professional or expert witnesses may be asked to see members of the family or another professional to clarify issues of possible contention and possibly resolve them. Generally, it is worthwhile agreeing with this, as it removes adversarial discussions from the courtroom and means the court can devote its time to deciding on the best interests of the child rather than which of the differing opinions they are going to act upon. Such discussions may result in differences being resolved or questions clarified so that it is not necessary to give evidence at all.

When called upon to give evidence, after taking the oath, the solicitor or barrister will lead the witness through the 'evidence in chief'. This is the easy bit and all that is necessary is to watch the judge and ensure they have finished writing before continuing giving evidence. Cross-examination can give cause for concern, so marshalling experience and knowledge in relation to the case is of supreme importance (Reder *et al*, 1994). Competent witnesses never make a statement beyond their expertise and never become angry or determined to win the point. The rules for the ethical witness are detailed in Box 27.2. Occasionally, taking a metaphorical step back and remembering the game-like qualities of the situation can offer an oasis of calm for the witness. This may seem to undermine the gravitas of the situation, but the child whose interests are being represented will be far better served by a thoughtful, measured presentation than an emotionally unpredictable, reactive diatribe (Wolkind, 1994). Tactics that facilitate taking a step back include sipping from a glass of water, asking for the question to be repeated or addressing the judge for clarification. In all cases, answers should be addressed to the judge rather than the examining solicitor or barrister.

When evidence is completed, the barrister or solicitor will usually request that the witness be given leave to go.

Training issues

Training for mental health work leads to the development of a different set of skills from legal training. If mental health professionals are to function

---

Box 27.2 Rules of court work for the ethical witness

The ethical expert will:

- not give evidence beyond their expertise
- undertake CPD to maintain their expertise
- have an awareness of the possibilities for the treatment or placement of those on whom they prepared reports when making their recommendations to the court
- declare any conflict of interests to the court (e.g. if a recommendation is made for the placement of a person in an establishment in which the expert has an interest or the child is or has been their own patient)
- prepare a report based on their opinions from the evidence and their specialist knowledge, uninfluenced by the exigencies of the litigation and regardless of who commissioned the report
- be cognisant of the funding arrangements of organisations such as the Legal Services Commission, so ensuring value for money; this may include questioning whether a psychiatric report is really necessary
- have the integrity to resist any pressure to 'adjust' their report to suit the needs of the instructing lawyer or their client
- be clear about timescales for the preparation of reports so that delay is minimised
- retain all their notes.

Reproduced from Royal College of Psychiatrists, 2008

---

effectively in the legal system, they must be trained, and maintain skills, in using and describing their expertise in mental health and disorder as well as ethical understanding. Those who undertake court work should be prepared to give the court evidence of their CPD in court work and the field in which they are giving evidence (Royal College of Psychiatrists, 2008). To increase the interest, knowledge and confidence of CAMHS professionals in undertaking court work affecting children and young people, it may be helpful for them all to:

- prepare a report for a child protection case conference
- attend at least one child protection case conference per year
- prepare a report for a statutory agency or the courts on a case with which they are involved
- visit a court hearing to watch an experienced witness
- attend a workshop on writing reports for court and courtroom skills
- work with colleagues from other disciplines to prepare a report on a child at risk
- spend some time in joint work with a member of a youth offending team
- become involved in a mini-pupillage scheme run by a local court.

If CAMHS professionals are regularly preparing reports for the courts, they should be part of a peer-review group of individuals with similar court work training requirements as part of their CPD.

Court work can be stressful. There is a hierarchy of regard present in how courts hear from different disciplines and this, along with the fact that the legal world is different to the clinical world, means that training is imperative. Court can be a minefield for the uninitiated and the unprepared. Box 27.3 lists the training needs for court work.

Conclusion

The idea of appearing in court is frightening to many mental health professionals, but it is occasionally necessary to ensure the welfare of a child. All mental health professionals should have a basic competence in report writing as they may be required to give evidence as a professional witness, particularly in relation to mental health tribunals. In the duty to the child, it will be necessary to understand how to prepare a clear and concise report that is helpful to the court and to those making decisions about the child's welfare. That duty may necessitate appearing in court, and preparation for this by referring to Lord Justice Wall's book (2007) or, if a psychiatrist, to doctor-specific recommendations (Friston, 2005;

Box 27.3 Training needs for court work

- To have a working knowledge of the legal frameworks affecting children and young people
- To know how to plan and undertake assessments for statutory authorities and the courts
- To have experience in preparing and writing court reports in an effective and acceptable way
- To develop confidence in courtroom skills
- To develop knowledge of how to access more detailed information on legal issues relating to children and young people
- To clarify understanding of legal instructions
- To plan and undertake assessments in both civil and criminal cases
- To develop a functional and understandable format for court reports
- To use a mental health knowledge base while working in legal proceedings
- To develop the capacity to represent children and their needs by understanding that the needs of the child are paramount, especially in an adversarial legal process
- To understand court structures and processes
- To understand the welfare checklist (White et al, 2004) and use it in the interests of the child
- To be involved in a peer-development group devoted to court practice

Royal College of Psychiatrists, 2008) should ensure the feared humiliation is avoided.

References

Adcock, M. & White, R. (1998) *Significant Harm*. Significant Publications.

Black, D., Harris-Hendricks, J. & Wolkind, S. (eds) (1998) *Child Psychiatry and the Law (3rd edn)*. Gaskell.

British Psychological Society (2000) *Managing Litigation Arising in Clinical Work with Children and Families*. BPS.

Brophy, J., Wale, C. J. & Bates, P. (1999) *Myths and Practices: A National Survey of the Use of Experts in Child Care Proceedings*. British Agencies for Adoption and Fostering.

Department of Health (1991) *Introduction to the Children Act 1989*. Stationery Office Books.

Donaldson, L. (2006) *Bearing Good Witness: Proposals for Reforming the Delivery of Medical Expert Evidence in Family Law Cases*. Department of Health.

Friston, M. (2005) Roles and responsibilities of medical expert witnesses. *BMJ*, **331**, 305–306.

Jones, D. P. H. (1992) *Interviewing the Sexually Abused Child. Investigation of Suspected Abuse*. Gaskell.

Reder, P., Lucey, C. & Fellow-Smith, E. (1994) Surviving cross examination in court. *Journal of Forensic Psychiatry*, **4**, 489–496.

Royal College of Psychiatrists (2008) *Court Work. Report of a Scoping Group. College Report CR147*. Royal College of Psychiatrists.

Tuffnell, G. (1993) Psychiatric court reports in child care cases: what constitutes good practice? *ACPP Review and Newsletter*, **15**, 219–224.

Tuffnell, G., Cottrell, D. & Giorgiades, D. (1996) Good practice for expert witnesses. *Clinical Child Psychology and Psychiatry*, **3**, 365–385.

Vizard, E. & Harris, P. (1997) *The Expert Witness Pack*. Family Law.

Wall, N. (2007) *A Handbook for Expert Witnesses in Children Act Cases*. Family Law.

Wolkind, S. (1994) Legal aspects of child care. In *Child and Adolescent Psychiatry: Modern Approaches* (eds M. Rutter, E. Taylor & L. Hersov), pp. 1089–1102. Blackwell Scientific.

CHAPTER 28

Tier 4 options

Tim McDougall, Anne Worrall-Davies, Lesley Hewson,
Rosie Beer and Greg Richardson

'Two roads diverged in a wood, and I–
I took the one less travelled by,
And that has made all the difference.'
>   Robert Frost (1874–1963)

Introduction

Tier 4 CAMHS aim to meet the needs of children and young people with the most complex, severe or persistent mental health problems. Tier 4 services include in-patient care (see Chapter 29), as well as a range of day care and intensive community home-based and outreach services for specific groups of children and young people.

Day services

Early descriptions of child and adolescent mental health day units emphasised 5-day 'milieu' provision with a strong emphasis on education and behaviour management (Brown, 1996), whereas now they frequently provide daily focused activities to which children and families are invited, depending on their needs. Currently, about half of UK day services are linked to in-patient units, and many in-patient units have a day programme (Green & Jacobs, 1998). It is impossible to classify day services owing to the enormous range in milieu and interventions provided (Green & Worrall-Davies, 2008). However, day services broadly offer:

- support and transition to community services following in-patient admission;
- intensive 5 days per week treatment packages for children and their families;
- treatment of disruptive behaviour, using multimodal treatment strategies with a combination of individual, family and psychopharmacological interventions;
- specialist management and programmes of care for younger children with developmental disorders such as autism, speech and language disorders or neuropsychiatric disorders;
- intensive intervention aimed at improving family functioning in situations of family breakdown or child maltreatment.

Provision and organisation

Day units can offer assessment and therapeutic services that are more specialised, complex and intensive than out-patient services, although they are still community-based and less disruptive than in-patient admission. Most also have the benefit of educational input. Close liaison with specialised education and Social Services is central to their work. There is general acceptance of the central importance of maintaining attachments and working with whole systems if the complex needs of children are to be met. Day units can work with children and young people individually and in groups, as well as with their families, while keeping the focus of concern within the community and avoiding the 'out of sight, out of mind' dilemma of in-patient services.

Day services can be diverse, flexible and responsive to local needs, and can provide a wide range of readily accessed programmes (Box 28.1). They may offer part-time attendance only to maximise the range of options available and enable continued school attendance or the involvement of other services. Other day services may be more specialised, providing for rarer or more complex difficulties, and may aim to offer an alternative to in-patient care or special education. Full-time provision (5 days per week) or the flexibility to offer this when needed is then usual. Day units can be stand-alone or combined with in-patient services; this often reflects the history of the resource and its influence upon the type of service offered.

There is an organisational and, to some extent, philosophical tension between day and in-patient provision. For example, a service organised for part-time attendance and structured individual/group programmes would struggle to meet a need for urgent assessment or more extended contact. Similarly, a service offering full-time attendance for young people with a wide range of complex disorders may have difficulty maintaining group and therapist consistency.

Box 28.1 Services offered by day units

- Specialised group work such as social skills, activity-based, psychodynamic, art or drama therapy and communication skills
- Programmes or groups for particular disorders such as Asperger syndrome, anxious school non-attendance, ADHD, moderate learning plus social skills difficulties, physical and emotional disabilities
- Parent groups focused on support and parenting skills
- Integrated programmes of individual, group, parenting and family work
- Assessment of complex neurodevelopmental, behavioural and parenting problems
- Maintenance in the community or rehabilitation after a period of in-patient care of young people with psychotic disorders

---

Although some day services work with the full age range, most specialise in working with either children or adolescents, the cut-off age being usually around 12 years. The target age group will tend to influence the type of service provided – for example, day units for children usually see extensive work with parents (and often siblings) as essential to their work with the referred child. The type of service will also reflect the geographical situation. Day services are limited by distance (i.e. time of travel). Services in rural areas are likely to be closely linked to the locality CAMHS and providing for their needs, whereas day services in large cities or conurbations may develop more specialised services and draw referrals from a number of neighbouring health districts.

The model of day service chosen should be clear to potential users (Box 28.2). Day services need to be integrated firmly with the full range of CAMHS both clinically and managerially so that young people can move smoothly between different parts of the service according to their needs. The role of the unit in relation to other services (especially education and Social Services) must also be clear, particularly if funding is inter-agency. Points of good practice for day units are listed in Box 28.3.

Staffing

Day services for children and young people with complex needs require an experienced, well-resourced and well-supported multidisciplinary team if they are to function effectively. Although the composition of teams varies, there is a common emphasis on the need for specialised training, regular skilled supervision and well-maintained inter-agency links. Skill mix is as important as multidisciplinary balance, and most day-unit teams should have members with higher training and qualifications in group work, creative therapies, psychodynamic psychotherapy, play therapy and family therapy, in addition to higher training in child and adolescent mental

---

Box 28.2 Referral protocol

- Clarity for managers, referrers, day-service staff, referred children/young people and parents about the type of service offered and for whom (including clarity about the catchment area)
- Clear routes of referral and stipulation of who can refer: CAMHS professionals only or also education or Social Services, or paediatricians
- How, when and by whom decisions are made about whether a referral has been accepted and when a place may be available
- Are urgent referrals ever accepted; moreover, if they are, what are the criteria
- Are management arrangements clear: are these arrangements in line with local CAMHS

Box 28.3 Good practice for day units

- Prompt feedback to a referrer as to whether the referral is suitable for the day service, and if not, possible other sources of help.
- Minimal waiting times between referral and beginning evaluation, unless referral is for a particular time-limited programme.
- An initial networking meeting and/or telephone contacts with previously involved professionals to exchange information and clarify the aims of admission to the day service. This meeting may also act as a consultation to the referring professionals to clarify needs, other possible sources of help and/ or other necessary actions (e.g. child protection planning).
- Initial meetings with the child or young person and family to reach a shared understanding of their needs, the aims of unit admission and expected input from staff and family.
- Regular reviews while the child or young person is attending the unit and close liaison with school, referrer and other professionals involved. Review meetings may usefully involve family and professionals, so that misunderstandings and 'splitting' can be avoided.
- Careful discharge planning to ensure continuity of provision by locality CAMHS or other community services.
- A system for regular feedback on levels of satisfaction with the service from all involved, and constructive evaluation of any complaints or suggestions for change.

---

health. Staffing levels and discipline mixes vary considerably, often as a reflection of the historical development of the particular service; ideally, staff should include professionals from nursing, occupational and creative therapies, psychotherapy, child and adolescent psychology and psychiatry, plus possibly physiotherapy and speech/language therapy. Teaching staff (funded by the education service) and social work input (funded by Social Services) are crucial to the type of service offered and to effective inter-agency liaison. Experienced administrative and secretarial support is critical to ensure clear and regular communication between the service and the outside world. Stability is aided by some staff working full time in the day service, whereas the presence in the team of members who also work part time in community services will help foster awareness of need and integrated working.

Staffing levels are difficult to stipulate as working practices and structures vary so widely, but child and adolescent day services are specialised and demanding; they are not a cheap option. Transport to and from the unit may need to be provided as a routine part of the service, for example for younger children and their parents, for those travelling long distances or where no suitable public transport exists, and for house-bound adolescents for whom attendance independent of their parents is a critical part of their treatment.

Evaluation

Audit and evaluation can present difficulties because multiple therapeutic approaches are often employed simultaneously, family, school and community influences are still active daily, and diagnostic categories may be less clear and less helpful than in other services. In addition, children, young people and parents may deny, distort or exaggerate their difficulties in ways that are integral to the decision to involve day services, but may render many assessment scales invalid. The diversity and patchy availability of day services may make it difficult to relate efficacy to the impact on other services locally and to make meaningful comparisons between units. Nevertheless, user, carer and referrer perspectives on the service should be continually assessed.

Although attempts have been made in the USA and Canada to assess the clinical effectiveness and cost-effectiveness of day attendance (Grizenko & Papineau, 1992; Zimet *et al*, 1994), there is a dearth of such reports in the UK (Creed *et al*, 1997; Goldberg & Collier, 1999). However, a number of accounts have begun to explore the planning, organisation and clinical potential of day services that offer a wide range of clearly defined specialised services (e.g. Place *et al*, 1990; Davison, 1996; McFadyen, 1999). There have been evaluation studies of day services (Weiner *et al*, 1999), referrer satisfaction surveys (Park *et al*, 1991), attempts to compare the costs and benefits of day services with those of other services (Zimet *et al*, 1994), and discussions of the complex inter-agency aspects of outcome that need to be addressed if the full value of day services is to be assessed (McFadyen, 1999; Weiner *et al*, 1999; Hayter, 2000). As with all services, clarity of aims is a prerequisite of evaluation. Liaison with a wide range of other services is an essential part of the work. A system to record workload must have a way of recognising and valuing time spent in liaison, including on the telephone and via emails. Controlled use of day services alone has shown that they are effective for preschool and school-age children with complex needs (Grizenko *et al*, 1993). Innovative examples of day services provide opportunities to transfer care and treatment from in-patient settings into the community and family environment (McCarthy *et al*, 2006), or meet the needs of children and young people with complex needs through multi-agency partnerships between health, education and Social Services.

Intensive community services

A range of alternatives to admission to a psychiatric ward for adults have been adapted for use with children and young people. These include assertive outreach, multisystemic therapy, treatment foster care and home-based services. The key components of intensive community services are:

- small case-loads for each professional or team
- the ability to provide a 24-hour rapid response

- multimodal treatment strategies
- close involvement of partner agencies
- individually tailored treatments
- flexible working practices
- systemic approaches to the young person's difficulties
- strong partnerships with young people and their families or carers.

Research evidence supports the use of alternatives to in-patient admission for certain groups of children and young people with mental health problems (Woolston, 1998). Intensive community services have been shown to produce positive outcomes for some groups of children and young people, particularly those who self-harm (Harrington et al, 1998) and those with conduct disorder or antisocial behaviour (Henggeler et al, 1998). In the UK there are numerous community services supporting young people with serious mental health problems at home, using a range of models of care, some loosely based on assertive outreach (Hewson, 2002; Street et al, 2005; Ahmed et al, 2006), others using specific or adapted models of multisystemic therapy (Jefford & Squire, 2004) and dialectical behaviour therapy (Miller et al, 1997). Many have been derived or adapted from intensive community services in Europe and the USA. Some home-based services are located within specialist CAMHS (Hewson, 2002), others are provided within adult mental health services (Street et al, 2005) and several are defined as multi-agency projects (Kelly et al 2003). Common to all services is same-day response, intensive community-based care and treatment, and transition to community CAMHS during recovery (Kelly et al, 2003; Street et al, 2005; Worrall-Davies & Kiernan, 2005).

Home-based treatment

Home treatment is an intensive service for young people with mental disorders who are in crisis and are otherwise eligible for admission to a residential setting. The key features are: availability 24 hours a day, 7 days a week; rapid response time; and the ability to work flexibly with young people, their families and carers, and a range of multi-agency services. Evidence from Germany (Lay & Schmidt, 2001; Mattajat et al, 2001) shows that young people with a range of mental disorders can be treated as safely and successfully at home as in an in-patient unit. The German studies and an RCT of the similar Family Preservation Program in the USA (Wilmshurst, 2002) also suggest that home-based treatment leads to longer maintenance of symptom and behaviour improvements.

Multisystemic therapy

Multisystemic therapy is an intensive family-based treatment that targets children and young people with severe behaviour problems, including chronic, serious and violent offenders, and their families (Henggeler et al, 1998). The primary aims are to reduce criminal activity, reduce antisocial behaviour such as substance misuse and violence, and decrease rates of incarceration, out-of-home placements and hospital admission. Whether such a provision properly belongs within CAMHS or should be provided on a multi-agency basis with input from CAMHS remains a matter for discussion.

Multisystemic therapy teams provide services 24 hours a day, 7 days a week for a case-load of 4–6 young people aged between 10 and 17. Each treatment lasts 4–6 months and there is an average of 60 hours of contact during the treatment period. During this time, the team provides a range of systemic interventions that address personality traits associated with the development of conduct disorder and antisocial personality disorder. The team will also provide interventions to tackle offending behaviour, reparation work, interpersonal skills and family support.

Multisystemic therapy does not have a unique set of intervention techniques; instead, intervention strategies are integrated from other pragmatic, problem-focused treatment models including strategic family therapy, structural family therapy and CBT. It is distinguished from other intervention approaches by its comprehensive conceptualisation of clinical problems and the multifaceted nature of its interventions.

Multidimensional treatment foster care

Multidimensional treatment foster care, which is based on social learning theory, comprises structured therapy within a foster family setting and is delivered within a multi-agency context. Treatment foster care services recruit, train, supervise and support foster families, who usually look after only one fostered child for a period of 6–9 months. Treatment foster care differs from standard foster care in several ways, including the provision of a detailed functional analysis with close monitoring of the child or young person's behaviour. Substantial training and supervision for foster parents by case managers emphasising therapy is provided.

The intervention appears to produce a reduction in symptoms and lowers rates of offending for mentally disordered and young offenders respectively compared with in-patient care groups (Chamberlain, 2002, 2003).

Case management

Case management encompasses a number of approaches including assertive outreach, assertive community treatment and wraparound services. Like all interventions for children and young people with mental health problems, case management lacks a strong evidence base in the UK. The coordination and responsibility of care for an individual child or young person is assigned to an individual practitioner or team. Case managers have the responsibility of assessing individual needs, providing intensive clinical or rehabilitative services and signposting young people to services that will meet their individually identified needs. Unlike home-based services that are time limited, case management is intended to be ongoing, providing young people with whatever they need, whenever they need it, for as long as necessary.

The assertive outreach/community treatment model is recommended as part of the national adult mental health policy (Department of Health, 2002). The key features are multidisciplinary interventions with small caseloads of young people, 24 hours a day, 7 days a week care and treatment, and the availability of crisis intervention services. There is a focus on promoting life skills development, social inclusion and the principles of recovery. There is a relatively good evidence base that assertive outreach is as effective and safe as in-patient care for young adults with early-onset psychosis. It is valued by service users and is cost-effective (Craig *et al*, 2004).

Wraparound services are designed to help families develop a plan to address their child's individual needs at home and at school. The services are provided through teams that implement comprehensive support plans. These aim to link children, families or carers and their support networks with health, Social Services, education and youth justice services. Outcomes suggest that this model of brokering services results in significant behavioural improvements, reduces time spent in hospital, and may be as effective, but cheaper than, treatment foster care (Burns *et al*, 2000).

Commissioning Tier 4 services

Historically, the commissioning of Tier 4 services has been locally driven and badly planned due to a lack of information about need and demand. Although Tier 4 services have previously been commissioned by local primary care trusts, increasingly they are being commissioned through collective arrangements at a subregional or regional level, and are provided by the NHS and independent sector. In-patient adolescent forensic services are commissioned nationally by the National Commissioning Group.

Despite Tier 4 CAMHS being targeted at the most challenged and challenging young people in our population, the lack of strategic commissioning to date has meant that the standards for success identified over 14 years ago by the NHS Health Advisory Service (1995) remain difficult to achieve. Factors contributing to the complexity of commissioning Tier 4 CAMHS include:

- increased referral rates to Tier 4 CAMHS
- highly variable accessibility in different geographical areas
- poor integration with community CAMHS
- limited inter-agency working
- little involvement of children and young people in planning services
- poor information for service users
- poor support after discharge.

At a regional level, a lack of systematic and robust information about Tier 4 services precludes year-on-year comparisons of activity and cost, so even need based on demand or use cannot be accurately calculated (Beecham *et al*, 2003). In addition, comparisons between regions are difficult as levels of information and systems for data collection are highly variable. For example, if a health authority wanted to compare and contrast Tier 4 provision, capacity or access for their population, there is currently no single data source that could provide this basic information. More sophisticated analysis, for example on the value of commissioned services in terms of outcome, quality and cost is even more elusive (Crofts & Corbett, 2006). Commissioners require good information on which to base decisions, commission competently and plan future service developments based on a range of properly evaluated Tier 4 services that improve outcomes for the children and young people who use them. Relying solely on the benchmark of beds per population gives an incomplete picture of current and potential future capacity to meet the needs of children and adolescents requiring comprehensive Tier 4 services.

We must develop commissioning mechanisms to support the growth of innovative alternatives to bed-based services, in terms of cost, reduction in length of treatment and, ultimately, outcomes for the children and young people who use such services. Child and adolescent mental health service mapping demonstrates some patchy growth in community-based Tier 4 services, particularly home-based services and outreach teams. Transition services between Tier 4 CAMHS and adult mental health remain variable, with some areas of the country providing excellent partnership working between CAMHS, early intervention psychosis services and adult mental health in-patient provision. However, partnerships working in other areas of the country are poorly developed, with older adolescents falling between services.

Conclusion

Most areas of the country do not have the recommended number of beds for children or adolescents with mental disorders. Indeed, there have been a small number of high-profile proposed and actual closures of in-patient beds, particularly of those for younger children. Supra-regional or national coordination of needs assessments may enable a more strategic approach to be taken, where long-term capacity planning and the development of a range of evidence based alternatives to in-patient provision are commissioned. All home-based treatment services appear to offer services for young people with a range of mental disorders including acute psychosis, eating disorders and suicidal behaviour, and seem largely to avert admission to in-patient services without a significant deterioration in mental health and social functioning (Worrall-Davies & Kiernan, 2005).

References

Ahmed, D., Salmon, G., Ahuja, A., *et al* (2006) Development and philosophy of a new service. *Child Psychology and Psychiatry*, **11**, 591–605.

Beecham, J., Chisholm, D. & O'Herlihy, A. (2003) Variations in the costs of child and adolescent psychiatric units. *British Journal of Psychiatry*, **183**, 220–225.

Brown, M. (1996) Day patient treatment. In *Child Psychiatric Units: At the Crossroads* (eds R. Chesson & D. Chisholm), pp. 45–52. Jessica Kingsley.

Burns, B., Schoenwald, S., Burchard, J., *et al* (2000) Comprehensive community based interventions for youth with severe emotional disorders: multisystemic therapy and the wraparound process. *Journal of Child and Family Studies*, **9**, 283–314.

Chamberlain, P. (2002) Treatment foster care. In *Community Treatment for Youth: Evidence Based Interventions for Severe Emotional and Behavioural Disorders* (eds B. J. Burns & K. Hoagwood), pp. 117–138. Oxford University Press.

Chamberlain, P. (ed.) (2003) Multidimensional treatment foster care program components and principles of practice. In *Treating Chronic Juvenile Offenders: Advances Made Through the Oregon Multidimensional Treatment Foster Care Model*, pp. 69–93. American Psychological Association.

Craig, T., Garety, P., Power, P., *et al* (2004) The Lambert Early Onset (LEO) Team: randomised controlled study of effectiveness of specialised care for early psychosis. *BMJ*, **329**, 1067–1072.

Creed, F., Mbaya, P., Lancashire, S., *et al* (1997) Cost effectiveness of day and in-patient psychiatric treatment: results of a randomised controlled trial. *BMJ*, **314**, 1381–1385.

Crofts, M. & Corbett, K. (2006) *Developing Strategic and Specialised Commissioning for Tier 4: Tier 4 Policy Implementation Guidance Development Group Discussion Paper 3*. Care Services Improvement Partnership.

Davison, I. (1996) Innovation and efficacy: the challenges of a new children's day resource. *Child Psychology and Psychiatry Review*, **1**, 26–30.

Department of Health (2002) *A National Service Framework for Mental Health*. Department of Health.

Goldberg, D. & Collier, P. (1999) Why are there so few adolescent day services? *Young Minds Magazine*, **40**, 14–15.

Green, J. & Jacobs, B. (1998) *In-patient Child Psychiatry: Modern Practice, Research and the Future*. Routledge.

Green, J. & Worrall-Davies, A. (2008) Provision of intensive treatment: in-patients units, day units and intensive outreach. In *Rutter's Child and Adolescent Psychiatry, Fifth Edition* (eds M. Rutter, D. Bishop, D. Pine, *et al*), pp. 1126–1142. Blackwell.

Grizenko, N. & Papineau, D. (1992) A comparison of the cost-effectiveness of day treatment and residential treatment for children with severe behaviour problems. *Canadian Journal of Psychiatry*, **37**, 393–400.

Grizenko, N., Papineau, D. & Sayegh, L. (1993) Effectiveness of a multimodal day treatment programme for children with disruptive behaviour problems. *Journal of American Academy of Child and Adolescent Psychiatry*, **32**, 127–134.

Harrington, R., Kerfoot, M., Dyer, E., *et al* (1998) Randomised trial of a home based family intervention for children who have deliberately poisoned themselves. *Journal of the American Academy of Child and Adolescent Psychiatry*, **37**, 512–518.

Hayter, J. (2000) Day therapy for adolescents: the evolution and practice of a day therapy service. *Young Minds*, **47**, 13–17.

Henggeler, S., Schoenwald, S., Borduin, C., *et al* (1998) *Multisystemic Treatment of Antisocial Behaviour in Children and Adolescents*. Guilford Press.

Hewson, L. (2002) Care begins at home: reducing the use of in-patient beds. *Young Minds*, **58**, 3–5.

Jefford, T. & Squire, B. (2004) Model practice. *Young Minds*, **71**, 17–18.

Kelly, C., Allan, S., Roscoe, P., et al (2003) The mental health needs of looked after children: an integrated multi agency model of care. *Clinical Child Psychology and Psychiatry*, **8**, 323–335.

Lay, B. & Schmidt, M. (2001) Effectiveness of home treatment in children and adolescents with externalizing psychiatric disorders. *European Child and Adolescent Psychiatry*, **10** (supp. 1), 180–190.

Mattajat, F., Hirt, B., Wilken, J., et al (2001) Efficacy of in-patient and home treatment in psychiatrically disturbed children and adolescents: follow up assessment of the results of a controlled treatment study. *European Child and Adolescent Psychiatry*, **10** (suppl. 1), 171–179.

McCarthy, G., Baker, S., Betts, K., et al (2006) The development of a new day treatment programme for older children (8–11 years) with behavioural problems: the go zone. *Child Psychology and Psychiatry*, **11**, 156–166.

McFadyen, A. (1999) Doubly disadvantaged: providing a psychotherapeutic and educational service to children with complex disorders and their families. *Clinical Child Psychology and Psychiatry*, **4**, 91–105.

Miller, A., Rathus, J., Linehan, M., et al (1997) Dialectical behaviour therapy adapted for suicidal adolescents. *Journal of Practical Psychiatry and Behavioral Health*, **3**, 78–86.

NHS Health Advisory Service (1995) *Together We Stand: Commissioning, Role and Management of Child and Adolescent Mental Health Services*. HMSO.

Park, M., Langa, A., Likierman, H., et al (1991) Setting up a new regional child and family psychiatry unit: the involvement of referrers. *Psychiatric Bulletin*, **15**, 142–144.

Place, M., Rajah, S. & Crake, T. (1990) Combining day patient treatment with family work in a child psychiatry clinic. *European Archives of Psychiatry and Neurological Science*, **239**, 373–378.

Street, C., Allan, B. & Saedi, K. (2005) *Benchmarking of Tier 4 services in the Eastern Region*. YoungMinds Consultancy and Training, YoungMinds.

Weiner, A., Withers, K., Patrick, M., et al (1999) What changes are of value in severely disturbed children? *Clinical Child Psychology and Psychiatry*, **4**, 201–213.

Wilmshurst, L. (2002) Treatment programs for youth with emotional and behavioral disorders: an outcome study of two alternate approaches. *Mental Health Services Research*, **4**, 85–96.

Woolston, J. (1998) Intensive, integrated, in-home psychiatric services: the catalyst to enhancing out-patient intervention. *Child and Adolescent Psychiatric Clinics of North America*, **7**, 615–633.

Worrall-Davies, A. & Kiernan, K. (2005) *Using a Virtual Team: An Evaluation of the Bradford CAMHS Intensive Home Treatment Approach. Research Report*. University of Leeds (http://www.leeds.ac.uk/medicine/psychiatry/reports/Home%20Treatment%20Report%20Cover%20Final%202005.doc).

Zimet, S. G., Farley, G. K. & Zimet, G. D. (1994) Home behaviours of children in three treatment settings: an out-patient clinic, a day hospital, and an in-patient hospital. *Journal of the American Academy of Child and Adolescent Psychiatry*, **33**, 56–59.

CHAPTER 29

In-patient psychiatric care

Angela Sergeant, Greg Richardson, Ian Partridge,
Tim McDougall, Anne Worrall-Davies and Lesley Hewson

> "'It all comes", said Pooh crossly, "of not having front doors big enough.'"
> A. A. Milne, *Winnie the Pooh*

Introduction

Despite the development of home treatment teams and early intervention psychosis services, the demand for in-patient child and adolescent beds remains. It is rare for young people with mental disorders to require in-patient services, but when they do, beds are few and far between. Reasons for admission include severity of illness, deterioration in psychological functioning despite community treatment, high risk to self or others, or family difficulties making treatment difficult, any of which may lead to the need for 24-hour care (Green & Worrall-Davies, 2008). In-patient care is a specialised field providing treatment for young people with serious psychiatric illness by skilled and experienced staff.

Who and what are in-patient units for?

There is a range of psychiatric, educational, social, criminal and societal indicators for admission to an in-patient service. It is usually impossible to separate the different aspects or contributors to the young person's disorder so that each can be provided by the different agencies responsible for it. Psychological disorders, because of adverse life experiences, are common and pure psychiatric disorders are rare, but they all have educational and social precursors and sequelae. Trying to compartmentalise children into unidisciplinary treatment pigeonholes is problematic as:

- admission to psychiatric in-patient units considerably disrupts education and the young person's functioning in the community
- education authorities have to meet young people's special educational needs but cannot isolate these from other social and mental health factors, which they often do not have the resources to address
- residential policies of Social Services departments tend to address young people's mental health and educational needs only as secondary considerations

- the Home Office and Ministry of Justice, which will provide care in a prison setting, have little investment in childhood preventative work for the large proportion of young people with conduct disorder and complex needs when they become adults.

Work on sharing residential responsibility and input requires considerable inter-departmental and inter-agency working, but each agency will be uncertain who is going to reap the most for investing in them, and the harvest is not guaranteed. A lack of clarity about the purpose and function of in-patient units is not surprisingly problematic owing to:

- a lack of clarity on the criteria for admission
- being seen as the last resort rather than a source of expertise
- the difficulty of maintaining young people's locality links during and after the period of stay
- a lack of clarity about the respite role
- the problems over the continuing education of the young people
- difficulties of rapid access, especially in emergencies (Cotgrove *et al*, 2007)
- a lack of inter-agency agreements on the placement of children for whom they are responsible, when they no longer require in-patient psychiatric care
- uncertainty over whether the in-patient service should provide out-patient follow-up or outreach
- limited information on outcomes and effectiveness
- problems with the recruitment, training and retention of staff
- uncertainty over the transition of young people to adult services or more specialist services.

In-patient units depend on referrals from a wide catchment area and numerous referring teams, their responsiveness being usually variable depending on bed availability and the dynamic mix of the young people placed on the unit at the time. This can result in poor mutual understanding and frustration for those trying to access in-patient treatment, particularly in an emergency. Haphazard geographical spread and limited responsiveness can make in-patient facilities appear inefficient and ineffective.

Admission criteria

Although experts in the USA have reached a reasonable degree of agreement on which adolescents require residential care (Strauss *et al*, 1995), namely those with conduct disorder and a history of substance misuse, few British CAMHS professionals consider that such young people would benefit from psychiatric admission. In the UK, it is felt that children with psychiatric disorder are best treated within their family environment, and only severity of disorder, an associated level of risk that cannot safely be managed in the community and lack of responsiveness to community interventions should dictate in-patient care in a safely monitored environment being considered.

There is therefore a need for in-patient facilities for psychiatrically ill adolescents, which has as its indications for admission:

- psychotic disorders
- major depressive disorders
- eating disorders unresponsive to other treatment
- emotional disorders that are incapacitating
- psychosomatic disorders that threaten life or development.

Those admitted to adolescent psychiatric in-patient care have complex needs, often with comorbidity. The reason for admission is to provide around-the-clock care from trained nursing staff and a specialist multidisciplinary team. However, admission must operate within a system of comprehensive treatment that involves the local community teams to avoid long protracted lengths of stay and loss of contact with the young person's family and community. Children under 11 years very rarely require psychiatric admission, and such admission should not be used to deal with extreme aggressive behaviour, bearing in mind that children are further damaged by prolonged distant removal from their home and community. Those under 8 years should probably not be admitted without their family in view of the importance of attachments at younger ages. Alternatives to in-patient admission are discussed in Chapter 28.

Adequacy of in-patient provision

The World Health Organization recognises that there should be separate in-patient facilities for child and adolescent mental healthcare, as children and adolescents can experience fear and intimidation if they are treated alongside adults (World Health Organization, 2005). This has been confirmed in two reports from the Children's Commissioner for England, *Pushed into the Shadows* (Office of the Children's Commissioner, 2007) and *Out of the Shadow's* (YoungMinds, 2008). Standard 9 of the *National Service Framework for Children, Young People and Maternity Services* (Department of Health, 2004) sets the expectation that children and young people should receive care and treatment in services that are suited to their age and development, recognising that insufficient adolescent in-patient beds are being commissioned to meet need. For the majority of young people requiring in-patient psychiatric care this will and certainly should be in child or adolescent in-patient units, but there will be occasions when placement on an adult mental health ward is the safest or least restrictive option. The *National Service Framework for Mental Health* (Department of Health, 1999a) states that:

'if a bed in an adolescent unit cannot be located for a young person, but admission is essential for the safety and welfare of the user and others, then care may be provided on an adult ward for a short while. As a contingency measure, Trusts are asked to set standards for developmentally appropriate care. This should include identifying wards or settings that would be better suited to meet the needs of young people; agreeing protocols between CAMHS and adult mental health services; and putting in place procedures to safeguard a young person's safety, welfare and dignity.'

The duty to ensure age-appropriate accommodation for young people under 18 is part of the Mental Health Act 1983 (amended in 2007) and revised Code of Practice (Department of Health, 2008). To ensure adherence to the Act, placement of children aged under 16 years of age on adult psychiatric wards is not permissible. Commissioners and hospital managers will need to ensure that young people aged 16 and 17 are treated in age-appropriate accommodation by April 2010.

In 1999 in England, the National In-patient Child and Adolescent Psychiatric Study (O'Herlihy *et al*, 2003) identified 72 child and adolescent psychiatric in-patient units providing 844 beds, 73% being managed by the NHS and approximately 12.5% operating on a 5-day week. The average length of stay was 74 (s.d. = 60) days. In the years to 2006, there had been an increase of 19 units and 284 beds, 69% of the increase in beds being provided by the independent sector (O'Herlihy *et al*, 2007). Some units specialise in treating young offenders, young people with eating disorders, learning disability, and neuropsychiatric and psychosomatic disorders, but most deal with the full range of psychotic, emotional, psychosomatic and eating disorders at the severe end of the range. Bed provision varies from 9.1 to 44.2 beds per million population, with an average of 23 (O'Herlihy *et al*, 2007). London, where there is still considerable difficulty accessing beds, is at the top end of the range, and Yorkshire and Humber at the bottom, having experienced a reduction in beds since 1999. Needs assessment would indicate that there are likely to be higher incidences of serious psychiatric disorder in deprived inner-city areas, but still the bed requirements are so small that estimates are difficult. The Royal College of Psychiatrists (1999) has recommended that between 8 and 16 in-patient beds per million population are required for children, but such beds are currently reducing well below that target. For adolescents, they recommend that between 16 and 24 beds per million population will be required, and certain English regions are now reaching that level (O'Herlihy *et al*, 2007).

Integrating in-patient treatment into a continuum of care

In the UK, community working has replaced much in-patient care and this trend is echoed in the decline of residential child care and residential education. A period of in-patient care is just one part of the care pathway, which starts and ends with care by community CAMHS. Admission must always be preceded by the comprehensive assessment of young people as soon as they encounter CAMHS, in order to avoid the demand-led in-patient services of the USA (Bickman *et al*, 1996). Discharge planning should occur well before a young person is admitted to an in-patient unit so that the in-patient care becomes a part of the total care package and not an isolated, short-term problem-solving, disruptive event in the young person's life. However, this is not always possible, particularly in emergencies. Discharge planning requires agencies to take responsibility for smoothing the care pathway so that the in-patient work with the young person is undertaken in the context of family and local professional networks. More recently, some in-patient teams are moving away from the model of in-patient or separate day-care provision to a 'stepped care' model in which in-patient stay is kept to the minimum required, reducing the risk of dependency on residential treatment and minimising disruption to home and school environments. By offering day, in- or out-patient programmes more flexibly, a graded return to the young person's community is provided. This flexible arrangement also allows services to respond in an emergency if there is a necessity to work more intensively, and promotes a collaborative approach with young people and their families. This also allows services to tailor modalities of treatment for each individual, and is well placed to assess levels of risk and judge the necessity for the correct level of intensity of treatment. The CHYPIE study (Green *et al*, 2007) demonstrated the expense to families of their child being in an in-patient unit, so support and assistance for the families of young people resident in in-patient facilities, especially with regard to transport, should be considered.

In-patient services should provide: written documentation to the referring community CAMHS on the findings and agreements arising from the pre-admission assessment; a report on the initial assessment review after the initial period of in-patient care; regular (e.g. six-weekly) reports; the notes of all discharge planning meetings; and a discharge summary.

In-patient services should take care not to disempower locality CAMHS by automatically offering follow-up care of in-patients and taking over the community and out-patient care of patients referred to them, unless this is clearly negotiated with the referring service. Equally, community CAMHS must recognise that in-patient care is part of a pathway of care, which begins and ends with them. Worryingly, Green *et al* (2007) demonstrated that at follow-up, a quarter of young people had not received any of the services recommended at discharge, and only 10% received the full discharge package. It may not be surprising that some young people relapse following discharge (Green *et al*, 2001). Discharge planning and aftercare based on the principles of the care programme approach are vital in helping to prevent relapse.

Consideration may be given to the appointment of in-patient link workers to community CAMHS, which develop close relationships with in-patient staff and help young people and their families in the transition to and from in-patient facilities. They might also be involved in the provision of therapeutic interventions (e.g. family therapy) with the young people for whom they are responsible at the in-patient unit.

Effectiveness of in-patient provision

Evidence is appearing that in-patient services are effective (Pfeiffer & Strzelecki, 1990; Blantz & Schmidt, 2000; Green *et al*, 2007) in terms of the outcomes arising from admission, with clinical improvement across a range of domains. The average cost of admission in the CHYPIE study (Green *et al*, 2007) was £24000 for 116 days, with an associated average cost to the family of £1180. There is, however, a lack of quality data that compare one model of in-patient care with another or the benefits of specialised, disorder-specific care *v*. generic adolescent in-patient services (York & Lamb, 2006). The use of routine outcome measures such as Health of the Nation Outcome Scales Child and Adolescent (HoNOSCA; Gowers *et al*, 1999), the Children's Global Assessment Scale (CGAS; Shaffer *et al*, 1983) or the Paddington Complexity Scale (Yates *et al*, 1999), as well as questionnaires specific to particular disorders, is increasingly required as good practice within in-patient services. Each in-patient service should have developed evidence-based protocols for the management of conditions that cause young people to be admitted to that service, which with robust admission and discharge policies should ensure as effective use as possible within the limits of current knowledge.

Organisation

The poor availability of adolescent in-patient provision has frequently led to young people being admitted to adult psychiatric beds, a practice that must now cease for those under 16. To work effectively, each in-patient service should:

- have a designated catchment area commensurate with its bed capacity
- a comprehensive operational policy
- a desirable bed occupancy rate of 80–85%
- operate for 7 days a week, 52 weeks a year, as the severity of disorder and level of dependence these young people experience when they are acutely ill is such that it is not safe to place them elsewhere at weekends.

How practical it will be to allow the preservation of beds in each unit for emergency admissions is uncertain (Cotgrove *et al*, 2007). However, psychiatric emergencies in young people are rare, so such young people should be thoroughly assessed locally by child mental health professionals as suffering from a psychiatric disorder before a referral is made. The only real psychiatric emergency is acute-onset psychosis. Young people cachectic from an eating disorder may best be cared for on a paediatric or medical ward in order to ensure their metabolic stability before being transferred to an in-patient facility, which should be achievable with some rapidity. In these cases, the period while the young person is on the medical ward gives the family time to become acquainted with an in-patient facility and its staff, and to decide whether they consider transfer to be helpful. Self-harm may provide a high-risk situation, but comprehensive community assessment and management should precede admission (which can often be unhelpful for young people who self-harm) and the young person and family or carers should be given ample opportunities to visit, talk about and discover the pros and cons of in-patient admission.

Substance misuse is increasingly common among young people and cannot be used as a reason for the exclusion of a young person from an in-patient service if their mental state justifies admission.

In-patient units of fewer than 10 or 12 beds become very expensive per bed because it is not possible to have proportionately fewer staff. For example, there will always need to be at least two staff on at night and three throughout the day, whether there are four or ten young people on the unit.

Whatever the local provision, there may still need to be an occasional very specialist placement for forensic or neuropsychiatric purposes, or when local services have not been able to manage the young person's illness successfully.

Each unit should then be able to respond to all requests for admissions in the following circumstances.

- The young person is suffering from a psychiatric disorder.
- The young person has been assessed by a senior CAMHS professional who is requesting the referral. This should ensure that the young person has been fully assessed as requiring psychiatric in-patient assessment, treatment or management, and that such assessment, treatment or management is not possible in the community.
- The young person meets the overt admission criteria of the in-patient unit.
- The unit has a contractual commitment to the relevant commissioning authority or primary care organisation, the commissioning authority having agreed how many in-patient psychiatric beds it requires for the young people for whom it is responsible. Such contracts are the only way the provision of in-patient services can be guaranteed.
- The place to where the young person will be discharged is clear. Discharge planning is an integral part of in-patient care: it is the vehicle that ensures the period of in-patient care is as short as possible, and is part of an integrated package of care. Community CAMHS, as well as local education and Social Services, must therefore give high priority to discharge planning meetings and Section 117 meetings held by the in-patient facilities. The care programme approach (Department of Health, 1999b) provides a useful model for this, which should be used with all young people hospitalised in a psychiatric ward.
- The local CAMHS has made a commitment to attend reviews and discharge planning meetings held on the young person at the in-patient facility.

- The problems of interface between the adolescent and adult services and the need for adolescent and adult psychiatrists to work together in providing transitional services for 16- to 19-year-olds so that provision from either service is most suited to their needs has been addressed.

In order to ensure these criteria are met, once the decision to assess a young person for in-patient treatment has been made, a comprehensive pre-admission assessment should be undertaken to allow the patient and family to make an informed decision about admission, and the service to determine whether it can be helpful to the young person. However, same-day admission is important for service users, referrers and commissioners (Street, 2004) when opportunities to complete a full pre-admission assessment are limited. Despite the need for crisis services, the majority of in-patient units do not offer same-day admission (O'Herlihy *et al*, 2003; Cotgrove *et al*, 2007).

Unique to in-patient units is the 'therapeutic milieu' that provides the foundation for the provision of care. This milieu creates a supportive and nurturing interpersonal environment that teaches, role models and reinforces constructive interaction. It should include a daily programme that is structured by well-defined service components with specific activities being performed by identified staff. Within the daily programme, the staff will be encouraging daily living skills, overseeing delivery of specific psychological treatments, dispensing medication, observing socialisation and the dynamics between young people and staff, as well as managing contact with families.

Unit programmes usually allow for community/business meetings that occur once a day to clarify the structure of each young person's day (i.e. school/therapies). In addition, there may be evening or weekly meetings to address issues pertinent to the continuity and effectiveness of the treatment milieu, as well as group work alongside education and components that occur outside the therapeutic milieu (e.g. family therapy, psychological individual work such as CBT).

Throughout admission on a weekly basis, consideration should be given to the length of stay. Regular (at least six-weekly) care programme approach meetings should be held with the referring teams, and if delays to discharge relating to accommodation or transition to adult services are experienced, they must be addressed and commissioners informed of the reasons for the prolonged stay. Prior to discharge, the final care programme approach meeting should ensure that the young person has an identified care coordinator to monitor their progress and provide a smooth transition back into the community. At this meeting, factors affecting prognosis and relapse prevention plans must be fully considered and documented, with the families central to this discussion. There is a risk of relapse following discharge from in-patient care, as the intensity of care is reduced and as the family readjust to living together again. This may be minimised if the unit operates a stepped care model and if there is negotiated, comprehensive community involvement.

In-patient pathway of care

The acceptance of a referral to an in-patient unit will depend on a discussion between the in-patient staff and the referring community CAMHS staff. Once such a referral is accepted an initial assessment meeting is arranged. This pre-admission assessment is an opportunity for the young person and their family to meet two or three representatives of the in-patient team and discuss with them the reasons that admission is being considered, their expectations of the admission, the likely treatment plan and to discuss whether all are agreed that the admission should take place. The family is able to familiarise themselves with the in-patient facility and is a partner in determining the necessity for and purposes of the admission. This pre-admission assessment should include a current risk assessment, childhood history, assessment of mental state and interventions already tried. There should be a clear discussion on the risks and benefits of in-patient treatment and an opportunity to discuss alternatives to such treatment. It must be emphasised that in-patient treatment is only part of the pathway of care from and to community care.

If it is agreed that in-patient intervention is required then clear aims for the admission need to be agreed with the family and referring agency. Planning for discharge should ensure involving the referring team, establishing the nature of ongoing involvement following discharge and exploring the possibility of joint therapeutic interventions. Prior to admission, families should receive written information and an explanation of why in-patient treatment is recommended, what are the benefits and risks associated with it, and what alternative treatments are available. In-patient teams must have clear aims to avoid 'therapeutic perfectionism', trying to resolve all the presenting problems that are evident on admission or emerge thereafter. It is often the case that young people and their families may have long-standing difficulties and therefore treatment aims need to be realistic and achievable.

Prior to admission, professionals need to consider the young person's capacity to consent to treatment, as a competent adolescent of 16 or 17 can no longer have their refusal of consent overridden by their parents, and refusal of consent needs to be taken seriously in competent younger adolescents. Staff need to be competent to assess such matters and be aware of the legal frameworks in which they are operating (see Chapter 3).

On admission, risk assessment will dictate observation levels operated by staff. Staff will begin to establish a therapeutic relationship, both with the young person and with their family or carers, encouraging autonomy and a collaborative approach. As well as having a nominated care coordinator, key worker or named nurse, young people should be allocated to a core team of multidisciplinary staff who will be responsible for coordinating the treatment plans and will work closely with the young person and their family. They will also have an allocated consultant psychiatrist who is medically responsible for them.

Families should be advised of what the goals of treatment will entail and the timescales expected to achieve these discussed. They will be given a clear explanation of the roles of the core team and information on lines of communication, and how progress will be monitored. This core team will be the focus for communication with the family and referring teams. Regular care programme approach reviews must be held at a minimum of six-weekly intervals with the families and referring teams to keep the momentum of working towards transition back to the community.

Families should also receive support in their own right in groups such as parents' support groups and advice/helplines, and be actively involved in the treatment offered by means of regular review meetings, family discussion and family therapy.

Each young person will have an individualised treatment plan based on the patient's perceived difficulties in biological, psychological and social functioning, in the development of which they are actively involved. This may be embedded into clinical practice by their involvement in 'core team meetings' attendance at clinical reviews, collaborative care planning, written feedback from the young person prior to treatment reviews, or feedback on weekend leave. A psychoeducational component enables the young person and their families to have a richer understanding of the evidence base for their treatment and their prognosis. They will need to understand triggers of potential relapse and support systems that will be available after discharge.

Staffing

The in-patient unit must be managed by an adequately staffed, multidisciplinary team (Royal College of Psychiatrists, 1999) who regularly review progress and provide multidisciplinary leadership and interventions. All staff must have clear lines of accountability and access to regular supervision, both managerial and clinical. In addition, all staff should be subject to annual individual performance reviews that will highlight professional training requirements. This should be part of the unit's annual review of knowledge and skills audit, to inform the next year's training plan. In-patient services need to be adequately resourced to offer safe, evidence-based treatments embedded into clinical practice.

Within in-patient CAMHS, effectiveness is largely dependent upon the work of the in-patient nursing team, both qualified and unqualified. They provide the day-to-day care, create the therapeutic milieu and provide all the background information that contributes to the 24-hour assessment and treatment of young people. For most services, the registered mental health nurse qualification is often the primary requirement, but registered sick children's nurses or double-qualified nurses are valuable, particularly in light of the paediatric-oriented presentation and needs of some young people. The Allitt Inquiry (Department of Health, 1994) recommended staff have a specialist qualification in children's nursing or specialist training in child and adolescent mental health. A key worker or primary nurse system should be in place to ensure that there is one member of staff who takes responsibility for the planning of the day-to-day care of the young person and who ensures that this is integrated with the treatment plan. The key worker is then the focus for communication by the young person, the family, the involved community professionals and other members of the in-patient team. The young person and family should always be informed who is standing in as key worker when the key worker is off duty.

Senior staff and culture carriers within the milieu should hold specialist experience within CAMHS. Qualities looked for in professionals by colleagues and service users within CAMHS are intuitive, warm-hearted and caring, with personal stability, a capacity to tolerate anxiety, and a sense of humour and playfulness (Brown *et al*, 1974). In addition to these qualities, the modern milieu demands a strong sense of resilience and an ability to remain professional in the face of adversity. They must also take responsibility for ensuring systemic discussion about the functioning of the service.

In-patient care requires highly skilled staff who are competent in the management of crisis situations and can contain potentially conflicting dynamics within the therapeutic milieu. There need to be adequate staffing levels not only to maintain a safe environment but to allow the young people the intensity of involvement that is expected within an in-patient service. When working with adolescents, the interactional style of communication differs from the style used within child or adult mental health settings. Adolescents often get easily bored, impatient or distracted, therefore the therapeutic relationship needs to be creative and dynamic. This will require staff to be spontaneous, flexible and opportunistic.

Staff must be trained adequately to deal with high-risk situations and in dealing with the conflicts that may arise within the clinical setting. Nurses should be trained in control and restraint techniques, and there should be protocols for rapid tranquillisation if required. They must be competent in clinical decision-making that is able to adapt to the rapid fluctuations in need between or even within shifts. Risk assessment is a vital requirement of in-patient services and staff need to be competent in managing risk. Staff must be able to cope with young people detained under the Mental Health Act and therefore be trained and have up-to-date knowledge of the Act.

The multidisciplinary team must meet regularly (probably weekly as a minimum) to discuss the progress of in-patients, and at a separate meeting discuss policy and operational issues.

All units must have robust clinical governance systems in place, constantly improving the standard of clinical practice and ensuring continuous improvement of service delivery. The senior clinical team should meet at least monthly to review service effectiveness and clinical governance. The Quality Network for In-patient CAMHS (2006) is a peer-review process that monitors standards across several aspects of in-patient functioning:

- environment and facilities
- staffing and training
- access, admission and discharge
- care and treatment
- information, consent and confidentiality
- rights, safeguards and child protection
- audit and policy
- location in a public health context.

After each peer review, QNIC produces individual service reports and publishes an annual report that brings together key themes facing all in-patient services.

Clinical supervision and reflection on practice presents crucial opportunities for professionals to explore the valuable elements of clinical practice promoting professional development through learning action plans. The problem of professional isolation in in-patient units has to be addressed by ensuring that these professionals work closely with community CAMHS so that they understand their work and circumstances.

An agenda for the future

1 Standardisation of the age ranges accepted by in-patient units in order that referrers and commissioners can have a clearer understanding of the function and capacity of their local units.

2 The admission criteria for general in-patient units need to be standardised so they can be understood by health professionals and by other agencies. Only then will unrealistic expectations be recognised and appropriate young people be referred for effective treatment.

3 In-patient units should develop strategies to meet the standards now being recognised nationally (Quality Network for In-patient CAMHS, 2006).

4 The establishment of permanent, finance-backed agreements that ensure guaranteed beds (when required) to those who have made a financial commitment to the existence of the in-patient unit. Such agreements should also ensure that commissioners influence service provision and standards. With such an agreement, the referring community service can develop relationships with the in-patient team over time, so improving transition for patients and families between community and in-patient care. From the providers' point of view, the viability of the unit is assured and they develop links with the community staff with whom they have an agreement.

5 Psychiatric illness meeting the criteria for admission detailed earlier is rare in prepubertal children. None the less, for such patients there may need to be a facility for family admissions. There are probably more contraindications than indications for the psychiatric admission of children under the age of 8 without a parent.

6   Specialist training of nurses in child and adolescent mental health is required to ensure that young people on in-patient units are cared for by staff who understand their illness in the context of their development and environment.

References

Bickman, L., Foster, E. M. & Lambert, E. W. (1996) Who gets hospitalised in a continuum of care? *Journal of the American Academy of Child and Adolescent Psychiatry*, **35**, 74–80.

Blantz, B. & Schmidt, M. (2000) Practitioner review: preconditions and outcome of inpatient treatment in child and adolescent psychiatry. *Journal of Child Psychology and Psychiatry*, **41**, 703–712.

Brown, S., Kolvin, I., Scott, D., *et al* (1974) The child psychiatric nurse: training for residential care. In *The Residential Psychiatric Treatment of Children* (ed. P. Barker). Granada.

Cotgrove, A., McLoughlin, R., O'Herlihy, A., *et al* (2007) The ability of adolescent psychiatric units to accept emergency admissions: changes in England and Wales between 2000 and 2005. *Psychiatric Bulletin*, **31**, 457–459.

Department of Health (1994) *The Allitt Inquiry: Independent Inquiry Relating to Deaths and Injuries on the Children's Ward at Grantham and Kesteven General Hospital during the Period February to April 1991.* HMSO.

Department of Health (1999a) *National Service Framework for Mental Health.* Department of Health.

Department of Health (1999b) *Effective Care Co-ordination in Mental Health Services: Modernising the Care Programme Approach.* Department of Health (http://www.dh.gov.uk/en/Publicationsandstatistics/Publications/PublicationsPolicyAndGuidance/DH_4009221).

Department of Health (2004) *National Service Framework for Children, Young People and Maternity Services.* TSO (The Stationery Office).

Department of Health (2008) *Mental Health Act 1983: Revised Code of Practice. Summary of Changes from Current Code.* TSO (The Stationery Office) (http://www.dh.gov.uk/prod_consum_dh/groups/dh_digitalassets/@dh/@en/documents/digitalasset/dh_084595.pdf).

Gowers, S. G., Harrington, R. C., Whitton, A., *et al* (1999) Brief scale for measuring the outcomes of emotional and behavioural disorders in children. Health of the Nation Outcome Scales for Children and Adolescents (HoNOSCA). *British Journal of Psychiatry*, **174**, 413–416.

Green, J. & Worrall-Davies, A. (2008) Provision of intensive treatment: in-patient units, day units and intensive outreach. In *Rutter's Child and Adolescent Psychiatry, Fifth Edition* (eds M. Rutter, D. Bishop, D. Pine, *et al*), pp. 1126–1142. Blackwell.

Green, J., Kroll, L., Imrie, D., *et al* (2001) Health gain and predictors of outcome in inpatient and related day patient child and adolescent psychiatry treatment. *Journal of the American Academy of Child and Adolescent Psychiatry*, **40**, 325–332.

Green, J., Jacobs, B., Beecham, J., *et al* (2007) In-patient treatment in child and adolescent psychiatry – a prospective study of health gain and costs. *Journal of Child Psychology and Psychiatry*, **48**, 1259–1267.

O'Herlihy, A., Worrall, A., Lelliott, P., *et al* (2003) Distribution and characteristics of in-patient child and adolescent mental health services in England and Wales. *British Journal of Psychiatry*, **183**, 547–551.

O'Herlihy, A., Lelliott, P., Bannister, D., *et al* (2007) Provision of child and adolescent mental health in-patient services in England between 1999 and 2006. *Psychiatric Bulletin*, **31**, 454–456.

Office of the Children's Commissioner (2007) *Pushed into the Shadows: Young People's Experience of Adult Mental Health Facilities.* 11 Million.

Pfeiffer, S. & Strzelecki, S. (1990) Inpatient psychiatric treatment of children and adolescents: a review of outcome studies. *Journal of the American Academy of Child and Adolescent Psychiatry*, **29**, 847–853.

Quality Network for In-Patient CAMHS (2006) *QNIC – Quality Network for Inpatient CAMHS: Service Standards*. Royal College of Psychiatrists.

Royal College of Psychiatrists (1999) *Guidance on Staffing of Child and Adolescent In-patient Psychiatry Units. Council Report CR76*. Royal College of Psychiatrists.

Shaffer, D., Gould, M. S., Brasic, J., *et al* (1983) A Children's Global Assessment Scale (CGAS). *Archives of General Psychiatry*, **40**, 1228–1231.

Strauss, G., Chassin, M. & Lock, J. (1995) Can experts agree when to hospitalize adolescents? *Journal of the American Academy of Child and Adolescent Psychiatry*, **34**, 418–424.

Street, C. (2004) In-patient mental health services for young people: changing to meet new needs? *Journal of the Royal Society for the Promotion of Health*, **124**, 115–118.

World Health Organization (2005) *Child and Adolescent Mental Health Policies and Plans*. WHO.

Yates, P., Garralda, M. E. & Higginson, I. (1999) Paddington Complexity Scale and Health of the Nation Outcome Scales for Children and Adolescents. *British Journal of Psychiatry*, **174**, 417–423.

York, A. & Lamb, C. (2006) *Building and Sustaining Specialist Child and Adolescent Mental Health Services. Council Report CR137*. Royal College of Psychiatrists.

YoungMinds (2008) *Out of the Shadows? A Review of Responses to Recommendations Made in Pushed into the Shadows: Young People's Experiences of Adult Mental Health Facilities*. 11 Million.

CHAPTER 30

Forensic services

Sue Bailey and Enys Delmage

'Only connect.'
> Edward Morgan Forster (1879–1970)

Introduction

Young people at the interface of the criminal justice system and mental health services face social exclusion, alienation and stigmatisation (Bailey, 1999). The definition of this group varies across and within agencies; their needs are diverse and require a range of mental health services that can be effective only if integrated with the services of other agencies.

Young people account for almost a quarter of all persons arrested in a single year (Home Office, 2007). The psychosocial and biological factors placing young people at risk of both offending and mental health problems are well established (Junger-Tas *et al*, 1994; Kazdin, 1995; Rutter & Smith, 1995; Shepherd & Farrington, 1996; Rutter *et al*, 1998; Rutter, 1999).

Definitions

Forensic mental health has been defined as an area of specialisation that involves the assessment and treatment of those who are both mentally disordered and whose behaviour has led or could lead to offending (Mullen, 2000). Defining forensic psychiatry in terms of the assessment and treatment of the mentally disordered offender delineates an area of concern that could engulf much of mental health.

Offending behaviour is common in the whole community and among adolescents it is approaching the universal, with just under 40% of all known offenders being under the age of 21, and 24% of all offenders being aged 10–17 (Home Office, 2007). Males are more likely to have committed an offence, with 30% of males saying they had committed an offence in the past year (Home Office, 2006).

Antisocial behaviour is also prevalent with 23% of all young people having committed at least one act of antisocial behaviour in the previous year (Home Office, 2006). In practice, patients often gravitate to forensic services when the nature of their offending or the anxiety and apprehension created by their behaviour is such as to overwhelm the tolerance or confidence of professionals in the general mental health services.

In part, these cases are also driven by the emerging culture of blame, in which professionals fear being held responsible for failing to protect their fellow citizens from the violent behaviour of those who have been in their care. Mullen (2000) stresses that mental health expertise should address the mental health component of social problems, and highlights the importance of rigorous risk assessments and management. There is a significant overlap between the risk factors for offending, poor mental health and substance misuse. The number of assessed risk factors increases as a young person moves further into the youth justice system (Youth Justice Board, 2005*a*).

Background

In England and Wales in particular, during the past 20 years there have been major changes in legislation that were meant to bring about an improvement in services to children. The Children Act 1989 reformed the law, and brought public and private law under one statutory system, and the Children Act 2004 (Chapter 31) created the post of the Children's Commissioner, who has access to young offenders' institutes to review the conditions within, and encourages safeguarding and promotion of welfare of young offenders.

Section 37 of the Crime and Disorder Act 1998 lays the statutory duty on services, including health, education, the police, probation and Local Authority Social Services, to prevent crime through effective inter-agency practice and appropriate forms of intervention. The Criminal Justice Act 2003 (Part 12) brought about tougher penalties for crime, including the controversial sentence of Imprisonment for Public Protection (or Detention for Public Protection in those under 18).

We await with interest the effects of the new Criminal Justice Bill 2007, which describes youth rehabilitation orders, extension to referral orders, youth conditional cautions for 16- and 17-year-olds, violent offender orders, antisocial behaviour measures and youth default orders. Certainly, remedies for high youth-offending rates are on the government agenda, with papers such as the Green Paper *Youth Matters* (HM Government, 2005) putting heavy emphasis on managing this group of young people in need.

Surveys of young people at different points in the criminal justice system, both in the UK and in the USA, show consistently high rates of psychiatric disorder, although rates vary widely by study, ranging from 50 to 100% (Atkins *et al* 1999; Shelton 2001; McCabe *et al* 2002; Teplin *et al* 2002; Vermeiren *et al* 2002; Wasserman *et al* 2002; Gosden *et al* 2003; Ruchkin *et al* 2003; Dixon *et al* 2004; Lederman *et al* 2004; Vreugdenhil *et al* 2004).

Despite some positive policy moves in the UK (Harding, 1999), a large number of young offenders still end up remanded or sentenced to custody, and this is illustrated by the rising number of young people and children who now find themselves in the new secure state provision. This includes an average of 2900 young people incarcerated at any one time in Local

Authority secure children's homes, young offender institutions, secure psychiatric units and secure training centres (Youth Justice Board, 2007). Detention for Public Protection sentences (Criminal Justice Act 2003) will almost certainly increase the number of young people in young offenders' institutions.

When young people become involved in the detention justice system, the focus on their offending behaviour tends to take precedence over developmental and mental health issues. The young offender with a mental health problem tends to fall into the gap between the organisational boundaries of different agencies such as Social Services, youth offending teams, educational provision and CAMHS. Some young offenders are not engaged in mainstream education and health services.

It is critical that these young people are supported to access the mainstream and specialist services they require while under the supervision of the youth offending team or in custody. Otherwise, once their service ends, they can and do become detached from services, their overall circumstances deteriorate, leading to both risk of more offending and great demands on specialist services as they become older.

The multidisciplinary youth offending teams established by the Crime and Disorder Act 1998 have aided the coordination and cooperation for offenders under 18 years, and are subject to Home Office reviews (youth offending team inspections) to help improve the services provided and aid multidisciplinary working. However, such cooperation can be effective only if there are resources within CAMHS and professionals trained and willing to do the job.

Problem profiles

The assessment of a young person whose mental health is called into question is the responsibility of the locality CAMHS. It should be the first port of call for those dealing with young offenders such as social workers or youth offending teams. Such work will require prioritising and resource allocation. Bailey & Kerslake (2008) stress the need for CAMHS to offer an integrated assessment with other agencies.

The aim is to work with young children with antisocial behaviour in a family context using parent management training strategies combined with individual interventions for the young person, which take into account subtyping of conduct disorder based on age at onset.

The long-term follow-up studies of young people in secure care appear to demonstrate five routes into offending (Bullock et al, 1998):

- young people in long-term care
- young people requiring prolonged special education
- young people whose behaviour suddenly deteriorated in adolescence
- one-off grave offenders
- serious and persistent offenders.

Broad and overlapping sets of problems associated with offending have been identified and will need to be addressed concurrently. Rutter *et al* (1998) stress the heterogeneity of antisocial behaviour in terms of the pervasiveness, persistence, severity and patterns of such behaviour. Comorbid factors with youth offending include the following:

- Attention-deficit hyperactivity disorder.
- Early onset of antisocial behaviour, which includes aggressive, violent, disruptive behaviour, coercive sexual activity, arson, and fluctuations in mood state and levels of social interaction.
- Sexual offences.
- Juvenile homicide.
- Drug use and misuse, which have increased rapidly over the past 10 years (the most recent British Crime Survey (Home Office, 2007) shows that the highest rates of drug use occur in the 20- to 24-year-old age group for males, and the 16- to 19-year-old age group in females).
- Repetitive high-risk behaviours such as female adolescents presenting with serious suicide attempts and self-mutilation interspersed with externalising destructive behaviours – such young people raise grave anxieties within existing service provision, but even here violent behaviour in girls is underestimated, partly owing to the non-specific and insensitive diagnostic criteria for conduct disorders in girls (Jasper *et al*, 1998).
- Sexual and physical abuse in the previous lives of offending boys who also go on to self-harm.
- Mental illness, which may have a lead-in period of 1–7 years to early-onset psychosis, during which time there is a marked variation in the degree of non-psychotic behaviour and disturbance (the importance of the accurate assessment of young offenders who show multiple high-risk episodes associated with a fluctuating mental state needs to be more fully recognised).
- Learning disability – in a recent study of 301 young offenders, Chitsabesan *et al* (2007) found that 20% of young offenders met the criteria for mental retardation (IQ <70) and 41% had a below average IQ (IQ 70–84).

Situations of particular vulnerability and risk are homelessness and penal remand detention. Interconnections between homelessness, mental disorders, substance misuse and offending are complex and remain poorly understood (Sleegers *et al*, 1998; Rumball & Crome, 2004).

The risk in adult life for both girls and boys is the development of personality disorder, particularly for young people who have been victims themselves with unaddressed PTSD. The full range of psychological therapies should be available to those vulnerable adolescents, particularly those leaving care and at risk of custody. Multisystemic therapy, with family- and community-based interventions, can be effective in terms of improved clinical outcomes and cost savings (Henggeler *et al*, 1999).

287

Addressing the problem

Young offenders require the following.

- A strategic approach to commissioning and delivering services for them (this approach must develop effective and predictable services that meet their current and future needs, build upon established concepts of service, and ensure that workforce planning issues are addressed and met by longer-term training).
- A better understanding of young offenders' needs across all involved agencies, which must also develop local inter-agency strategies, such as flexible working in court diversion schemes with innovative partnerships with the voluntary sector.
- Access to primary healthcare.
- Speedy access to CAMHS, as their needs are unlikely to be met by adult mental health services.
- An overcoming of the reluctance to accept them into services, despite the fear of stigmatising the young people.
- Speedy access to drug and alcohol education and treatment centres (intensive forms of intervention for drug users with complex care needs would involve specialist residential services and mental health teams closely linked to CAMHS and forensic services).
- Speedy access to HIV testing.
- Improved inter-agency training of non-health professionals in identifying the indicators of mental vulnerability in young people, thus strengthening the communications with professionals in the mental health services.
- Recognition that adolescents with intellectual disability will have a slower pace of developing coping strategies and changing, which must always be balanced against their risk to others.
- Awareness by all agencies of gaps in the capacity of existing services.
- The establishment, on a regional basis, of adolescent forensic mental health teams (Box 30.1).

There is also a need for social regimes that help to promote the health of young people in prison. Girls and young people from ethnic minority groups are recognised to be particularly vulnerable to aversive prison regimes. The Youth Justice Board (2005b) have now commissioned four units for young women to provide specialist services for this group.

There is a drive for the specialist assessment, management and treatment of adolescents who display the criminal behaviours of interpersonal violence, arson and sexual offences. The focus should be on developmental issues, in contrast to the past tendency to apply adult treatment models to young people (Vizard & Usiskin, 1999).

Young people should be referred to a specialist forensic service only if they have been assessed locally to require such resources. Local multi-agency interventions must take priority.

> Box 30.1 Purposes and aims of an adolescent forensic mental health team
>
> - Improved outreach services
> - The extension of court psychiatric schemes and pre-court diversion to youth courts
> - The development of programmes for young people before they reach the courts and custody including adolescent in-patient services and access to secure forensic facilities, and liaison with local youth offending teams
> - Post-custodial rehabilitation and support for young offenders
> - A shared approach to risk assessment and management together with agreed protocols for better information exchange between the health service and criminal justice agencies
> - An awareness of professional practice and service developments and research

Interventions via liaison with local youth offending teams can prove efficacious, and many CAMHS now offer regular mental health input to these agencies – many have developed screening tools to detect mental health difficulties and which allow earlier intervention.

Progress and solutions

Ways to develop services have been described from assessments of need, commissioning exercises and clinical experience (Bailey & Farnworth, 1998; Kurtz *et al*, 1998; Audit Commission, 1999; Knapp & Henderson, 1999).

For those with the most complex mental health needs, a review of the adolescent forensic service at Salford's Prestwich Hospital (NHS Health Advisory Service *et al*, 1994) concluded that the greatest immediate need was for an increase in secure NHS-funded provision for:

- mentally disordered offenders
- sex offenders and abusers
- adolescents at severe risk of suicide and self-harm
- very severely mentally ill adolescents
- adolescents who need to begin psychiatric rehabilitation in secure circumstances
- brain-injured adolescents and those with severe organic disorders.

A framework for services

A strategic framework for youth offender mental health services would be a four-tier model in which local generic and regional specialist services allow for the multidimensional problems encountered by these young people to be tackled by local CAMHS in conjunction with other agencies. The four tiers would comprise the following.

1   Local CAMHS provision for young offenders, while ensuring resources for the rest of the locality CAMHS are not depleted by this work.
2   Local CAMHS augmented by advice and training offered by a peripatetic outreach team that is based in and works from specialised centres of expertise in forensic child and adolescent mental health. These patients are highly mobile, as their families frequently move from one Local Authority to another and their residential placements often change. Funding and services must follow the child and not be obstructed by agency and geographical boundaries to ensure continuity of care.
3   Peripatetic specialised forensic services in which the young people are seen directly by members of an outreach service from a specialised centre of expertise, sharing responsibility with the locality CAMHS. Such a forensic service may work directly with young offenders or provide advice and supervision to the CAMHS service.
4   Tier 4 centres of specialist forensic expertise, which deliver services directly to patients and their families. This may involve open units, high-dependency units and intensive assessment and care units, with security between medium and high, and considerable emphasis being placed on staff training and the dissemination of expertise.

Such a strategic framework is ambitious and requires:

- staff wanting to work in this area
- comprehensive training systems
- evidence-based interventions
- an international forensic child and adolescent mental health research and development network, which has now been established (www. europe.efcap.org/), to ensure that what is learnt from research is put into practice.

Since April 2000, there has been central commissioning (by the National Commissioning Group) for developed and developing adolescent forensic secure psychiatric in-patient units in England, with a strengthening of an adolescent forensic practitioner network. The Royal College of Psychiatrists now has its own Adolescent Forensic Psychiatry Special Interest Group (since November 2002), providing further support for practitioners in this field.

Conclusion

The government strategy for modernising mental health services (Department of Health, 1998) put forward a health strategy with risk assessment and public protection as top priorities. Child and adolescent mental health professionals have traditionally been involved at the interface between the law and the welfare of children, but historically this has often been via the need for their professional opinion on children in the childcare system rather than in forensic matters.

Child and adolescent mental health services are important in helping professionals in other agencies to recognise developmental and interactional influences on offending behaviour, and it is often the case that input from CAMHS is greatly sought after by services such as youth offending teams and other diversionary or early intervention services. Close liaison with other mental health teams is also vital, including general adult, forensic and addictions psychiatrists.

References

Atkins, D., Pumariega, A. J., Rogers, K., *et al* (1999) Mental health and incarcerated youth. I: Prevalence and nature of psychopathology. *Journal of Child and Family Studies*, **8**, 193–204.

Audit Commission (1999) *Children in Mind: Child and Adolescent Mental Health Services.* Audit Commission.

Bailey, S. (1999) Young people, mental illness and stigmatisation. *Psychiatric Bulletin*, **23**, 107–110.

Bailey, S. & Farnworth, P. (1998) Forensic mental health services. *Young Minds*, **34**, 12–13.

Bailey, S. & Kerslake, B. (2008) The process and systems for juveniles and young persons. In *Handbook of Forensic Mental Health* (eds K. Soothill, P. Rogers & M. Dolan), pp. 89–123. Willan Publishing.

Bullock, R., Little, M. & Millham, S. (1998) *Secure Treatment Outcomes: The Care Careers of Very Difficult Adolescents.* Ashgate Publishing.

Chitsabesan, P., Bailey, S., Williams, R., *et al* (2007) Learning disabilities and educational needs of juvenile offenders. *Children's Services*, **2**, 4–16.

Department of Health (1998) *Modernising Mental Health Services. Safe, Sound and Supportive.* TSO (The Stationery Office).

Dixon, A., Howie, P., & Starling, J. (2004) Psychopathology in female juvenile offenders. *Journal of Child Psychology and Psychiatry*, **45**, 1150–1158.

Gosden, N. P., Kramp, P., Gabrielsen, G., *et al* (2003) Prevalence of mental disorders among 15-17-year-old male adolescent remand prisoners in Denmark. *Acta Psychiatrica Scandinavica*, **107**, 102–110.

Harding, R. (1999) Prison privatisation: the debate starts to mature. *Current Issues in Criminal Justice*, **11**, 109–118.

Henggeler, S. W., Rowland, M. D., Randall, J., *et al* (1999) Home-based multisystemic therapy as an alternative to the hospitalization of youths in psychiatric crisis: clinical outcomes. *Journal of the American Academy of Child and Adolescent Psychiatry*, **38**, 1331–1339.

HM Government (2005) *Youth Matters.* TSO (The Stationery Office).

Home Office (2006) *Young People and Crime: Findings from the 2005 Offending, Crime and Justice Survey.* TSO (The Stationery Office).

Home Office (2007) *Crime in England and Wales 2006/07.* TSO (The Stationery Office).

Jasper, A., Smith, C. & Bailey, S. (1998) One hundred girls in care referred to an adolescent forensic mental health service. *Journal of Adolescence*, **21**, 555–568.

Junger-Tas, J., Terlouw, G. & Klein, M. (1994) *Delinquent Behaviour Among Young People in the Western World.* Kugler.

Kazdin, A. E. (1995) *Conduct Disorder in Childhood and Adolescence (2nd edn).* Sage.

Knapp, M. & Henderson, J. (1999) Health economics perspectives and evaluation of child and adolescent mental health services. *Current Opinion in Psychiatry*, **12**, 393–397.

Kurtz, Z., Thornes, R. & Bailey, S. (1998) Children in the criminal justice and secure care systems: how their mental health needs are met. *Journal of Adolescence*, **21**, 543–553.

Lederman, C. S., Dakof, G. A., Larrea, M. A., *et al* (2004) Characteristics of adolescent females in juvenile detention. *International Journal of Law and Psychiatry*, **27**, 321–337.

McCabe, K. M., Lansing, A. E., Garland, A., *et al* (2002) Gender differences in psychopathology, functional impairment, and familial risk factors among adjudicated delinquents. *Journal of the American Academy of Child and Adolescent Psychiatry*, **41**, 860–867.

Mullen, P. E. (2000) Forensic mental health. *British Journal of Psychiatry*, **176**, 307–311.

NHS Health Advisory Service, Mental Health Act Commission & Social Services Inspectorate (1994) *A Review of the Adolescent Forensic Psychiatry Services Based on the Gardener Unit*. Prestwich Hospital, Manchester.

Ruchkin, V., Koposov, R., Vermerien, R., *et al* (2003) Psychopathology and age at onset of conduct problems in juvenile delinquents. *Journal of Clinical Psychology*, **64**, 913–920.

Rumball, D. & Crome, I. (2004) Social influences. In *Young People and Substance Misuse*. (eds I. Crome, A. H. Ghodse & E. Gilvarry), pp. 62–71. Gaskell.

Rutter, M. & Smith, D. J. (1995) *Psychosocial Disorders in Young People: Time Trends and Their Causes*. John Wiley and Sons.

Rutter, M., Giller, H. & Hagell, A. (1998) *Antisocial Behavior by Young People*. Cambridge University Press.

Rutter, M. L. (1999) Psychosocial adversity and child psychopathology. *British Journal of Psychiatry*, **174**, 480–493.

Shelton, D. (2001) Emotional disorders in young offenders. *Journal of Nurse Scholarships*, **33**, 263.

Shepherd, J. P. & Farrington, D. P. (1996) The prevention of delinquency with particular reference to violent crime. *Medicine, Science and the Law*, **36**, 334.

Sleegers, J., Spijker, J., van Limbeek, J., *et al* (1998) Mental health problems among homeless adolescents. *Acta Psychiatrica Scandinavica*, **97**, 253–259.

Teplin, L. A., Abram, K. M., McClelland, G. M., *et al* (2002) Psychiatric disorders in youth in juvenile detention. *Archives of General Psychiatry*, **59**, 1133–1143.

Vermeiren, R., Schwab-Stone, M., Ruchkin, V., *et al* (2002) Predicting recidivism in delinquent adolescents from psychological and psychiatric assessment. *Comprehensive Psychiatry*, **25**, 174–182.

Vizard, E. & Usiskin, J. (1999) Providing individual psychotherapy for young sexual abusers of children. In *Children and Young People who Sexually Abuse Others: Challenges and Responses* (eds M. Erooga & H. Masson), pp. 104–123. Taylor & Frances/Routledge.

Vreugdenhil, C., Doreleijers, T. A. H., Vermeiren, R., *et al* (2004) Psychiatric disorders in a representative sample of incarcerated boys in the Netherlands. *Journal of the American Academy of Child and Adolescent Psychiatry*, **43**, 97–104.

Wasserman, G. A., McReynolds, L. S., Lucas, C. P., *et al* (2002) The voice DISC-IV with incarcerated male youths: prevalence of disorder. *Journal of the American Academy of Child and Adolescent Psychiatry*, **41**, 314–321.

Youth Justice Board (2005a) *Risk and Protective Factors*. Youth Justice Board.

Youth Justice Board (2005b) *Strategy for the Secure Estate for Children and Young People: Plans for 2005/06 to 2007/08*. Youth Justice Board.

Youth Justice Board (2007) *Youth Justice Annual Workload Data 2006/07*. Youth Justice Board.

CHAPTER 31

Neuropsychiatry and neuropsychology services

Tom Berney

'... good practice requires not simply the collection of test data and observation, but the interpretation of these data in the context of age, developmental stage, injury/insult severity, and psychosocial context.'
Vicki Anderson (2002)

What are neuropsychiatry and neuropsychology?

We have come to appreciate the biological underlay to mental health over the past 30 years; the extent to which central nervous system dysfunction, whether innate or acquired, affects mental functioning in ways that range from a varied mix of intellectual deficits through to altered emotion, behaviour and motivation. Clinicians have moved towards models that see disorder as the result of an interaction between brain biology and the environment, dumping the *tabula rasa* and the nature–nurture dichotomies with concepts such as 'endogenous' and 'reactive'.

This shift in thinking has brought neuropsychiatry and neuropsychology into their own, focusing on the dysfunction in the brain as the origin from which psychological difficulties stem both directly and also indirectly from its interaction with the environment. The dysfunction has an immediate, direct effect on the way a child thinks and feels. However, it also will affect those around the child, which, in turn, shapes their response. The upshot is a complex, ever-changing mix of factors that will determine the child's vulnerability to environmental stress. For example, a child might start with a specific difficulty in processing spoken language which leaves them struggling to understand what people are saying to them; a difficulty that goes unrecognised as their speech sounds fluent. The child's apparent inattentiveness is irritating, making those around impatient and leading them to treat the child as if there is a learning disability. The child gets a sense of failure, a resentful disregard for rules, and diagnoses of ADHD and conduct disorder. Management requires that these interacting issues are teased apart; something that can take high-level, cutting-edge psychometry by more than one discipline: it will need the skills of a speech and language therapist in addition to those of the neuropsychologist and psychiatrist. This is biological psychiatry at its most florid and, to treat children effectively, their clinicians not only need to understand what is happening but also must have a knowledge of the limitations as well as of the utility of potential therapies.

Childhood imposes its own stamp on neurological disorder, preventing extrapolation from adult conditions; the younger anyone is, the less clear-cut the link between anomaly and behaviour with an effect that is less focal and a cognitive result more diffuse to the extent of being generalised. On top of this are compensatory mechanisms and relatively fast developmental changes that will reduce or amplify its effect and lead to delayed ('latent' or 'sleeper') effects.

What kind of disorder?

Although neuropsychiatry and neuropsychological services are potentially available for a wide range of problems, their actual remit will depend on local resources, rules and routes of referral. There is a pressing demand for the assessment and management of the developmental disorders – innate, genetically driven problems that unfold or improve over time – to follow their own, characteristic, developmental trajectory. For example, after appearing in early childhood, a disorder such as autism or epilepsy may improve in the early years of schooling only to return or intensify in adolescence before, once again, improving as the person moves into adulthood. The actual pattern varies but will shape the need for services, setting priorities for different ages and stages of educational and occupational placement.

In addition to these innate disorders, other events such as infections and injuries damage the brain. These secondary disorders also vary with time and development and, although not classed as developmental disorders, can mimic them.

Some of the more prominent groups requiring services are the following.

- Complex learning disabilities that may start simply with specific, often subtle impairments. An example is the language difficulty described earlier which, unrecognised and untreated, had a far-reaching impact on the child and the family. However, such disabilities tend to come in clusters, combining with problems in perception, movement and coordination, which make it difficult to identify individual elements let alone to give them due weight. Not uncommonly, the confusion, the lack of any better category and the shortage of services encourage clinicians to lump such cases into a rag-bag diagnosis of autism.

- The syndrome of autism is a genetic disorder in its own right but can result from any of the medical disorders that cause learning disability. It comes in all shades of severity and across a wide range of ability. Autism-spectrum disorder acknowledges this protean presentation as well as the difficulty in judging the point at which autism crosses the boundary into neurotypical normality or into a thicket of other disabilities. Neuropsychology goes behind the label to pick out the difficulties the child actually has to cope with.

- Other developmental disorders such as Tourette (tic) disorder and ADHD, which are linked to intellectual and emotional characteristics that are poorly described and therefore often unrecognised, and which can give rise to as much difficulty as the core disorder.
- Epilepsy, another developmental disorder, which is more than simply about having seizures, as its effect can represent contributions from:
  - the lack of function by the underlying area of brain abnormality that is the source of the epileptic activity;
  - the disruptive effect of its electrical discharges;
  - the effects, both good and bad, of antiepileptic medication;
  - the attitudes and perceptions of the child, their family and the community in which the child lives;
  - comorbid pathology in the shape of other developmental disabilities and emotional disorder.

  The extent of the emotional and cultural baggage that goes with epilepsy can lift it out of the neurological clinic for closer scrutiny, although this may take a very violent child or very assertive parents. Dissecting out this complicated bundle can take not only assessments of the child and the family but also trials of different treatments and needs a multidisciplinary group that functions as a team rather than a loose-knit network (Stokes *et al*, 2004).

- Brain injury, which may come from infection, biochemical adversity (notably hypoxia), cardiovascular accident, trauma (including perinatal trauma) or tumour. It may come very early in life during pregnancy (including birth) as a congenital anomaly, or later, after a period of normal development, as acquired brain injury; the contrast highlights the different responses of the brain and those around at different stages of development. However, particularly in early childhood, early normality may be inferred rather than obvious and the distinction between congenital and acquired insult is not clear-cut (British Psychological Society, Division of Neuropsychology, 2006).
- Neurodegenerative disorders, including dementia.
- Some systemic disorders that bring psychological disturbance in their wake. Although both tics and obsessive–compulsive symptoms are rife in child mental health practice, it is only in the past decade that they have been recognised as the occasional after-effect of bacterial infection in a small number of prepubertal children. Separately classed as Paediatric Autoimmune Neuropsychiatric Disorders Associated with Streptococcal Infection (PANDAS), they have a characteristic, explosively sudden onset, followed by an episodic relapsing–remitting course, very different to the gentler rise and fall that is the more usual pattern of disorder (Swedo *et al*, 2004). Although it is probable that this disorder occurs rarely, the consequences can be severe for a child in whom the condition is not recognised.
- Legal issues, both civil and criminal, require a more precise answer in a variety of areas including a child's mental capacity to make a decision

or be responsible for an offence. These can bring their own distinct sources of funding, allowing the child access to resources that would be unavailable otherwise.

- The emphasis on the investigation or treatment of physical disorder equips neuropsychiatry to determine their place in other, more apparently psychogenic problems such as conversion disorders.

What kind of services?

The shape of a service is determined to a considerable extent by its context, by what is available from other local services, as well as by the personality and enthusiasm of individual professionals. It is only one part of a mosaic of services that identify, define and manage problems that range from acute assessment and treatment through to medium-term rehabilitation and longer-term support: a network of care that should ensure continuity between hospital and community, health and other agencies, and from childhood into adolescence and beyond. Although many disorders improve over time and with age, most are long term and, as there is nothing magical about the 18th birthday, the network has to extend into adulthood to accompany the person as they move on to further education, adult neurorehabilitation or general psychiatry (Berney, 2009). This aspiration, expressed in the mantra of a seamless, well-integrated service, is rarely achieved.

With so many components, referrals to neuropsychiatry/neuropsychology services risk falling foul of demarcation disputes around the child's age and ability. The aim therefore should be to blur the boundaries with other areas of CAMHS while ensuring that they are a central element of paediatric neurology, neurosurgery and neurorehabilitation. The attempt to be all things to all people may leave the service an undeveloped orphan unless it has a powerful champion.

The most relevant complementary services are likely to be those for children with an intellectual disability which traditionally have come from either specialist learning disability services or community child health rather than from mainstream CAMHS, a distinction encouraged by several factors. First, even where psychological problems do not result directly from the medical disorder underlying a disability, they will be coloured by it, giving the psychopathology a strong biological emphasis, with autism and epilepsy particularly prevalent. Second, a behavioural tradition and the child's limited communication mean that its style is to put the emphasis on working with the family, carers and teachers rather than directly with the child; the more so, the greater the degree of disability. Third, is the presence of the specialist learning disability services from other agencies, notably education. This compartmentalisation on the basis of ability does not lend itself to the development of good comprehensive services and, in the UK, it has left neuropsychiatry and neuropsychology restricted to children of more normal ability and with the limited resources of a niche market. Their specialist needs tend to be overlooked in the competitive development of CAMHS, with services growing in an *ad hoc* fashion out of personal interests and research to operate on a supra-regional level. Lacking local services, referrals are often made to other clinicians who, working with adults or in other areas of CAMHS, apply their own, not always well-informed, models.

The focus on biological psychiatry and inclusion effectively removes some of these distinctions making a case for learning disability services to expand to the broader remit of developmental psychiatry.

One hallmark of a service is the effectiveness of its liaison with other services and agencies, including the following.

- Child health services, notably community child health and oncology.
- Education:
  - schools, colleges and special education resources, all of which can provide the core for a rehabilitation programme as well as remedial services;
  - educational psychology, which has a central role in the reconciliation of school and the child to the advantage of both. Depending on resources, activities range from the assessment and remediation of specific intellectual difficulties through to facilitating an extensive school-based rehabilitation programme that includes the development of self-help and social skills, confidence and emotional maturity.
- Social Services, whose provisions range from counselling through to short-break and residential care.
- Connexions – a personal advisor can support a young person not just through school but also beyond (up to the age of 25 years): a central element in the transition through the various stages of moving from school into adulthood.
- Employment services, which make special provision for those with a disability.
- Voluntary services. Many have been developed by parents around a particular disorder such as epilepsy, physical disability, autism, and Tourette/tic disorder (the internet encouraging the growth of a group for nearly every genetic syndrome). These serve a wide variety of functions, but of especial value is their provision of:
  - mutual support between individuals and families facing common problems. The networks range from local to national and international; for example, in the UK, Contact a Family (www.cafamily.org.uk/) is a useful starting point for parents and professionals;
  - specialist education which, as Local Authorities provide better specialist resources, tends to deal with those who are very disabled or very complex, or else are very able but unable to cope with mainstream services;
  - out-of-home care whether for a short break, as a part of residential schooling or even as a long-term home.

297

What kind of work?

A multidisciplinary approach is fundamental to an effective service, any work that is not part of a coordinated approach being inefficient with short-lived results. It requires close liaison and often joint work with a variety of specialties (paediatrics, neurology, psychiatry) and with practitioners of different disciplines (psychologist, language therapist, occupational therapist, physiotherapist), of whom many will have a special interest and expertise in the field.

Neuropsychiatry and neuropsychology have distinct areas of expertise each complementing the other, but they also overlap to a substantial degree. Psychiatry, with its medical background, places an emphasis on organic pathology and the use of physical and pharmacological treatments, in contrast to psychology, which deals with the areas of psychometric assessment and psychological (especially behavioural) management. However, there is considerable role diffusion and both disciplines work in areas such as psychotherapy, whether with individuals, groups or families, and in both hospital and community (particularly school) settings (British Psychological Society, Division of Neuropsychology, 2004).

Assessment is a basic function of the neuropsychology service that gives a description of their child that might include the following.

- Intellectual ability – the child's cognitive strengths and deficits. This draws on a range of psychometric instruments that go beyond the standard IQ tests to measure not just the presence of a general intellectual disability but also pick out other, more specific disabilities, as well as identifying contributory factors such as the different components that allow memory, calculation or communication. Such elements may contribute to additional, more global disabilities such as social impairment or problems in executive function. Analysis of these requires skill and experience in order to focus the investigation rather than falling back on a routine and wasteful battery of tests.

- Functional ability – here, a discrepancy with the intellectual ability might reveal over- or underachievement.

- The presence of primary or comorbid disorder such as ADHD, anxiety and depression.

- Mental capacity – the ability that determines the extent to which a child may take part in making decisions or can understand and recount what they have seen or heard.

- The level of risk (e.g. of harm to self or to others) in certain circumstances (e.g. if the child goes on living at home or attending a given school).

- The psychodynamics of the situation that might affect the outcome. For example, the adjustment of the child and family and their adherence to treatment will depend on their premorbid state, the timing and nature of any injury or anomaly, their relationships, and external factors such as monetary benefits and compensation.

- The resources and coping capacity of the child and of their family as well as those resources that will be required as part of rehabilitation (e.g. special education or input from the community mental health team) – an important element, as those families who most need help can be the most reluctant to ask for it.

The more formal, clinic-based interview is supplemented with information about the child's behaviour across different settings and from different informants – usually at home and at school, the latter providing a standardised setting within which a child can be compared with their peers – to give the clinician a global perspective of the child's level and form of function.

Assessment may be a one-off, a baseline measure, or something that happens serially to evaluate change, such as a child's response to a therapeutic trial. Neuropsychometry is part of a range of neurodiagnostic services, including neurophysiology and neuroimaging, that help in understanding the impact of a specific anomaly, a particular drug or an operation on the brain.

What does a service require?

A number of points are relevant to the commissioning of a service.

- The service requires a core team of specialist clinicians (psychologist, psychiatrist, nurse and social worker) whose key skills must include the ability to work well with others. This group, if it is to function efficiently and as a coherent team, has to be supported by a dedicated secretary/administrator.
- Many of the disorders have a low frequency of occurrence but a high level of need. In order to develop and maintain their specialist expertise, a team needs to work across several health districts at a Tier 4 level.
- An operational plan must define the service's referral priorities clearly. It should include the status of work done for the independent sector and the courts, which, as they bring separate funding, can be an important factor in determining a service's viability.
- The recruitment and retention of good-calibre staff will be affected not only by the nature of the work required but also by matters such as their affiliation, the time set aside for academic activities and the location of the service. Although an academic affiliation can help recruitment, it must include adequate academic resources rather than simply be an empty title.
- There is some flexibility in selecting a base for a service whose function extends from the hospital into the community where it works with other specialist services (e.g. epilepsy nurse, special education or the head injury team). However, the base (where the secretary and records are housed and where the team meets) will determine the identity of

the service, whether as part of CAMHS, paediatric neurosciences or community services.

- This is an area of work that is changing rapidly. The credibility of assessment and management depends on their underpinning evidence. They have to be based in research and use all the tools of clinical governance with the allocation of sufficient resources to keep them out of the realm of fortune-telling.

Conclusion

Neuropsychiatric and neuropsychological services are needed but they cannot just be left to develop in response to local clinical need. Fragments will emerge as a result of individual enthusiasm, but they have to be supported by collaborative commissioning across a large area if they are to develop into an informed, coherent specialist service that will replace referrals to national centres.

References

Anderson, V. (2002) Child neuropsychology. *Brain Impairment*, **3**, 89–91.

Berney, T. (2009) Developmental disorders come of age. *Psychiatric Bulletin*, **33**, 1–3.

British Psychological Society, Division of Neuropsychology (2004) *Commissioning Child Neuropsychology Services*. British Psychological Society.

British Psychological Society, Division of Neuropsychology (2006) *Clinical Neuropsychology and Rehabilitation Services for Children with Acquired Brain Injury*. British Psychological Society.

Stokes, T., Shaw, E. J., Juarez-Garcia, A., *et al* (2004) *Clinical Guidelines and Evidence Review for the Epilepsies: Diagnosis and Management in Adults and Children in Primary and Secondary Care*. Royal College of General Practitioners.

Swedo, S. E., Leonard, H. L. & Rapoport, J. L. (2004) The pediatric autoimmune neuropsychiatric disorders associated with streptococcal infection (PANDAS) subgroup: separating fact from fiction. *Pediatrics*, **113**, 907–911.

CHAPTER 32

Mental health provision for deaf children: study of a low-incidence service provision

Mandy Barker, Sophie Roberts and Barry Wright

'What matters deafness of the ears when the mind hears? The one true deafness, the incurable deafness, is that of the mind.'

Victor Hugo

Introduction

There are a handful of specialist national resources for children who have low-incidence conditions. These tend to be in London and offer out-patient and in-patient assessment and treatment. The service may be excellent but such centralisation raises issues of inequality of access for young people who live at a distance and find the travel problematic.

These services include gender dysphoria services, severe OCD, body dysmorphic disorders, autism assessment teams and neuropsychiatry. All of these are based at South London and Maudsley Hospital. There are also centrally funded adolescent secure forensic services around the country, as described in Chapter 30. These services are commissioned by the National Commissioning Group (NCG).

The role of the NCG is to commission services on a national basis for the population of England. In order to be eligible for funding by the NCG, the total number of patients in need of the service must be less than 400 per year nationally.

It is accepted that by concentrating the resources for these services on a national basis, it is possible to develop expertise in how best to commission them, to ensure safety and quality through a concentration of skills in a few centres, and to mitigate the risk to individual primary care trusts of unpredictable episodes of very expensive treatment.

The NCG was established in April 2007, following the recommendations of an independent review chaired by Sir David Carter (Department of Health, 2006). National commissioning is a responsibility of strategic health authorities and the NCG is hosted by NHS London on behalf of all 10 strategic health authorities. There are two elements to the NCG: an expert group whose role it is to advise Ministers on which services should be nationally commissioned; and the National Specialised Commissioning Team who support the NCG and implement its recommendations.

Specialist CAMHS for deaf children are also commissioned and funded centrally. This chapter aims to describe the development of CAMHS for deaf children as an example of how highly specialist CAMHS can be provided for low-incidence populations in an accessible way.

Background

Prior to 2004, the only specialist in-patient and out-patient mental health service for deaf children in England was in London. This meant that deaf children and their families who managed to access this service often had to travel great distances for assessment and locally based intervention strategies were hard to arrange.

Recommendations in the report *Towards Equity and Access* (Department of Health, 2005) recognised this inequality, and in response the National Specialist Commissioning Group (NSCAG) set up a pilot project, funded for 3 years (January 2004–December 2006). This project involved two specialist CAMHS teams – one in York and one in Dudley – linking closely with the established London service to provide improved geographical access to a national service and to develop provision for a greater range of problems. An innovative part of this service is to utilise teleconferencing facilities to provide consultation, training, supervision and direct therapy across large distances.

This was achieved by placing these facilities into CAMHS teams and residential schools for the deaf. A comprehensive evaluation of these pilot services was carried out independently by the Social Policy Research Unit at York University using qualitative and quantitative methodologies. They found that the outcomes were good, consistent and the service was highly valued by users (Greco *et al*, 2009).

Policy context

National specialist services have the best opportunity to develop when there is a combination of identified need and professional expertise, and when legislation can support the need for a service. The establishment of mental health services for deaf children comes at a time when attention is being focused on ensuring the mental health needs of all children are better met. The publication of *National Service Framework for Children, Young People and Maternity Services* (Department of Health, 2004) establishes standards with regard to meeting the mental health needs of children. Standard 9 (mental health and psychological well-being of children and young people) stipulates that all children and young people who have 'mental health problems have access to timely, integrated, high quality mental health services' (Department of Health, 2004: p. 6). More specifically, within Standard 8 (disabled children and young people and those with complex health needs), Local Authorities, primary care trusts and CAMHS are charged with ensuring that disabled children have equal access to CAMHS (Department of Health, 2004: p. 15).

Standard 8 also states that services for low-incidence conditions need to be coordinated on a regional or national basis.

The report *Towards Equity and Access* (Department of Health, 2005) suggests best practice guidance as a response to the consultation document *A Sign of the Times* (Department of Health, 2002), which made a number of recommendations for local services for deaf children and adults. At present, the profile of the issues surrounding mental health and deafness is high at governmental level.

Understanding the problem

Epidemiology

An estimated 840 children are born in the UK every year with moderate to profound deafness (National Deaf Children Society, 2003). Although vaccination programmes mean fewer babies are born deaf as a result of their mothers having rubella during pregnancy, this fall has been offset by more babies being born deaf from other causes such as premature birth or lack of oxygen during birth. Furthermore, more babies survive with multiple disabilities than used to be the case. The National Deaf Children's Society suggest that there are more than 35000 deaf children and young people in the UK (www.ndcs.org.uk/about_us/ndcs/index.html). About 1 in every 1000 children is deaf at 3 years old. This rises to 2 in every 1000 children aged 9–16 years. The government has recently initiated a national screening programme for all newborn children, and diagnosis will now be made soon after birth.

Many deaf children grow up to use British Sign Language (BSL). However, more than 90% of these children will be born into hearing families with no previous experience of deafness (National Deaf Children Society, 2003). Thus, most deaf children will experience difficulties in communicating with their own families, with hearing peers, and in school.

The education of deaf children has been the subject of extremely polarised views. The issue centres on whether it is preferable for a deaf child to learn oral communication to enable integration into a predominantly hearing world or whether to emphasise signing, which in the right environment can produce much more effective communication among those who share signing language.

There is evidence that some children who achieve good hearing gained through cochlear implantation or hearing aids can progress well in an auditory environment. Equally, there is convincing evidence that those who do not achieve a good result from these interventions will do much better educationally in a signing environment.

Putting the needs of the child first and helping parents make a well-informed choice is most important, and the national deaf child and family services all offer a service in the mode of communication preferred by the children.

Prevalence of mental health problems

Communication problems, subsequent difficulties with peer relationships and family dynamics, and a high incidence of central nervous system damage are some of the main reasons why deaf children are approximately 1.5 times more likely to develop mental health problems than their hearing peers (Hindley, 1997). The likely prevalence of child mental health problems (ranging from emotional and behavioural disorders to major mental illnesses) among deaf children and young people is approximately 40% (Hindley, 1997). The NHS Health Advisory Service (1998) report on deafness and mental health estimates that the prevalence of disabling mental health problems in deaf children (requiring referral to a specialist mental health service for deaf children) is 3.4%.

Additional considerations when working with deaf children

Deaf children and their families require access to the same range of mental health services as their hearing counterparts. In any geographical area, the numbers of deaf children will be relatively low and therefore they have a range of special needs for which ordinary mental health services would find it hard to develop the skills needed to provide an appropriate service. In particular, generic mental health services may not be geared up to having an adequate understanding of the following issues.

Communication needs

A child's method of communication is heavily influenced by the communication method used to provide their education. It is possible that this may not necessarily be their preferred way of communicating. For some deaf children, not being able to understand or be understood in speech could be seen as failing. The heart of all mental health assessment and treatment is based upon communication: any difficulties with this immediately influences the experience of the session. It is crucial to be able to offer a range of communication methods.

It is not always clear to those not used to working with this population which is the best means of communication. Many children who are educated orally prefer to use BSL in therapeutic settings. Using an interpreter doesn't mitigate the need for staff to be aware of deaf issues and culture. Staff need to have deaf awareness training to be aware of how to maximise communication. For those children who choose to communicate through speech and lip reading, staff need to recognise when a child or young person is saying they have understood but haven't fully understood the conversation.

Development

Deaf children tend to be socio-emotionally developmentally delayed because of a lack of social experiences and poverty of incidental social learning. Their development of language (Quigley & Paul, 1984) is different to that of hearing children, especially as they are potentially learning spoken language as a second language. This is particularly important with emotional language and literacy. Deaf children find it difficult to appreciate the range of emotions.

Locus of control

Deaf children grow up with a poorly developed internal locus of control and tend to show empathy skills delay. They tend to have a limited range of coping strategies to manage the frustration implicit in poor communication.

Self-belief

Deaf children tend to have developed a negative attributional bias over many years of low expectations. Society, schools and parents can add to this when discussing possible careers for a deaf young person.

Deaf culture

Deaf children, particularly from deaf families, will be heavily involved in the deaf community and have a strong sense of deaf culture. This sees deafness not as a disability but as a strength.

Resources

A lot of the resources and information on mental health and support such as CBT need significant changes for this population. Deaf children appreciate the world visually and need predominantly visual resources. English is for many a second language, or a language that is significantly delayed. As a result, many children who have permanent severe or profound bilateral deafness and have mental health problems will have difficulty in accessing and effectively using mainstream mental health services (Hindley, 1997).

Developing a specialist service

Service models

All services that form the national network have evolved differently, but all have developed ways of working in the specialist residential and mainstream schools that emphasise consultation and collaboration with the other skilled professionals and parents. The services all offer consultation clinics and meetings to a range of professionals such as teachers of the deaf, Social Services staff, and residential care staff. They have also developed links with audiologists and paediatricians. Children who are at residential school live all over the UK, making a traditional clinic model difficult and often inappropriate to implement. Owing to a lack of existing services, many referrals are complex as the issues have developed in seriousness over time. Engaging families who have historically had a poor experience of support from services can be difficult. It is particularly helpful to travel to meet them for assessment. The teams offer a range of interventions depending on the need and what is practical and sustainable. Some interventions will be entirely provided by the specialist team and others will be provided by local services with support and advice from the team (e.g. local family therapy to support residential school-based individual work).

Use of new technology: telelink screens

The national specialist mental health service for deaf children has installed video link screens in York, Birmingham, London and the three residential schools that use the service. To date, the screen has been used in a number of different ways.

- Direct clinical work: assessments, individual therapy, family work, post-discharge support (e.g. ongoing contact with schools, follow-up of children discharged from the in-patient unit in London), and facilitating multifaceted team involvement in cases.
- Professional practice and multidisciplinary working: consultation between teams, training and supervision, sharing and spreading clinical expertise, and business meetings.

New ways of working have been needed and will continue to be developed to fully utilise this new technology. In addition, the ways the technology is used by the service has changed and, it is envisaged, will continue to develop and change over time. The teams are now exploring the use of webcams to have more regular contact with families and deaf young people from their own home.

The teams use the telelink screen in a variety of ways to enhance service provision as outlined above. One major use has been in enabling young people who want to access psychotherapy with a BSL-using deaf clinician. It has been found that there need for half-termly face-to-face meetings, and that any issues of risk and communication between families, school and care staff need to be very carefully managed. It has, however, been well evaluated by some young people who almost prefer the use of the technology.

Evaluation

A key part of the development of these supra-regional services has been an external evaluation of the services provided. The Social Policy Research Unit at the University of York undertook this. The following findings suggest that in terms of quantitative and qualitative data, the services provide a clinically beneficial service to families and young people (Greco *et al*, 2009).

- Overall, the evidence from children and young people, parents and referrers shows that the service is meeting its aim of providing a mental health service that meets the specific needs of deaf children and young people. In particular, the service is able to meet the child/young person's communication needs and it is staffed by people with an expertise in deafness and mental health. The presence of deaf staff in the teams is important and valued. In addition, the positive accounts of the service from the children and young people suggest the service is 'child-/young person-friendly'. Referrers and parents are very clear that generic services cannot meet the mental health needs of deaf children and young people.

- One solution to the issue of access suggested by referrers was to increase the use of and access to the telelink. Overall, young people who had used the telelink were very positive about it and believed it should be more widely available.

Service developments

Following on from the successful pilot projects and within the growing policy drivers, the NCG has now agreed to fund a new national deaf CAMHS with bases in Dudley, London, York and Taunton. The first three will have outreach staff embedded in generic CAMHS at geographically spread locations to give national coverage. The model will see these centres adding to the landscape of services at the specialist end, while providing comprehensive support to generic CAMHS workers. This also includes the continued use of telemedicine equipment and widening of deaf awareness.

Conclusion

Services for low-incidence complex disorders can be provided and commissioned on a national basis. Specialist services by their nature will never be available in every location, but by utilising new technologies and when necessary going to the young person and their family, a person-centred service can be achieved. Technology can be used in an innovative way to support professionals and enable young people to have access to culturally and linguistically appropriate mental health services.

Belief in the need for change and persistence and creativity can see a change in traditional service provision or the development of new services.

References

Department of Health (2002) *A Sign of the Times – Modernising Mental Health Services for People who are Deaf*. TSO (The Stationery Office).

Department of Health (2004) *National Service Framework for Children, Young People and Maternity Services, Child and Adolescent Mental Health (CAMHS)*. TSO (The Stationery Office).

Department of Health (2005) *Mental Health and Deafness – Towards Equity and Access: Best Practice Guidance*. TSO (The Stationery Office).

Department of Health (2006) *Review of Commissioning Arrangements for Specialised Services*. Office of Public Sector Information.

Greco, V., Beresford, B. & Sutherland, H. (2009) Deaf children and young people's experiences of using specialist mental health services. *Children and Society*, **23**, 455–469.

Hindley, P. (1997) Psychiatric aspects of hearing impairment. *Journal of Child Psychology and Psychiatry*, **38**, 101–117.

National Deaf Children Society (2003) *Factsheet: Statistics on Childhood Deafness in the UK*. NDCS (http://www.ndcs.org.uk/document.rm?id=719).

NHS Health Advisory Service (1998) *Forging New Channels: Commissioning and Delivering Mental Health Services for People who are Deaf*. British Society for Mental Health and Deafness.

Quigley, S. P. & Paul, P. V. (1984) *Language and Deafness*. College Hill Press.

CHAPTER 33

Chief Executives – what do they want and how do they get it?

Chris Butler

'He who has never learnt to obey commands cannot be a good commander.'
Aristotle, 4th century BC

A little on structure

The concept of the Chief Executive is still relatively new in the 60-year-old NHS. Arguably, the role is merely another stage in how services are developed, led and delivered as it has evolved from different types of management systems.

The first model was the medical control of services through medical superintendents supported by matrons. This changed with the establishment of co-equal 'hospital management teams' – comprised of a doctor, a nurse and an administrator. This was followed by general management, with the implementation of the Griffiths (1983) report. Finally, for the moment at least, the development of the concept of corporate management through the Boards of Directors of NHS trusts and primary care trusts. The emergence of NHS foundation trusts has seen, alongside Boards of Directors, the requirement of foundation trusts to have a membership drawn from the communities they serve. Foundation trusts also have a Board of Governors, the majority of whom are elected from the membership. The Board of Governors, among other things, hire (or fire) the non-executive directors of the Board of Directors. Foundation trusts are set up as 'mutual' organisations such as those in the cooperative movement. They receive their 'terms of authorisation' from Monitor, an independent regulator of foundation trusts set up by Parliament. The terms of authorisation describe each foundation trust as a public benefit corporation. Foundation trusts are outwith the control of the Department of Health and their local strategic health authority. They report quarterly to Monitor against a number of indicators. If these indicators indicate good organisational performance, foundation trusts are left alone to manage their own affairs.

The wider landscape

All NHS Chief Executives are the 'accountable officer' of the organisation in which they work (Monitor, 2008). To this effect, a memorandum is signed by each Chief Executive describing their personal responsibilities and obligations. Chief Executives are therefore responsible for the overall performance of their organisation. Things can go wrong, sometimes suddenly. In extreme circumstances, the Chief Executive is the first to walk the plank, often followed by the rest of the Board of Directors. When this happens, it is rare for others such as senior clinicians to get a P45 as quickly. Being a Chief Executive is therefore a risky business. The reality of life for all Chief Executives is that they are only as good as their last game. This goes some way to explaining why Chief Executives can come across as being obsessed by organisational performance. However, for the overwhelming majority of Chief Executives, their primary driver is that of working in an organisation that is the best it can be at what it does. Where they differ is in the techniques they use to make this a reality.

National Health Service Chief Executives always operate simultaneously in multiple environments. The first is the complex internal environment of their own workplace. In the case of Leeds Partnerships NHS Foundation Trust, this means trying to relate personally to service users and carers, in addition to some 2500 staff, across 48 sites spanning the metropolitan district of Leeds. It also means being responsible for £108 million of public money.

At the same time, a Chief Executive operates in large health and social care community, sometimes referred to as a 'local health economy'. In this context, the Chief Executive represents the broader issues of their organisation. The total investment in England alone in adult mental health services in 2008/09 is reported as being £5.892 billion, or £181 per head of the weighted working age population (Department of Health, 2009). In this context, it is surprising that mental health and learning disability receive little airtime compared with the rest of the NHS either locally or nationally. The Chief Executive is often the sole voice of mental health and learning disability services in their local health economy. In this context, a Chief Executive needs resilience and persistence in getting the importance of their interests across. Sometimes this means enduring what can feel like interminable meetings in order to seize a short-term tactical advantage and to deliver progress in the medium term. At other times, it means making themselves a bit unpopular with their colleagues in the local health economy when they only really want to discuss other things such as waiting times in emergency departments or 18-week waiting times in the acute sector.

Outwith the local health economy, Chief Executives also interact with their peers regionally and nationally. They seek to exert influence on and sometimes positively change the external environment in which services operate, for example in the development of national priorities for the NHS, and most recently the legislative framework for the care of service users.

The art and science of management and leadership

We all have had experience of leaders we have loved and also those we have loathed.

Everybody, in all cultures and ages, has had views on management and leadership. The common denominator across these commentators focuses on the impact of the personality traits of the 'leader' and how these play themselves out, rather than anything related to the conscious execution by the leader of a scientific method. The best leaders, therefore, seem to be able to mesh together intellect, an understanding of the impact of emotions – both their own and those of others – and a clarity of purpose both on their own part and a wider system.

Numerous people have attempted to describe theoretical frameworks about management and leadership. These range from work process models based around industrial systems (Taylor, 1911; Mayo, 1945; Fayol, 1949) to a psychoanalytic understanding of what makes organisations tick (Ferenczi, 1916; Freud, 1922; Bion, 1968).

In the NHS in 2003, the Leadership Qualities Framework was promoted by the then NHS Leadership Centre, which was part of the NHS Modernisation Agency, both of which have been assimilated into the NHS Institute for Innovation and Improvement (NHS Institute for Innovation and Improvement, 2006).

The Leadership Qualities Framework is a model designed around the evidence for what makes effective leaders. It described three core leadership characteristics:

- setting direction
- personal qualities
- delivering the service.

Each of these in turn had a number of subcharacteristics as indicators for deployment of the three. For example, in setting direction – intellectual flexibility; in personal qualities – personal integrity; and in delivering the service – empowering others.

Although the world of the NHS continues to evolve, the Leadership Qualities Framework is still relevant. Recruitment processes for Chief Executives sometimes feature the assessment of candidates against this model.

Thinking continues to evolve. One example is the work of Paul Plsek and his work on Directed Creativity™ (www.directedcreativity.com; Plsek, 1997). In summary, some of Plsek's work describes how managers and leaders have to pay constant attention to structures, processes and behaviours, the most volatile element, not surprisingly, being behaviours.

My work as a manager is influenced by the theoretical frameworks of the psychoanalysts who have studied the application of psychoanalytic theory in organisations, in particular the role of the manager as dealing with anxiety, which, they argue, is present in complex systems.

Many Chief Executives have an understanding of such theoretical models. Some Chief Executives in their day-to-day dealings with people use different aspects of them in practice.

However, what is intriguing about these and other theories is that they all desire to establish a scientific and/or behavioural understanding of the vagaries of the human heart and mind. The reality is that people often identify good or great leadership in others in an instinctual rather than rational way.

Characteristics of a good leader

What are my top tips for effective leadership? They are, in no particular priority order, the following.

- Service: leaders have a sense of people and a world outside of themselves. They want to do the right thing in a good way.
- Optimism, celebrating success, and saying thank you: good leaders are confident in the altruistic intentions of the vast majority of their colleagues. They actively acknowledge, recognise and nurture this. They always do their best to say thank you to those people who go the extra mile, from the catering department to the nurse on the ward. They are able to describe the journey that people are on. They have a sense of and are hopeful for the future, and communicate this actively.
- Decide less, listen more: the more leaders take decisions, the less personally effective they are. The job is to help others closest to the heart of an issue to find the solution for themselves. There will be times, however, when a leader has to decide. The trick is to create a system in which this is the exception not the rule.
- Owning up: good leaders say that it is OK to be a human being. They tell people that they do not have a magic wand to solve their difficult problems and that they, in common with everyone else, will make mistakes. When they make a mistake they take it on the chin and address it. They are not afraid to say sorry.
- The truth: good leaders want to know what people really think. They are always appreciative of those people who really tell them what is on their mind.
- Beyond getting the basics right: good leaders never believe their own or others propaganda about how good their organisation is. They know that things can always be done in a better way and are unapologetic about wanting the best for everyone. They are clear about and react appropriately to unacceptable behaviour.
- Co-leadership: no one can do it all on their own. Good leaders pay time and attention to selecting their team. Good leaders want people on their team who are different; people who will challenge their colleagues, themselves, and their boss. It is essential that senior clinicians are active participants at all levels of a health organisation,

from the boardroom to front-line services. Healthcare organisations will struggle when there is not a full and equal partnership between clinicians and managers.

- Presence and engagement: good leaders have a good understanding of the experience of their colleagues and, as importantly, service users and carers. Good leaders give this as much priority as meetings of the Board of Directors. They drop by a lot as well as having planned opportunities to engage with people. In business language, they have a good understanding of whatever their 'product' is. Good leaders lead from the front, particularly when things are tough. They do not ask others to do what they would not themselves, and their colleagues know this.
- Checking assumptions and new possibilities: good leaders never take things at face value. They always check assumptions while listening for or sensing new possibilities or alternative scenarios. They engage, listen, challenge, and desire to be challenged by others.
- Championing: good leaders are relentless and cheerful in championing their convictions. They do this in season and out of season.
- Humane and compassionate: good leaders know that despite their best efforts, people will not always come up to the mark. They are receptive and respond positively to people's difficulty and distress. They do their best to treat others how they themselves want to be treated.
- Humour: able to make and take a joke!

Why is this important?

The best Chief Executives do their utmost to safeguard and develop the services for which they are responsible, as well as having a broader interest and advocacy role in their area of work.

Chief Executives simply want the best possible service for service users and carers, as well as being the best employer they can be. This is easy to say but extremely hard to do. In this regard, they are the natural allies of clinicians, service users and carers. At the same time, I have never met a Chief Executive who takes things at face value, and you can expect to be probed and challenged. This can sometimes feel like an interrogation.

Virtually all of the Chief Executives I have known have been highly motivated people from a variety of backgrounds who want to engage clinicians, service users and carers, find out what their issues are and what progress looks like, and work with people to see change happen.

References

Bion, W. R. (1968) *Experiences in Groups*. Tavistock Publications.

Department of Health (2009) *2008/09 National Survey of Investment in Adult Mental Health Services*. Department of Health (http://www.dh.gov.uk/en/Publicationsandstatistics/Publications/PublicationsPolicyAndGuidance/DH_088701).

Fayol, H. (1949) *General and Industrial Management*. Pitman.

Ferenczi, S. (1916) *Contributions to Psychoanalysis*. Richard Badger.

Freud, S. (1922) *Group Psychology and the Analysis of the Ego*. International Psycho-Analytic Press.

Griffiths, E. R. (1983) *NHS Management Inquiry Report*. Department of Health and Social Security.

Mayo, E. (1945) *The Social Problems of an Industrial Civilisation*. Harvard University Press.

Monitor (2008) *NHS Foundation Trust Accounting Officer Memorandum*. Monitor (http://www.monitor-nhsft.gov.uk/sites/default/files/publications/Accounting_Officer_Memorandum_April_2008.pdf).

NHS Institute for Innovation and Improvement (2006) *NHS Leadership Qualities Framework*. NHS Institute for Innovation and Improvement (http://www.nhsleadershipqualities.nhs.uk/portals/0/the_framework.pdf).

Plsek, P. E. (1997) *Creativity, Innovation, and Quality*. ASQ Quality Press.

Taylor, F. W. (1911) *Principles of Scientific Management*. Harper.

Index

Compiled by Linda English